Fundamentals of
PEDIATRIC
RADIOLOGY

Fundamentals of
PEDIATRIC
RADIOLOGY

Lane F. Donnelly, M.D.
Associate Professor of Radiology and Pediatrics
Children's Hospital Medical Center
University of Cincinnati College of Medicine
Cincinnati, Ohio

W.B. SAUNDERS COMPANY
A Harcourt Health Sciences Company
Philadelphia   London   New York   St. Louis   Sydney   Toronto

W.B. SAUNDERS COMPANY
A Harcourt Health Sciences Company

The Curtis Center
Independence Square West
Philadelphia, Pennsylvania 19106

Library of Congress Cataloging-in-Publication Data

Donnelly, Lane F.
Fundamentals of pediatric radiology/Lane F. Donnelly—1st ed.

p.   cm.

ISBN 0–7216–9061–0

1. Pediatric radiology.   2. Pediatric diagnostic imaging.   I. Title.   [DNLM:
  1. Technology, Radiologic—methods.   2. Diagnostic Imaging—Child.
  3. Diagnostic Imaging—Infant.   WN 240 D685f2001]

RJ51.R3 D66 2001

618.92′00754—dc21   00–066122

Acquisitions Editor: Lisette Bralow
Manuscript Editor: Jodi von Hagen
Production Manager: Norman Stellander
Illustration Specialist: Bob Quinn
Book Designer: Matt Andrews

FUNDAMENTALS OF PEDIATRIC RADIOLOGY   ISBN 0–7216–9061–0

Printed in the United States of America.

Last digit is the print number: 9   8   7   6   5   4   3   2   1

Foreword

Lane Donnelly has created a wonderful treatise on pediatric radiology that will help thousands of radiologists grasp a difficult and oftentimes confusing area of radiology. There are numerous reference books on pediatric radiology, but few are truly "readable." Lane's book is readable.

"The essence of genius is brevity." I don't know who to attribute that quote to, but I think it has a lot of merit. Plenty of scholars can produce a text that is all-encompassing. Only a few can produce a work that is succinct, yet comprehensive enough to be useful. It is a difficult task to reduce a mass of knowledge, such as exists in pediatric radiology, to a single volume, but Lane has done so.

I had the privilege of working with Lane for two years at Duke University Medical Center. He is one of the most prolific writers I have ever encountered. He has an uncanny ability to grasp a complex set of ideas quickly and reduce them to a common denominator. Even more uniquely, he is able to articulate the results of his research in a simple, understandable fashion. He is well suited for the task of producing a book on the fundamentals of pediatric radiology. I am flattered that he would style his work after my book, *Fundamentals of Skeletal Radiology*. I am honored to be able to write the foreword for a book that will one day be a classic in radiology.

CLYDE A. HELMS, M.D.

Preface

The intention of this book is to serve as a basic introductory text on pediatric radiology. The emphasis is on commonly encountered imaging scenarios and pediatric diseases, rather than on obscure diagnoses. Brief and practical differential diagnoses are included, rather than long and complete differential lists. The book is intended to be readable over a weekend or several nights and to serve as an excellent introduction or review for a resident or medical student who is about to begin a rotation in pediatric radiology or prepare for radiology oral boards. I know that as a resident, I retained more useful information when I read fundamental books over and over than when I read longer, more detailed texts once. This book may also serve as a review for a general radiologist who wishes to brush up on pediatric radiology. Pediatric residents or pediatricians who want to learn more about pediatric radiology may also benefit from reading this book.

Like other books in the W.B. Saunders Fundamental Series, such as Clyde Helms' *Fundamentals of Skeletal Radiology,* the style of the book is informal. The format is prose rather than outline. Each chapter emphasizes the commonly encountered imaging scenarios, pertinent normal variants, and likely diagnoses. The topics included reflect questions that I am commonly asked by residents on the pediatric radiology service, important issues that the rotating residents often seem not to know, and commonly made mistakes. Certainly, because of restriction in length, all diseases that affect children are not covered, and the book is in no means meant to serve as a reference text. Processes that have a similar appearance in children and adults are de-emphasized or not included, even if they occur commonly. The chapters are organized in a variable manner—sometimes by anatomic feature, sometimes by type of disease process, sometimes by diagnoses that are made at a particular age, and sometimes by disease processes that present with similar imaging findings. This type of organization was chosen so that the text could be more flexible in communicating which diseases and imaging findings are more likely to be encountered.

LANE F. DONNELLY, M.D.

Acknowledgments

Most of the information in this book represents the summation of what I have been taught by numerous radiologists. Many of these radiologists not only were good teachers but also inspired me to pursue a career in academic radiology. Although the list is too long to thank them all, I would like to mention a few by name: George S. Bisset, III, M.D.; Janet L. Strife, M.D.; Donald P. Frush, M.D.; Jerome F. Wiot, M.D.; Harold B. Spitz, M.D.; Joel E. Lichtenstein, M.D.; Robert L. Lukin, M.D.; J. Fred Johnson, III, M.D.; William S. Ball, M.D.; Neil D. Johnson, M.D.; Rendon C. Nelson, M.D.; and Clyde A. Helms, M.D. I thank Glenn G. Minano for contributing the diagrams and Blaise V. Jones for his help with Chapter 8. Finally, I would like to thank my wife, Jill, and children, Piper and Griffin, for being understanding when I am doing things like writing this book.

LANE F. DONNELLY, M.D.

Contents

1

Introduction: Special Considerations in Pediatric Imaging

There are many issues that are unique to the imaging of children when compared with imaging in adults. Many examinations that are easily carried out in adults require special adjustments in children. The resident on a pediatric imaging rotation and the radiologist who is accustomed to imaging adults but occasionally images children must be prepared to deal with these issues and adjust techniques so that the imaging examination is obtained safely and successfully. In this introductory chapter, several general issues that often arise when imaging children are briefly addressed.

INABILITY TO COOPERATE

Infants and young children are often unable to cooperate and fulfill requirements that are typically easily met by adults. For example, children are often unable to keep still, remain in a certain position, concentrate for more than a brief moment, or hold their breath. Different aged children often have unique limitations. Infants and toddlers are unable to stay still, whereas a 3-year-old child is more apt to refuse to cooperate. These limitations affect almost all pediatric imaging examinations: radiography, fluoroscopy, ultrasonography, computed tomography (CT), magnetic resonance imaging (MRI), and nuclear imaging. There are a number of potential solutions and tricks that can be helpful in these situations. Commonly used solutions include distracting the child, providing child friendly surroundings, and using immobilization or sedation.

Distracting the child is often a simple and easy tactic. The radiology department at the Children's Hospital Medical Center keeps a stock of rattles and noise-making toys to distract infants. Talking to older children about school and other activities can be helpful. Videotape players are provided in all the ultrasonography rooms. It is amazing how cooperative many children will be when they are able to watch television.

Providing child friendly surroundings may help ease a young child's anxiety and cause him or her to be more cooperative. Paintings on the walls and equipment as well as cartoonish figures in the examination rooms can be helpful. Eliminating or minimizing painful portions of the examination can also be helpful in keeping a young child cooperative. Placing an intravenous (IV) line often causes a great deal of anxiety and renders the patient uncooperative for the subsequent imaging study. Using a topical analgesic to decrease the pain of the IV placement often makes this portion of the examination less traumatic.

Immobilization is also a helpful technique. Infants who are bundled or "papoosed" in a blanket are more apt to stay still than are infants who are not. This may make the difference in needing or not needing sedation in order to perform a computed tomographic examination. There are also a number of commercially available immobilization devices that are helpful in performing certain examinations. Many pediatric radiologists use an octagon board for immobilization when performing fluoroscopic studies in young children. Many devices are also available for obtaining specific radiographic studies, such as chest radiographs. Imaging departments in which children are imaged should have such equipment available.

In certain situations, distraction and immo-

1

bilization may not be successful and conscious sedation of the child may be necessary in order to obtain an imaging study. Most children younger than 7 years of age require sedation for MRI studies. This is related to the prolonged nature of the examination and the need for the patient to be completely still. Sedation is needed less often now than in the past for children undergoing CT because newer CT scanners are faster. However, a number of children still need sedation for computed tomographic examinations. Other procedures that often require sedation include some nuclear medicine studies and most interventional procedures.

Standards of care for conscious sedation are required by the Joint Commission of Accreditation of Health Care Organizations (JCAHO) and are based on standards published by several organizations, including the American Academy of Pediatrics Committee on Drugs. Any imaging department in which children are sedated must have a defined sedation program that is in accordance with these guidelines. The sedation program must have protocols for presedation preparation, sedative agents used, monitoring during sedation and during postsedation recovery, and discharge criteria.

VARIABLE SIZE AND PHYSIOLOGY

Because of the variability of infant to adult-sized children, many adaptations in relation to size must be considered for pediatric imaging studies. The doses of contrast and drugs used in imaging examinations need to be adapted for the child's size, often on a per weight (milligram per kilogram) basis. For example in CT, the standard dose of IV contrast is 2 mL/kg. Oral contrast dosing is also based on patient weight or age (Table 1–1). To continue using CT as an illustrative example, other variables may also be affected by patient size. In

TABLE 1–1. **Single Dose of Oral Contrast for Computed Tomography in Relation to Patient Age**

Age (Yr)	Diatrizoate Meglumine (Hypaque)	Diluent
<1	4 mL	120 mL
1–5	8 mL	240 mL
6–12	12 mL	360 mL
12	16 mL	480 mL

TABLE 1–2. **Tube Current (Milliampere) for Body Imaging Application for Single-Slice Helical Computed Tomography**

Weight (kg)	Chest	Abdomen and Pelvis
4.5–8.9	40	60
9.0–17.9	50	70
18.0–26.9	60	80
27.0–35.9	70	100
36.0–45.0	80	120
45.1–69.0	100–120	140–150
>70	≥140	≥170

small children, the largest possible IV placed may be very small, often 22 or 24 gauge; the IV may be in the foot or hand; the length of the region of interest to be imaged is variable; and the length of the patient's veins is variable. Physiologic parameters, such as cardiac output, are more variable in children than in adults. These factors affect parameters such as the time between contrast injection and the onset of scanning as well as choices in contrast administration technique (hand bolus versus power injector). The thickness of the slice should be less in younger children because of their smaller anatomy. Similar adjustments must be considered in all imaging modalities performed in children.

Some of the more important parameters that need special attention in children are those that affect radiation dose. Because of their long potential life span, it is particularly important to keep radiation exposure to a minimum in children. When performing radiography, appropriate shielding of radiosensitive tissues (gonads, thyroid) and appropriate collimation are paramount. For CT, the tube current (in milliamperes [mA]) can be greatly reduced in small children because of their relatively small size and the reduced attenuation of the x-ray beam. Table 1–2 demonstrates the weight-based mA measurement that is used at the Children's Hospital Medical Center in Cincinnati, Ohio.

AGE-RELATED CHANGES IN IMAGING APPEARANCE

Another factor that makes imaging in children different from that in adults is the continuous change in the imaging appearance of multiple organ systems in relation to normal development during childhood. The normal imaging appearance of certain aspects of all the organ systems is different at different ages during childhood and also between children and adults. The ultrasonographic appearance of the kidneys is different in a neonate than in a 1-year-old child. The developing brain demonstrates differences in signal at different ages on MRI, which is related to changes in myelination. A large mediastinal shadow related to the thymus may be normal or severely abnormal, depending on the child's age. The skeleton demonstrates marked changes at all ages of childhood in relation to maturation of the apophyses and epiphyses and the progressive ossification of structures. Knowledge of the normal age-related appearance of these organ systems is vital to appropriate interpretation of imaging studies; lack of this knowledge is one of the more common causes of mistakes in pediatric radiology.

AGE-RELATED DIFFERENTIAL DIAGNOSES

The types of diseases that affect children are vastly different from those that commonly affect adults. Therefore, the differential diagnosis for and significance of a particular imaging finding in a child is dramatically different than are those for the identical imaging finding in an adult. In addition, the diseases that affect specific age groups of children are often very different. Therefore, as in comparing children and adults, the differential diagnosis and significance of a particular imaging finding in a 2-month-old infant may be dramatically different than that for the identical imaging finding when seen in a 10-year-old child.

RELATIONSHIP BETWEEN IMAGER AND PARENTS

In both pediatric and adult patient care situations, there are family members with whom the imager must interact. However, in the pediatric setting, there are several unique features in the relationships among imager, patient, and family. When caring for children, communication is often more between the radiologist and parent than between the radiologist and patient. In addition, the degree of interaction between the imager and the child-parent unit may be greater in the pediatric setting than in the adult setting because of associated issues, such as the potential need for sedation, the need for consent from the parent rather than from the child (if the child is a minor), and the need for a thorough explanation of the procedure to both the child and the parent on a level they can understand. People are also much more inquisitive and protective when their children, rather than others, are involved. Therefore, descriptions of what to expect during the visit to the imaging area may need to be more detailed when dealing with pediatric patients and their parents.

The stress level for a parent when their child is or may be ill is immense, and such stresses often bring out both the best and worst in people. Because of the intense bonds between most parents and their children, the relationship between imager and parent is most successful when the radiologist exercises marked empathy and patience. Those used to imaging adults should consider the issues discussed in this chapter when imaging children.

Suggested Reading

American Academy of Pediatrics Committee on Drugs. Guidelines for monitoring and management of pediatric patients during and after sedation for diagnostic and therapeutic procedures. Pediatrics 1992;89:1110–1115.

Chung T, Kirks DR. Techniques. In: Kirks DR, ed. Practical Pediatric Imaging of Infants and Children. 3rd ed. Philadelphia: Lippincott-Raven, 1998.

Frush DP, Bisset GS III. Pediatric sedation in radiology: the practice of safe sleep. AJR 1996;167:1381–1387.

Frush DP, Donnelly LF. State of the art. Spiral CT: technical considerations and applications in children. Radiology 1998;209:37–48.

Poznauskis L. Immobilization. In: Godderidge C, ed. Pediatric Imaging. Philadelphia: WB Saunders, 1995:145–158.

2

Airway

It has been said that one of the differentiating features between a pediatric radiologist and a general radiologist is that a pediatric radiologist remembers to look at the airway. Problems with the airway are much more common in children than in adults. For practical purposes, abnormalities of the airway can be divided into those that are acute and those that are chronic and into those that affect the upper airway and those that affect the lower airway. Clinically, children with upper airway obstruction (above the thoracic inlet) present with inspiratory stridor, whereas children with lower airway obstruction (below the thoracic inlet) are more likely to present with expiratory wheezing. However, the categorization of a child with noisy breathing into one of these two groups is often more difficult that we are led to believe. The primary imaging evaluation of the pediatric airway should include frontal and lateral high-kilovolt radiography of the airway and frontal and lateral views of the chest.

ACUTE UPPER AIRWAY OBSTRUCTION

The presentation of a young child with acute stridor is the most common indication for imaging the airway in children. The most frequent causes include inflammatory disorders and foreign bodies. Common inflammatory causes of acute upper airway obstruction include croup, epiglottitis, exudative tracheitis, and retropharyngeal cellulitis and abscess. Caustic ingestion is another cause. The following anatomic structures are especially important to evaluate on radiographs of children with acute upper airway obstruction: epiglottis,

aryepiglottic folds, subglottic trachea, and retropharyngeal soft tissues.

Croup

Croup (acute laryngotracheobronchitis) is the most common cause of acute upper airway obstruction in young children. Its cause is viral, and it is usually a benign, self-limited disease. Most children with croup are managed supportively as outpatients, and the parents are "managed" with reassurance. The children present with a barky ("croupy") cough and intermittent inspiratory stridor. It usually occurs after or during other symptoms of lower respiratory tract infection. Croup is a disease of infants and young children, with the peak incidence occurring between 6 months and 3 years of age. In children older than this, other causes of airway obstruction should be suspected.

The purpose of obtaining radiographs in a patient with suspected croup is not to document the diagnosis as much as it is to exclude other causes of upper airway obstruction that require intervention, such as a foreign body. However, the radiographic findings of croup are characteristic. On the frontal radiograph, there is loss of the normal shoulders (lateral convexities) of the subglottic trachea secondary to symmetric subglottic edema. The appearance has been likened to an inverted V or a "church steeple" (Fig. 2–1). The subglottic trachea becomes long and thin, with the narrow portion extending more inferiorly than the level of the piriform sinuses. Normally, the subglottic trachea appears rounded with "shoulders" that are convex outward (Fig. 2–2). Lateral radiographs may demonstrate narrowing or loss of definition of the lumen of

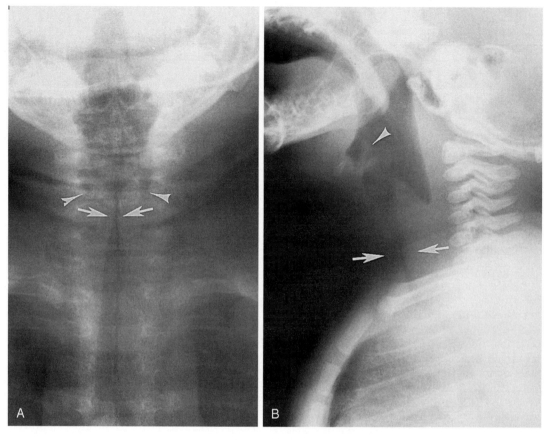

Figure 2–1. Croup in a 5-month-old girl. *A,* Frontal radiograph shows symmetric subglottic narrowing *(arrows),* with loss of normal shouldering. The narrowing extends more inferiorly than the piriform sinuses *(arrowheads). B,* Lateral radiograph shows subglottic narrowing *(arrows).* Note the normal-appearing epiglottis *(arrowhead).*

the subglottic trachea (see Fig. 2–1) or hypopharyngeal overdistention. The epiglottis and aryepiglottic folds appear normal.

Epiglottitis

In contrast to croup, epiglottitis is a life-threatening disease that requires potential emergent intubation. The arrival of a child with epiglottitis to a deserted radiology department used to be a constant cause of anxiety for on-call radiology residents. However, since most cases of epiglottitis are secondary to *Haemophilus influenzae,* which is now preventable by immunization, the incidence of epiglottitis has dramatically decreased. Children with epiglottitis usually appear toxic and present with an abrupt onset of stridor, dysphagia, fever, and restlessness, and an increase in respiratory distress when recumbent. The patients are typically older than those with croup, with the

peak incidence of presentation being 3½ years. Because of the risk of complete airway obstruction and respiratory failure, maneuvers that make the patient uncomfortable should be avoided. If the diagnosis is not made on physical examination, a single lateral radiograph of the neck should be obtained, usually with the patient erect or in whatever position breathing is comfortable. On the lateral radiograph, there is marked enlargement of the epiglottis and thickening of the aryepiglottic folds (Fig. 2–3). The aryepiglottic folds are the soft tissues that extend from the epiglottis anterosuperiorly to the arytenoid cartilage posteroinferiorly; they are normally convex inferiorly. When they become abnormally thickened, they appear convex superiorly. An obliquely imaged, or so-called omega-shaped, epiglottis may artifactually appear wide because both the left and right sides of the epiglottis are being imaged adjacent to each other. This should not be confused with a truly enlarged epiglottis. The presence or absence of thickening of the aryepiglottic folds can be helpful in this differentiation.

Exudative Tracheitis

Exudative tracheitis (also known as *bacterial tracheitis, membranous croup,* or *membranous laryngotracheobronchitis)* is another uncommon but potentially life-threatening cause of acute upper airway obstruction. The disorder is characterized by a purulent infection of the trachea in which exudative plaques form along the tracheal walls (much like those seen in diphtheria). Affected children are usually older and more ill than those with standard croup. Although initial reports described most cases to be secondary to *Staphylococcus aureus,* others have reported multimicrobial infections. It is

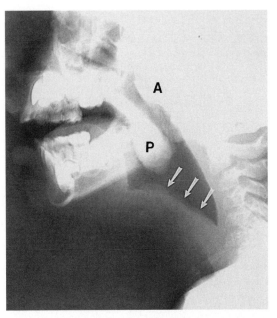

Figure 2–3. Epiglottitis in a 5-year-old girl. Lateral radiograph shows marked thickening of the epiglottis and prominence and convexity of the aryepiglottic folds *(arrows).* There is ballooning of the hypopharynx. Also, note the marked enlargement of the palatine tonsils (P) and adenoids (A).

unclear whether the disease is a primary bacterial infection or a secondary bacterial infection following damage to the respiratory mucosa from a viral infection. A linear soft tissue filling defect (a membrane) seen within the airway on radiography is the most characteristic finding. A plaque-like irregularity of the tracheal wall is also highly suspicious (Fig. 2–4). Other suspicious findings include symmetric or asymmetric subglottic narrowing in a child who is too old to have croup typically and irregularity or loss of definition of the tracheal wall.

If one of these exudative "membranes" is sloughed into the lumen, it can lead to airway occlusion and respiratory arrest. Therefore, children who are suspected of having exudative tracheitis are evaluated endoscopically, the exudative membranes are stripped, and elective endotracheal intubation is performed.

Retropharyngeal Cellulitis and Abscess

Retropharyngeal cellulitis is a pyogenic infection of the retropharyngeal space that usually

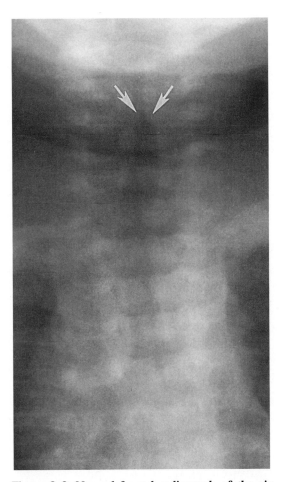

Figure 2–2. Normal frontal radiograph of the airway. The subglottic airway demonstrates rounded shoulders *(arrows)* that are convex.

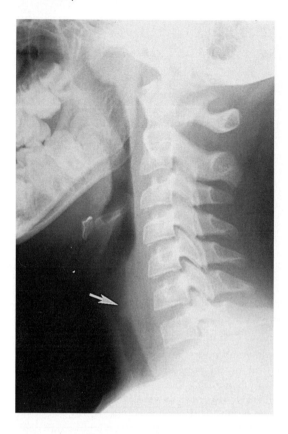

Figure 2–4. Exudative tracheitis in an 11-year-old boy. Lateral radiograph shows irregular plaque-like membrane (arrow) along posterior tracheal wall. Again, note the normal appearance of the non-thickened epiglottis in this patient.

follows recent pharyngitis or upper respiratory tract infection. Children present with sudden onset of fever, stiff neck, dysphagia, and occasionally stridor. Most affected children are young, with more than half of cases occurring between 6 and 12 months of age. Cellulitis alone is more common than a discrete abscess. On lateral radiography, there is thickening of the retropharyngeal soft tissues (Fig. 2–5). In an infant or young child, the soft tissues between the posterior aspect of the aerated pharynx and the anterior aspect of the vertebral column should not exceed the anteroposterior diameter of the cervical vertebral bodies. However, in infants (who have short necks), it is common to see "pseudothickening" of the retropharyngeal soft tissues when the lateral radiograph is taken without the neck being well extended. Supportive evidence that there is true widening of the retropharyngeal soft tissues includes apex anterior convexity of the retropharyngeal soft tissues (Fig. 2–6). If it is unclear on the initial lateral radiograph whether the soft tissues are truly artifactually widened, it is best to repeat the lateral radiograph with the neck placed in full extension (Fig. 2–7). The only radiographic feature that can differentiate abscess from cellulitis is the

identification of gas within the retropharyngeal soft tissues. In suspicious cases, computed tomography (CT) is performed to define the extent of disease and help predict cases in which a drainable fluid collection is present. On CT, a low-attenuation, well-defined area with an enhancing rim is suspicious for a drainable fluid collection.

Foreign Body

Most aspirated foreign bodies end up in the bronchi and these lower airway foreign bodies will be discussed further on. Laryngeal or tracheal foreign bodies are far less common than bronchial foreign bodies and usually present with abrupt stridor or respiratory distress. Radiographic findings include a radiopaque foreign body (Fig. 2–8), soft tissue density within the airway, and loss of visualization (silhouetting) of the airway wall contours. Foreign bodies lodged within the proximal esophagus may also present with airway compression.

CHRONIC UPPER AIRWAY OBSTRUCTION

In children who present with less abrupt, more chronic symptoms of upper airway obstruc-

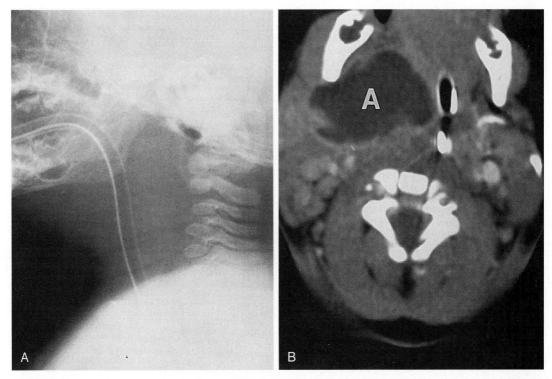

Figure 2–5. Retropharyngeal abscess in a 4-month-old girl with stridor and fever. *A,* Lateral radiographs shows marked thickening of the retropharyngeal soft tissues. No gas is present in the soft tissues. The patient is intubated. No aerated pharynx is present secondary to the marked swelling. *B,* Contrast-enhanced computed tomography (CT) shows a low-attenuation region, with enhancing rim (A) displacing the endotracheal tube.

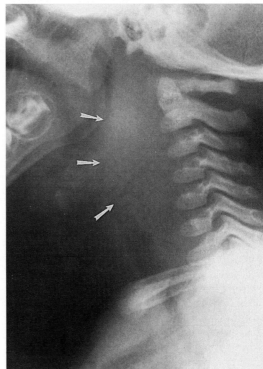

Figure 2–6. Retropharyngeal cellulitis in a 1-year-old boy. Lateral radiograph shows increased thickness of the retropharyngeal soft tissues *(arrows)*, which have an anterior convex appearance.

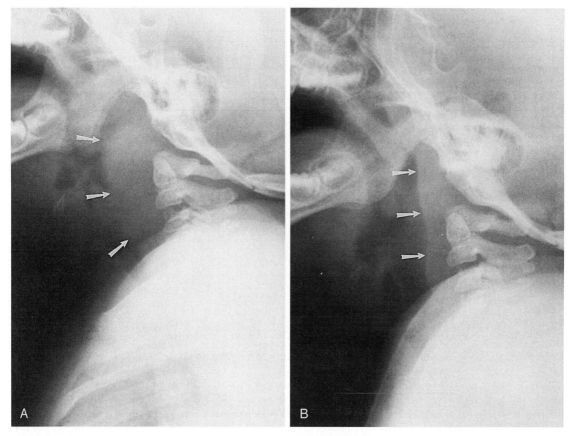

Figure 2–7. Pseudoretropharyngeal soft tissue thickening secondary to extended neck positioning in a 3-month-old infant. *A,* Initial lateral radiograph shows apparent thickening of retropharyngeal soft tissues *(arrows).* *B,* Repeat lateral radiograph with neck extended shows normal thickness *(arrows).*

tion, there is a separate list of differential considerations. These children may present with chronic stridor but may also manifest sleep apnea or snoring. Any space-occupying mass or fixed narrowing of the airway at any level can lead to such symptoms. Diagnostic considerations include inflammatory conditions, congenital disorders, and neoplastic masses. Obstruction within the nasal cavity can be secondary to things such as adenoid enlargement, choanal atresia, or juvenile angiofibroma. Obstruction within the posterior oropharynx can be secondary to micrognathia with posterior displacement of the tongue or macroglossia. Obstruction at the level of the larynx can be secondary to laryngeal malacia or congenital cysts.

The most common cause of chronic upper airway obstruction is enlargement of the palatine and adenoid tonsils. The palatine tonsils are easily evaluated on physical examination. However, because the adenoid tonsils are difficult to see on physical examination, lateral radiographs are often obtained to evaluate the adenoids for enlargement. On radiography, enlarged adenoids appear as a convex soft tissue mass in the posterior nasopharynx measuring greater than 2 cm in diameter. Markedly enlarged adenoid tissues may completely obstruct the nasopharynx. Enlarged palatine tonsils appear as a large soft tissue mass projecting over the posterior aspect of the soft palate on lateral radiography (Fig. 2–9).

LOWER AIRWAY OBSTRUCTION

The most common causes of wheezing in children include conditions of small airway inflammation such as asthma and viral illness (bronchiolitis). When the wheezing persists, presents at an atypical age for asthma, or is refractory to treatment, other reasons for lower airway obstruction are entertained. Causes of lower airway obstruction can be divided into those that are intrinsic to the

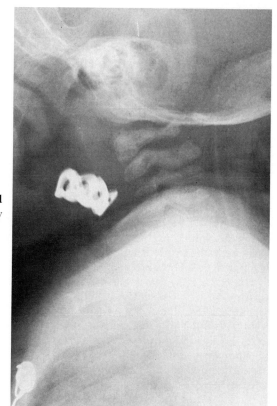

Figure 2–8. Laryngeal foreign body in a 6-month-old girl. Lateral radiograph shows radiopaque crown (toy part) perched on aryepiglottic folds.

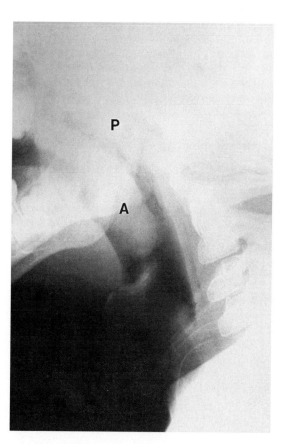

Figure 2–9. Enlargement of the adenoid and palatine tonsils in a 6-month-old girl. Lateral radiograph shows enlargement of the palatine (P) and adenoid (A) tonsils, with nearly complete obstruction of the nasopharynx.

airway—such as bronchial foreign body, tracheal malacia, or intrinsic masses—and those that cause extrinsic compression of the trachea, such as vascular rings. The initial screening procedure is frontal and lateral radiography of the airway and chest. Radiographs are used to exclude acute causes of upper airway obstruction, evaluate for other processes that can cause wheezing, such as heart disease, and help categorize the abnormality as more likely to be an intrinsic or extrinsic airway process. Important findings to look for on the radiographs include evidence of tracheal narrowing, position of the aortic arch, asymmetric lung aeration, radiopaque foreign body, and lung consolidation.

If the radiographs suggest an intrinsic abnormality, bronchoscopy is the next procedure of choice. If the radiographs suggest extrinsic compression, cross-sectional imaging is performed. There has been much debate over what constitutes the best imaging study to evaluate extrinsic airway compression: magnetic resonance imaging (MRI) or CT. MRI offers high intrinsic contrast between the airway and adjacent structures and is not dependent on contrast administration. Disadvantages include the need for sedation, which is of particular concern in an infant with a tenuous airway, and poor visualization of the lung. Contrast-enhanced CT provides nearly identical information, and often infants can be imaged without sedation, particularly when using the currently available rapid helical scanners. The lung is well visualized with CT. This modality is dependent on intravenous contrast and if

the bolus is missed when imaging a small child, a very suboptimal scan results. I think more institutions are moving toward using CT over MRI to evaluate the pediatric airway.

Extrinsic Lower Airway Compression

Almost any process that causes either a space-occupying mass within the mediastinum or enlargement or malposition of a vascular structure can lead to compression of the airway. The classically described vascular causes of lower airway compression include double aortic arch, anomalous left pulmonary artery, and innominate artery compression syndrome. However, other causes of airway compression include enlargement of the ascending aorta (Fig. 2–10), such as seen with Marfan syndrome; enlargement of the pulmonary arteries (Fig. 2–11), such as seen with congenital absence of the pulmonary valve; malposition of the descending aorta, as is seen in midline-descending aorta-carina-compression syndrome, enlargement of the left atrium; or abnormal chest wall configuration, such as a narrow thoracic inlet (Fig. 2–12). When differentiating causes of lower airway compression on radiography, it is important to note both the superior to inferior level of the tracheal compression and whether the compression is from the anterior or posterior aspect of the trachea (Fig. 2–13).

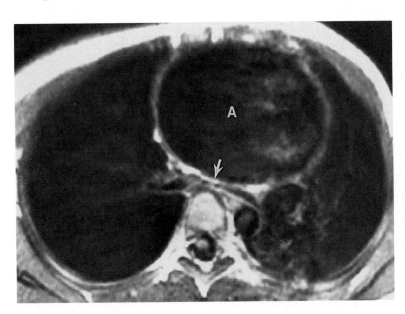

Figure 2–10. Giant aneurysm of the ascending aorta causing airway compression in a 7-year-old boy. Axial, T1-weighted MR image shows massive dilatation of ascending aorta (A), with resulting compression of tracheal carina *(arrow)*. (From Donnelly LF, Strife JL, Bisset GS III. The spectrum of extrinsic lower airway compression in children: MR imaging. AJR Am J Roentgenol 1997; 168:59–62.)

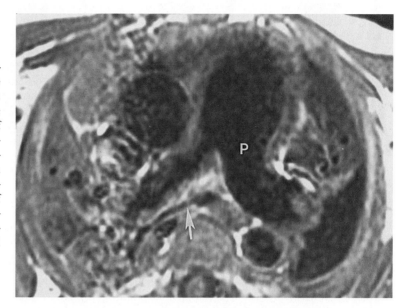

Figure 2–11. Enlarged pulmonary arteries compressing the airway in a 7-month-old boy. Axial, T1-weighted MR image shows massive dilatation of pulmonary artery (P), with resulting compression of tracheal carina *(arrow)*. (From Donnelly LF, Strife JL, Bisset GS III. The spectrum of extrinsic lower airway compression in children: MR imaging. AJR Am J Roentgenol 1997;168:59–62.)

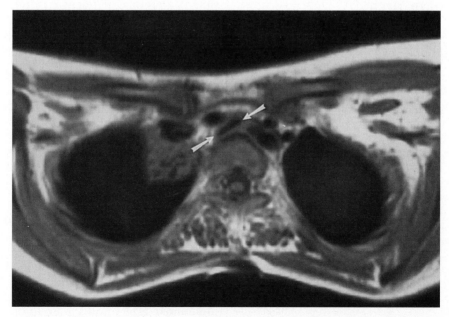

Figure 2–12. Narrow anteroposterior chest configuration with resulting airway compression. Axial, T1-weighted MR image shows narrow thoracic inlet with nearly complete occlusion of the trachea *(arrows)* between the innominate artery and the anterior aspect of the vertebral body. (From Donnelly LF, Strife JL, Bisset GS III. The spectrum of extrinsic lower airway compression in children: MR imaging. AJR Am J Roentgenol 1997;168:59–62.)

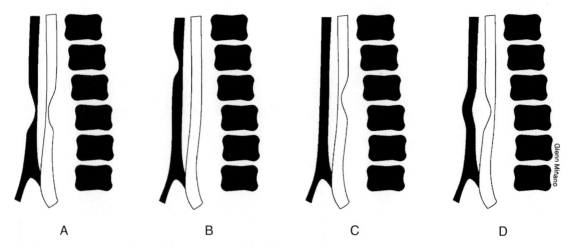

Glenn Miñano

A   B   C   D

Figure 2–13. Patterns of compression of the trachea and esophagus in common vascular rings. These diagrams are drawn as would be seen on a lateral radiograph of the chest. The trachea is black and the esophagus is white. *A,* Double aortic arch. The trachea is compressed from its anterior aspect, and the esophagus is compressed from its posterior aspect. *B,* Innominate artery compression. The trachea is compressed at its anterior aspect. The level of compression is just below the thoracic inlet, higher than other vascular causes of compression. *C,* Left arch with aberrant right subclavian artery or right arch with aberrant left subclavian artery. There is compression of the posterior aspect of the esophagus. The trachea is not compressed. *D,* Aberrant left pulmonary artery (pulmonary sling). The trachea is compressed at its posterior aspect, and the esophagus is compressed from its anterior aspect.

Double Aortic Arch

Double aortic arch is a congenital arch anomaly related to persistence of both the left and right fourth aortic arches. It is usually an isolated lesion and typically presents with symptoms early in life. It is the most common symptomatic vascular ring. Typically, the right arch is dominant, being both larger and more superiorly positioned (Fig. 2–14). In such cases, the left arch is ligated through a left thoracotomy. When the left arch is dominant, a right thoracotomy is performed and the right arch is ligated. Determining the dominant arch is one of the goals of performing cross-sectional imaging. Anatomically, the two arches surround and compress the trachea anteriorly and the esophagus posteriorly. The level of compression is the middle to lower intrathoracic trachea.

Pulmonary Sling

With anomalous origin of the left pulmonary artery (pulmonary sling), the left pulmonary artery arises from the right pulmonary artery rather than the main pulmonary artery and passes between the trachea and the esophagus as it courses toward the left lung. The resultant sling compresses the trachea. Pulmonary sling is the only vascular anomaly to course between the trachea and the esophagus (Fig. 2–15). Therefore, compression of the posterior aspect of the trachea and anterior aspect of the esophagus on lateral imaging is characteristic. It is the only vascular anomaly that is associated with asymmetric lung inflation on chest radiographs (Fig. 2–16). Pulmonary sling can be associated with congenital heart disease and with complete tracheal rings (see Fig. 2–16), which is an additional cause of airway problems.

Innominate Artery Compression Syndrome

The innominate artery passes immediately anterior to the trachea just inferior to the level of the thoracic inlet. In infants, in whom the innominate artery arises more to the left than it does in adults and in whom the mediastinum is "crowded" by the relatively large thymus, there can be narrowing of the trachea at this level. There is a spectrum from normal to severe narrowing, with the syndrome classification being reserved for patients who are symptomatic. The compression and resultant symptoms decrease with time as the child

Text continued on page 19

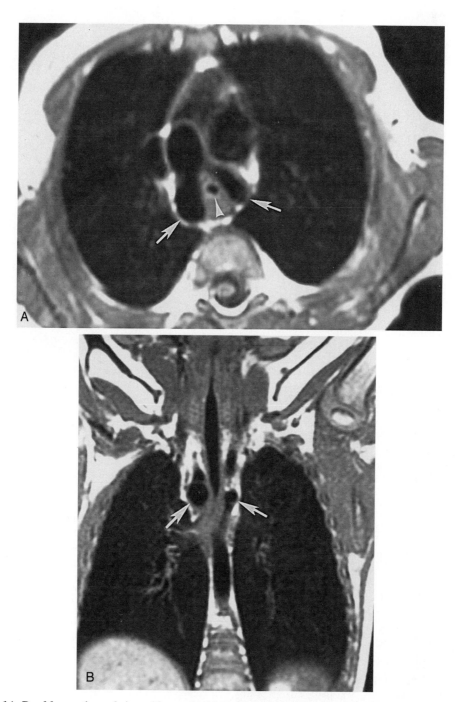

Figure 2–14. Double aortic arch in a 13-month-old girl. *A*, Axial, T1-weighted MR image shows right and left arches *(arrows)* surrounding small compressed trachea *(arrowhead)*. *B*, Coronal, T1-weighted MR image shows right and left arches *(arrows)* surrounding compressed trachea. Note typical configuration, with right arch being larger and more superiorly positioned than left arch.

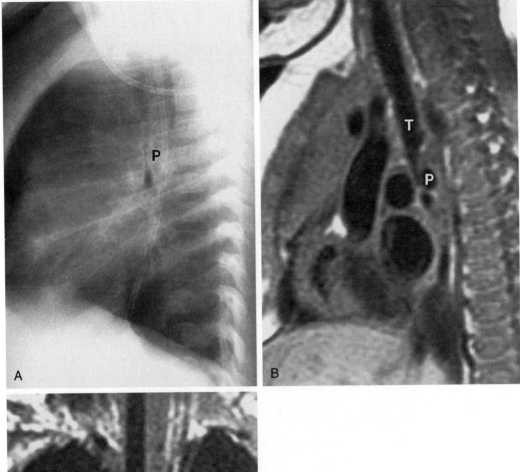

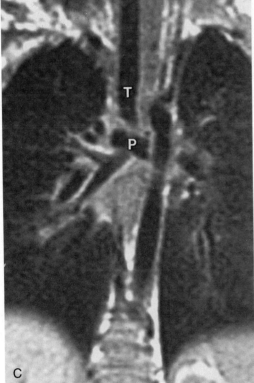

Figure 2–15. Pulmonary sling in a 12-week-old girl. *A,* Lateral radiograph shows soft tissue density (P) compressing the trachea from its posterior aspect and the esophagus (demonstrated by presence of feeding tube) from its anterior aspect. *B* and *C,* Sagittal (B) and coronal (C) T1-weighted MR image show anomalous left pulmonary artery (P) compressing the posterior trachea (T) as it passes from right to left.

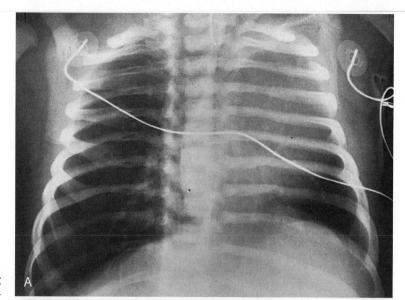

Figure 2–16. Pulmonary sling in a 1-month-old girl. *A,* Frontal radiograph shows asymmetric aeration of the lungs, which is often seen with pulmonary sling but rarely with other causes of extrinsic tracheal compression. *B,* Axial, T1-weighted MR image shows anomalous origin of left pulmonary artery *(arrows)* from right pulmonary artery rather than main pulmonary artery (P). The pulmonary sling wraps around and compresses the trachea *(arrowhead)* as it passes into the left hemithorax. *C,* Axial, T1-weighted MR image more superiorly shows trachea to be round and small in caliber at this level. These findings are suspicious for a complete cartilaginous tracheal ring.

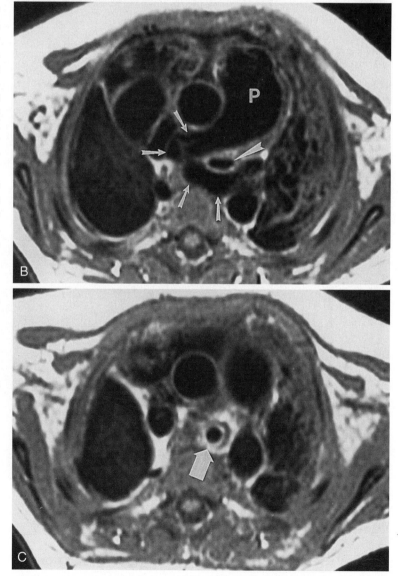

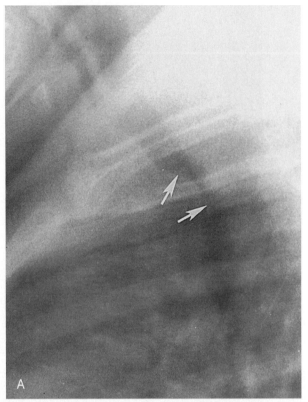

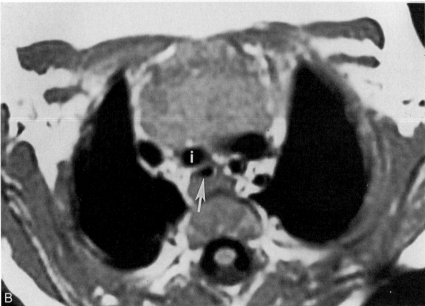

Figure 2–17. Innominate artery compression syndrome in a 4-month-old boy. *A,* Lateral radiograph shows anterior compression of the trachea *(arrows)* just below the level of the thoracic inlet. *B,* Axial, T1-weighted MR image shows innominate artery (i) compressing the trachea *(arrow)*. The trachea is oblong. Normally, the trachea is round at this level.

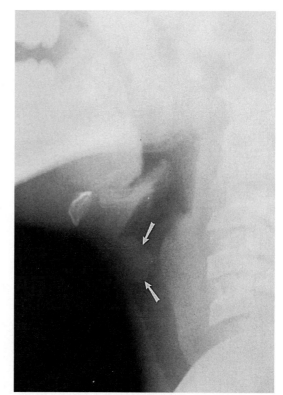

Figure 2–18. Subglottic granuloma in a 7-year-old boy. Lateral radiograph shows a round, well-defined subglottic mass *(arrows).*

grows, and surgical therapy is reserved for patients in whom symptoms are severe. On lateral radiography, there is indentation of the anterior aspect of the trachea at or just below the thoracic inlet (Fig. 2–17). Cross-sectional imaging demonstrates the abnormality and excludes other causes of the airway compression.

Intrinsic Lower Airway Obstruction

Intrinsic abnormalities of the lower airway include dynamic processes such as tracheomalacia, tracheal stenosis, foreign body obstruction, or focal masses. Tracheomalacia consists of tracheal wall softening related to an abnormality of the cartilaginous rings of the trachea. It can be a primary or secondary condition and results in intermittent collapse of the trachea. The diagnosis cannot be made on a single static radiograph. However, lateral fluoroscopy or endoscopy can demonstrate dynamic changes in the caliber of the trachea, which are diagnostic.

The most common soft tissue masses of the trachea include hemangiomas, which most commonly occur in the subglottic region and can cause asymmetric subglottic narrowing,

tracheal papilloma, and tracheal granuloma (Fig. 2–18).

Bronchial Foreign Body

Infants and toddlers explore their environment with their mouths and will stick almost anything in them. When such foreign bodies are aspirated, the bronchus is the most common site of lodgment. Often, the aspiration is not witnessed, and symptoms may be indolent, leading to an occult presentation. Radiographic findings of bronchial foreign bodies include asymmetric lung aeration, hyperinflation, oligemia, atelectasis, lung consolidation, pneumothorax, or pneumomediastinum. The vast majority of bronchial foreign bodies (as many as 97%) are nonradiopaque. Inspiratory films alone can be normal in up to one third of patients with bronchial foreign bodies. Because the volume of the affected lung segments can be normal, increased, or decreased, the key radiographic feature is a lack of change in lung volume demonstrated at different phases of the respiratory cycle (Fig. 2–19). Evaluation at different phases of the respiratory cycle is easily accomplished with expir-

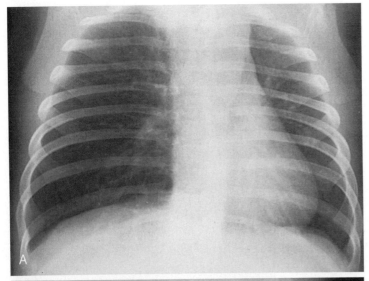

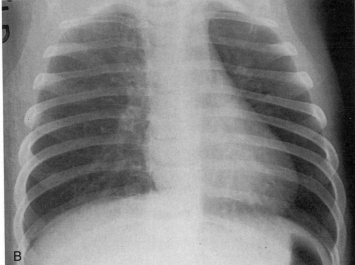

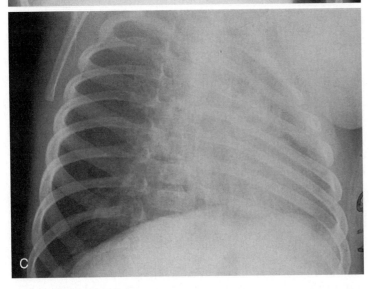

Figure 2–19. Bronchial foreign body in a 1-year-old boy who presented with wheezing that was refractory to therapy. *A,* Initial frontal radiograph shows slight asymmetry in lung volumes, with the right being greater than the left. *B,* Chest radiograph obtained with patient in right lateral decubitus (right side down) position shows no interval change in the right lung volume. *C,* Chest radiograph obtained with patient in left lateral decubitus (left side down) position shows collapse of the left lung, as expected. Therefore, there is a static right lung volume, and a right bronchial obstruction was suspected. Endoscopy showed a piece of mulch occluding the right main bronchus.

atory and inspiratory films in cooperative children. In uncooperative infants and children (the population most at risk for foreign body aspiration), air trapping can be detected with bilateral decubitus views of the chest or fluoroscopy. The differential diagnosis for an asymmetric, lucent lung includes a bronchial foreign body, the Swyer-James syndrome, and pulmonary hypoplasia.

Suggested Reading

Berdon WE, Baker DH. Vascular anomalies and the infant lung: rings, slings, and other things. Semin Roentgenol 1972;7:39–63.

Capitanio MA, Kirkpatrick JA. Obstruction of the upper airway in infants and children. Radiol Clin North Am 1968;6:265–277.

Donnelly LF, Frush DP, Bisset GS III. The multiple presentations of foreign bodies in children. AJR Am J Roentgenol 1998;170:471–477.

Donnelly LF, Strife JL, Bisset GS III. The spectrum of extrinsic lower airway compression in children: MR imaging. AJR Am J Roentgenol 1997;168:59–62.

Dunbar JS. Upper respiratory tract obstruction in infants and children. AJR Am J Roentgenol 1970;109:227–246.

Esclamado RM, Richardson MA. Laryngotracheal foreign bodies in children: a comparison with bronchial foreign bodies. Am J Dis Child 1987;141:259–262.

John SD, Swischuk KE. Stridor and upper airway obstruction in infants and children. RadioGraphics 1992; 12:625–643.

3

Chest

Chest radiography is one of the most commonly performed examinations in pediatric imaging. It is also the most likely examination to be encountered by radiology residents, pediatric residents, general radiologists, and pediatricians. Therefore, topics such as chest imaging in neonates and the evaluation of suspected pneumonia are discussed in detail.

NEONATAL CHEST

The causes of respiratory distress in newborn infants can be divided into those that are secondary to diffuse pulmonary disease (medical causes) and those that are secondary to a space-occupying mass that is compressing the pulmonary parenchyma (surgical causes).

Diffuse Pulmonary Disease in the Newborn

Diffuse pulmonary disease is a much more common cause of respiratory distress in the newborn than are surgical causes, particularly in premature infants, who make up the majority of cases of respiratory distress in the newborn. A simple way to evaluate these patients and try to offer a limited differential diagnosis is to evaluate the lung volumes and characterize the pulmonary opacities.

Lung volumes can be categorized as high, normal, or low. Normally, the apex of the dome of the diaphragm can be expected to be at the level of approximately the 10th posterior rib. Lung opacity, if present, can be characterized as streaky perihilar (central) densities that have a linear quality or as diffuse, granular opacities that have an almost sand-like character. Classically, cases fall into one of

the following two categories: (1) those with high lung volumes and streaky perihilar densities and (2) those with low lung volumes and granular opacities (Table 3–1). Obviously, this is a helpful guideline rather than a rule, because many patients have normal lung volumes. The differential diagnosis for patients with high lung volumes and streaky perihilar densities is meconium aspiration, TTN, and neonatal pneumonia. Most of these neonates will be born at term. The differential diagnosis for patients with low lung volumes and granular opacities is surfactant deficiency or β-hemolytic streptococcal pneumonia. Most of these neonates are premature.

Meconium Aspiration Syndrome

Meconium aspiration syndrome occurs secondary to intrapartum or intrauterine aspiration of meconium. It is usually secondary to stress, such as hypoxia, and more often occurs in term or postmature neonates. The aspirated meconium causes obstruction of small airways secondary to its tenacious nature as well as a chemical pneumonitis. The degree of respiratory failure can be severe. Radiographic findings include hyperinflation (high lung vol-

TABLE 3–1. **Differential Diagnosis of Diffuse Pulmonary Disease in the Newborn**

High lung volumes, streaky perihilar densities
  Meconium aspiration syndrome
  Transient tachypnea of the newborn
  Neonatal pneumonia

Low lung volumes, granular opacities
  Surfactant deficiency
  β-hemolytic streptococcal pneumonia

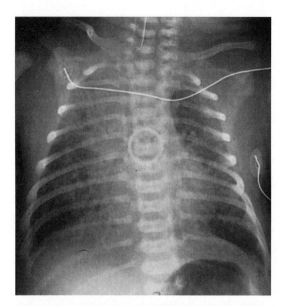

Figure 3–1. Meconium aspiration syndrome in a newborn boy with respiratory distress. Chest radiographs shows large lung volumes and coarse, ropy bilateral perihilar markings.

umes) that may be asymmetric and patchy and asymmetric lung densities that may have a ropy perihilar distribution (Fig. 3–1). There are often areas of hyperinflation alternating with areas of atelectasis. Pleural effusions can be present. Because of the obstruction of the small airways by the meconium, airblock complications are common, with pneumothorax occurring in 20 to 40% of cases.

Transient Tachypnea of the Newborn

Transient tachypnea of the newborn (TTN) is also referred to by a variety of other names, including *wet lung disease* and *transient respiratory distress*. It occurs secondary to delayed clearance of fetal pulmonary fluid. Physiologically, clearing of fetal pulmonary fluid is facilitated by the "thoracic squeeze" during vaginal deliveries, and most cases of TTN are related to cesarean section in which the thoracic squeeze is bypassed. Maternal sedation is another cause, and the condition is also seen in infants of diabetic mothers. The hallmark of TTN is a benign course. Respiratory distress develops by 6 hours of age, peaks at 1 day of age, and is resolved by 2 to 3 days. The radiographic findings are similar to those seen with the spectrum of mild to severe pulmonary edema. There is a combination of airspace opacification, coarse interstitial markings, prominent and indistinct pulmonary vasculature, fluid in the fissures, pleural effusion, and cardiomegaly (Fig. 3–2). Lung volumes are normal to increased.

Neonatal Pneumonia

Neonatal pneumonia can result from a large number of infectious agents that can be acquired in the uterus, during birth, or soon after birth. With the exception of β-hemolytic

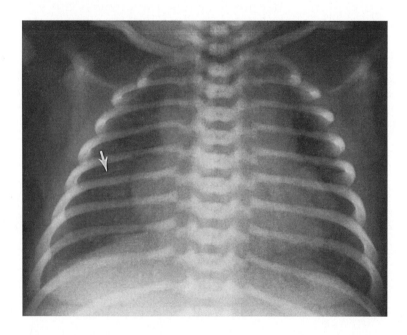

Figure 3–2. Transient tachypnea in a newborn boy. Chest radiograph shows normal lung volumes, cardiomegaly, indistinct pulmonary vascularity, and fluid in the minor fissure *(arrow)*. Within 24 hours, the patient was asymptomatic.

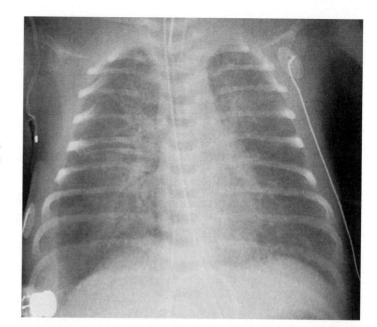

Figure 3–3. Neonatal pneumonia in a newborn boy. Chest radiographs shows large lung volumes and coarse, bilateral perihilar markings. There is a right pleural effusion.

streptococcal pneumonia, which will be discussed separately, the radiographic appearance of neonatal pneumonia is that of patchy, asymmetric perihilar densities and hyperinflation (Fig. 3–3).

Surfactant-Deficient Disease

Surfactant-deficient disease (SDD) (also referred to as *respiratory distress syndrome* or *hyaline membrane disease*) is the most common cause of death in newborns. It is a disease of premature infants and is related to the inabil-

ity of premature type II pneumocytes to produce surfactant. Normally, surfactant coats the alveolar surfaces and decreases surface tension, allowing the alveoli to remain open. As a result of the lack of surfactant, there is alveolar collapse, resulting in noncompliant lungs. The radiographic findings reflect these pathologic changes (Fig. 3–4). Lung volumes are low, and there are bilateral granular opacities that represent collapsed alveoli interspersed with open alveoli. Because the larger bronchi do not collapse, there are prominent air bronchograms. When the process is severe enough and the majority of alveoli are collapsed, there may be

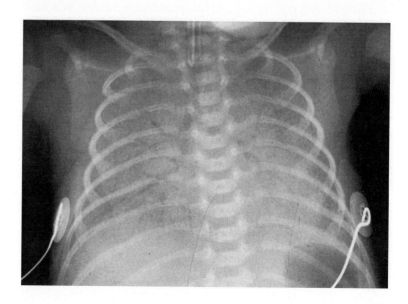

Figure 3–4. Surfactant-deficient disease in a newborn girl. Chest radiograph shows low lung volumes, granular opacities, and prominent air bronchograms.

coalescence of the granular opacities, resulting in a diffuse lung opacity. A normal film at 6 hours of age excludes the presence of SDD.

One of the therapies for SDD is surfactant administration. Surfactant can be given in nebulized and aerosol forms. It is released into the trachea via a catheter or adapted endotracheal tube. The administration of surfactant in neonates with SDD has been shown to be associated with decreased oxygen and ventilator setting requirements, decreased airblock complications, a decreased incidence of intracranial hemorrhage and BPD, and a decreased death rate. However, there is an increased risk of the development of patent ductus arteriosus or pulmonary hemorrhage, and there can be an acute desaturation episode in response to surfactant administration. Radiography may show complete (Fig. 3–5), central, or asymmetric clearing of the findings of SDD. There is usually an increase in lung volume. Patients without radiographic findings of a response to surfactant have a poorer prognosis than do those with such radiographic evidence. A pattern of alternating distended and collapsed acini may create a radiographic pattern of bubble-like lucencies that may mimic PIE.

β-Hemolytic Streptococcal Pneumonia

β-hemolytic (group B) streptococcal pneumonia is the most common type of pneumonia

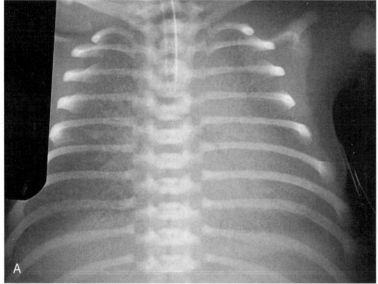
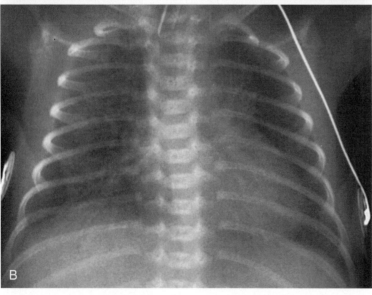

Figure 3–5. **Surfactant-deficient disease responding to surfactant therapy in a newborn girl.** *A,* Radiograph obtained shortly after birth shows low lung volumes, confluent densities, and prominent air bronchograms. *B,* Radiograph obtained immediately after surfactant administration shows increased lung volumes and decreased lung opacities.

seen in neonates. The infection is acquired during birth, and at least 25% of women in labor are colonized by the organism. Premature infants are infected more often than are term infants. In contrast to the other types of neonatal pneumonias, the radiographic findings of β-hemolytic streptococcal pneumonia include bilateral granular opacities and low lung volumes, findings identical to those of SDD. The presence of pleural fluid is a helpful differentiating factor. It is uncommon in surfactant deficiency and present in up to 67% of cases of β-hemolytic streptococcal pneumonia.

Persistent Pulmonary Hypertension of the Neonate

Persistent pulmonary hypertension of the neonate, also referred to as *persistent fetal circulation* is a term often used in neonatal intensive care units (NICUs) and is addressed here because it can be a source of confusion. The high pulmonary vascular resistance that is normally present in the fetus typically decreases during the newborn period. When such a decrease fails to occur, the pulmonary pressures remain abnormally high, and the condition is referred to as *persistent pulmonary hypertension.* It is a physiologic finding rather than a specific disease. It can be a primary phenomenon or can occur secondary to causes of hypoxia, such as meconium aspiration syndrome, neonatal pneumonia, or pulmonary hypoplasia associated with congenital diaphragmatic hernia. These patients are often quite ill. The radiographic patterns are variable and often are more reflective of the underlying cause of hypoxia rather than the presence of persistent pulmonary hypertension.

Neonatal Intensive Care Unit Support Apparatus

One of the primary roles of chest radiography in the NICU is to monitor support apparatus. This includes endotracheal tubes, orogastric tubes, central venous lines, umbilical arterial and venous catheters, and extracorporeal membrane oxygenation (ECMO) catheters. The radiographic evaluation of many of these tubes is the same as that in adults and will not be discussed. When evaluating the position of endotracheal tubes in small premature neonates, it is important to consider that the

length of the entire trachea may be only about 1 cm. Keeping the endotracheal tube in the exact center of such a small trachea is an impossible task for caregivers, and phone calls and reports suggesting that the tube needs to be moved 2 mm proximally may be more annoying than helpful. Phone calls may be more appropriately reserved for when the tube is in the main bronchi or above the thoracic inlet. There is an increased propensity for esophageal intubation in neonates compared with adults. Although it would seem that esophageal intubation would be incredibly obvious clinically, this is not always the case. I have seen cases in which it was seen in retrospect that a child has been esophageally intubated for over 24 hours. Therefore, the radiologist may be the first to recognize esophageal intubation. Obviously, when the course of the endotracheal tube does not overlie the path of the trachea, esophageal intubation is suspect. Supporting evidence includes low lung volumes, gas within the esophagus, and gaseous distention of the bowel (Fig. 3–6).

Umbilical Arterial and Venous Catheters

Umbilical arterial and venous catheters are commonly used in the NICU. Umbilical arterial catheters pass from the umbilicus inferiorly into the pelvis via the umbilical artery to the iliac artery. The catheters then turn cephalad within the aorta. These catheters can be associated with thrombosis of the aorta and its branches. Therefore, it is important not to leave the tip of the catheter at the level of the branches of the aorta (celiac, superior mesenteric, and renal arteries). There are two types of desired catheter position: *high lines,* which have their tips at the level of the descending thoracic aorta (T8-10) and *low lines,* which have their tips below the level of L3 (Fig. 3–7). The catheter tip should not be positioned between T10 and L3.

The pathway of the umbilical venous catheter goes from the umbilical vein to the left portal vein to the ductus venosus to the hepatic vein to the inferior vena cava (IVC). In contrast to umbilical arterial catheters, the course is in the superior direction from the level of the umbilicus. The ideal position of an umbilical venous catheter is with its tip at the junction of the right atrium and the IVC at the level of the hemidiaphragm (see Fig. 3–7). The umbilical venous catheter may deflect into the portal venous system rather than passing into the ductus venosus. Complications of such positioning can include hepatic hematoma or abscess (Fig. 3–8).

Extracorporeal Membrane Oxygenation

ECMO is a therapy of last resort that is usually reserved for respiratory failure that fails to respond to other treatments. It is reserved for patients who have reversible disease and a chance for survival. The majority of neonates who are treated with ECMO have meconium aspiration, persistent pulmonary hypertension from whatever cause, or congenital diaphragmatic hernia. ECMO is essentially a prolonged form of circulatory bypass of the lungs. For arteriovenous ECMO, the right common carotid artery and internal jugular veins are sacrificed. The arterial catheter is placed via the

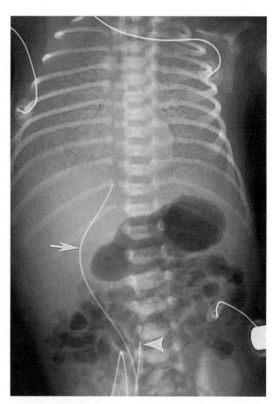

Figure 3–7. Expected location of umbilical catheters in a newborn boy. Radiograph demonstrates the umbilical arterial catheter *(arrowhead)* to pass initially inferiorly and have its tip positioned at the level of L4 (expected position of a *low line*). The umbilical venous catheter *(arrow)* passes directly superior to the umbilicus and has its tip positioned at the level of the right hemidiaphragm. Findings of surfactant deficiency are seen in the chest.

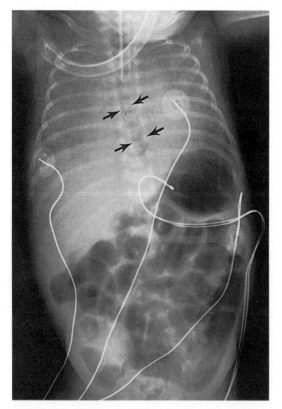

Figure 3–6. Esophageal intubation in a 6-day-old girl. Chest radiograph obtained after reintubation shows the endotracheal tube overlying the expected location at the midtrachea. However, there are low lung volumes, gas within the esophagus *(arrows)*, and multiple air-filled and distended bowel loops.

carotid artery and positioned with its tip overlying the aortic arch. The venous catheter is positioned with its tip over the right atrium (Fig. 3–9). Because of decreased ventilator settings and third space shifting of fluid, it is common to see white-out of the lungs soon after a patient is placed on ECMO (see Fig. 3–9). Patients receiving ECMO undergo anticoagulation and are at risk for hemorrhage.

Types of Ventilation—High-Frequency Oscillator Versus Conventional Ventilation

High-frequency oscillators are commonly used to treat neonates in the NICU. In contrast to conventional ventilation, high-frequency oscillators use supraphysiologic rates of ventilation

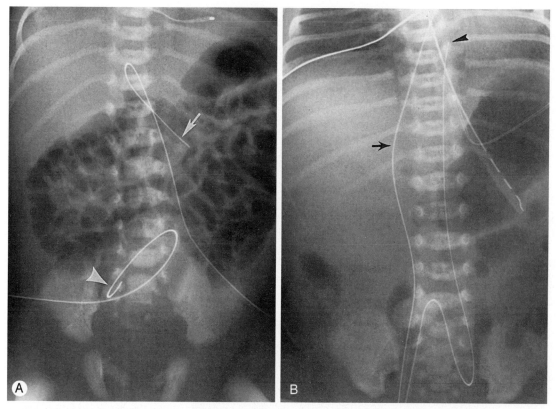

Figure 3–8. Nonacceptable positioning of umbilical catheters. *A,* Radiograph demonstrates the umbilical venous catheter *(arrow)* to be within the superior mesenteric vein. The tip of the umbilical arterial catheter is within the region of the internal iliac artery *(arrowhead). B,* Radiograph shows the umbilical venous catheter *(arrow)* to extend off the superior aspect of the film, passing through the right atrium, most likely exiting a patent foramen ovale. The umbilical arterial catheter *(arrowhead)* is within the region of the descending aorta, an expected position for a *high line.*

with very low tidal volumes. Conventional ventilation has been likened to delivering a cupful of air approximately 20 times per minute. In contrast, high-frequency oscillation is like delivering a thimbleful of air approximately 1000 times per minute. The air is vibrated in and out of the lung. The mechanism by which these oscillators work is poorly understood. In contrast to conventional ventilation, in which the diaphragm moves up and down, with high-frequency oscillators, the diaphragm is maintained at a certain anatomic level. This level can be adjusted by varying the mean airway pressure of the oscillator. Caregivers use the chest radiograph as a gauge to adjust the mean airway pressure up or down. They like to have the diaphragm approximately at the level of 10 1/2 posterior ribs. In general, the radiographic appearance of neonatal pulmonary diseases is not affected by whether the patient is being ventilated by conventional or high-frequency ventilation.

Complications in the Neonatal Intensive Care Unit

Like in adult intensive care units, major complications detected by chest radiographs are most commonly related to airblock complications, lobar collapse, or acute diffuse pulmonary consolidation. Another type of complication seen in neonates is the development of BPD. Imaging findings of lobar collapse and airblock complications such as pneumothorax, pneumomediastinum, and pneumopericardium are similar in neonates and adults. One type of airblock complication that is unique to neonates is PIE.

Pulmonary Interstitial Emphysema

In patients with severe surfactant deficiency, ventilatory support can result in marked increases in alveolar pressure, leading to perfo-

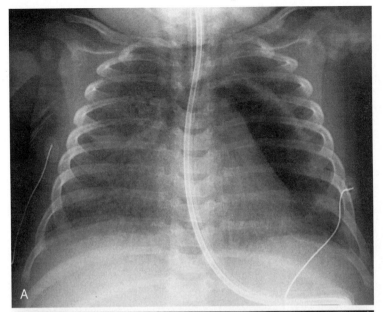

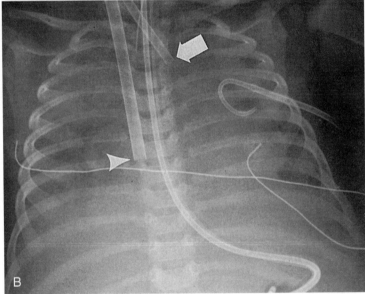

Figure 3–9. Extracorporeal membrane oxygenation (ECMO) catheter placement in a 6-month-old boy with acute respiratory distress syndrome (ARDS) secondary to burns. *A,* Chest radiograph before ECMO therapy has begun shows aerated lungs and medial left pneumothorax. *B,* Chest radiograph after ECMO therapy has been started shows decreased lung volumes and increased lung opacity, findings that are not uncommon after ECMO therapy is started because of fluid shifts and decreased ventilator settings. The venous catheter enters the right neck and has its tip *(arrow)* overlying the expected location of the right atrium. The arterial catheter has its tip *(arrowhead)* overlying the aortic arch.

ration of alveoli. The air that escapes into the adjacent interstitium and lymphatics is referred to as pulmonary interstitial emphysema (PIE) (Fig. 3–10). PIE appears on radiographs as bubble-like or linear lucencies and can be focal (Fig. 3–11) or diffuse. The involved lung is usually noncompliant and a static lung volume can be seen on multiple consecutive films. The finding is typically transient. The importance of detecting PIE is that it serves as a warning sign for other pending airblock complications such as pneumothorax, and its presence can influence caregivers regarding

decisions such as switching from conventional to high-frequency ventilation.

I think it can be very difficult to differentiate diffuse PIE from the bubble-like lucencies that are associated with developing BPD. When encountering this scenario, I rely on the patient's age to help me decide which condition is more likely. Most cases of PIE occur in the first week of life, at which time BPD is unlikely. In patients older than 2 weeks of age, BPD is more likely. Also, in patients who have a series of daily films, PIE tends to occur abruptly, whereas BPD tends to occur gradually.

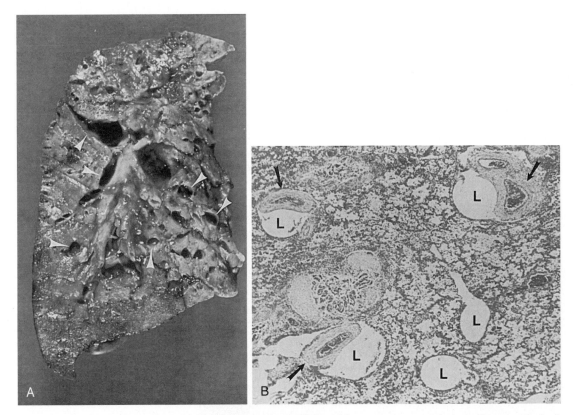

Figure 3–10. Pulmonary interstitial emphysema in a 20-day-old premature neonate. *A,* Gross pathologic specimen shows abnormal airspaces *(arrowheads)* within pulmonary interstitium. Interstitial emphysema surrounds and extends along bronchovascular structures. *B,* Photomicrograph shows collection of gas within lymphatics (L) adjacent to arterial structures *(arrows).* (*A* and *B* from Donnelly LF, Frush DP. Localized lucent chest lesions in neonates: causes and differentiation. AJR Am J Roentgenol 1999;172:1651–1658.)

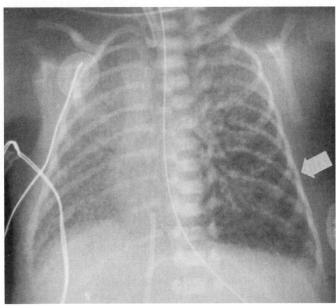

Figure 3–11. Pulmonary interstitial emphysema in a 3-day-old premature neonate. Chest radiograph shows bubble-like lucencies *(arrow)* within the left lower lobe.

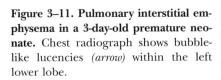

Causes of Acute Diffuse Pulmonary Consolidation

The occurrence of acute diffuse lung consolidation is nonspecific in neonates, as it is in adults, and can represent blood, pus, or water. In the neonate, the specific considerations include (Table 3–2) edema, which may be secondary to development of patent ductus arteriosus (Fig. 3–12); pulmonary hemorrhage, to

which surfactant therapy predisposes; worsening surfactant deficiency (during the first several days of life but not after); or developing neonatal pneumonia. Diffuse microatelectasis is another possibility. Neonates have the propensity to demonstrate diffuse lung opacity artifactually on low lung volume films (Fig. 3–13). This should not be mistaken for another cause of consolidation; such films offer little information concerning the pulmonary status of the patient and usually should be repeated.

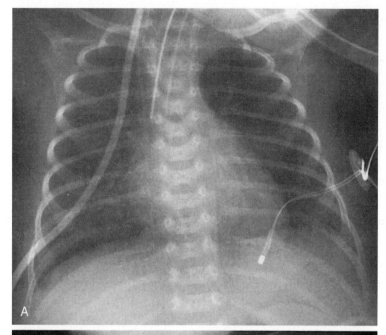

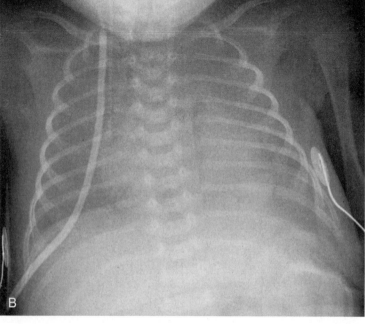

Figure 3–12. Patent ductus arteriosus leading to congestive heart failure in a 1-week-old premature neonate. *A,* Before the development of patent ductus arteriosus, radiograph shows normal-sized heart and clear lungs. *B,* After the development of patent ductus arteriosus, radiograph shows cardiac enlargement and bilateral lung consolidation.

TABLE 3–2. **Causes of Acute Diffuse Pulmonary Consolidation in Neonates**

Edema—patent ductus arteriosus
Hemorrhage
Diffuse microatelectasis—artifact
Worsening surfactant deficiency (only during first days of life)
Pneumonia

Bronchopulmonary Dysplasia

BPD is also referred to as *chronic lung disease of prematurity*. It is a common complication seen in premature infants and is associated with significant morbidity. It is related to injury to the lungs thought to result from some combination of mechanical ventilation and oxygen toxicity. Although four discrete and orderly stages in the development of BPD were originally described, they are not often seen and are probably not important to know. BPD typically occurs in a premature infant who requires prolonged ventilator support. At approximately the end of the second week of life, persistent hazy density appears throughout the lungs. Over the next weeks to months, a combination of coarse lung markings, bubble-like lucencies, and asymmetric aeration can develop (Fig. 3–14). Over years in children who survive, many of these radiographic findings decrease in prominence, and only hyperaeration may be present. The radiographic find-

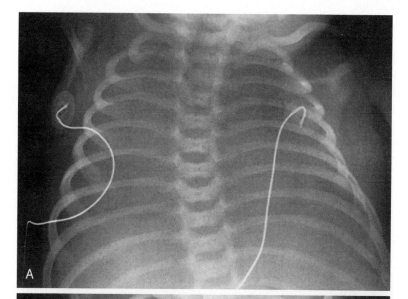
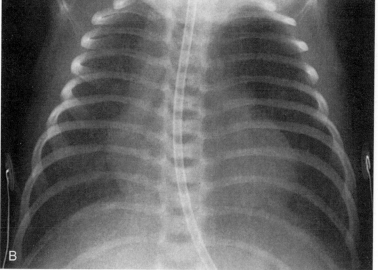

Figure 3–13. Expiratory chest radiograph mimicking diffuse lung consolidation in an 8-day-old infant girl. *A*, Initial radiograph shows bilateral diffuse lung opacity associated with low lung volumes. *B*, Repeat radiograph obtained immediately after that shown in *A* shows clear lungs.

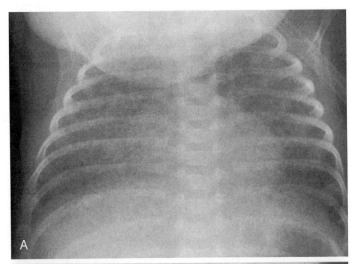

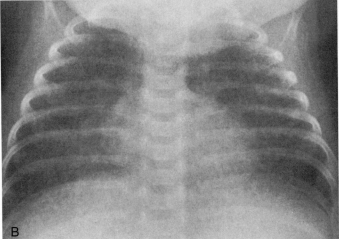

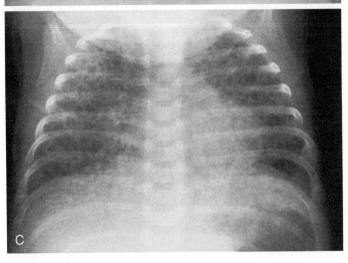

Figure 3–14. Bronchopulmonary dysplasia in a premature neonatal girl. *A,* Chest radiograph at 14 days of life shows persistent bilateral lung opacities. *B,* Chest radiograph at 20 days of life shows increased coarsening of the lung markings. *C,* Chest radiograph at 28 days of life shows development of increased coarse lung markings and diffuse bubble-like lucencies.

ings may completely resolve. Clinically, many children with severe BPD during infancy may develop normal pulmonary function over years or may only have problems such as exercise intolerance, predisposition to infection, or asthma.

Wilson-Mikity syndrome is a confusing and controversial term. It refers to the development of BPD in the absence of mechanical ventilation. Some debate whether this disease exists, whereas others think it is a variant of BPD. Certainly, there are cases in which findings of BPD develop with minimal ventilator support or develop earlier than is typically expected.

Focal Pulmonary Lesions in the Newborn

In contrast to diffuse pulmonary disease in newborns, focal mass can present with respiratory distress from compression of an otherwise normal lung. The differential diagnosis for a focal lucent lung lesion can be determined on the basis of whether the lesion is lucent or solid-appearing on chest radiography (Table 3–3). The most likely considerations for a lucent chest lesion in a newborn include congenital lobar emphysema, CCAM, persistent PIE, and congenital diaphragmatic hernia. Computed tomography (CT) may be helpful in differentiating among these lesions by demonstrating whether the abnormal lucency is related to air in distended alveoli, in the interstitium, or within abnormal cystic structures. Lesions that typically appear solid and not lucent during the neonatal period include sequestration and bronchogenic cyst. Many of these lesions can present in children beyond the neonatal period; those aspects of these entities will also be discussed.

TABLE 3–3. **Focal Lung Lesions in Neonates**

Lucent lesions
  Congenital lobar pneumonia
  Congenital cystic adenomatoid malformation
  Persistent pulmonary interstitial emphysema
  Congenital diaphragmatic hernia
Solid lesions
  Sequestration
  Bronchogenic cyst
  Congenital cystic adenomatoid malformation

Congenital Lobar Pneumonia

Congenital lobar emphysema is related to overexpansion of alveoli. The cause is debated. Most patients present during the neonatal period with respiratory distress. There can be associated anomalies, usually cardiac, but they occur in the minority of patients. There is a lobar predilection, with the most common site being the left upper lobe (43%), followed by the right middle lobe (32%) and right lower lobe (20%). On chest radiography, a hyperlucent, hyperexpanded lobe is seen. On initial radiographs, the lesion may appear of soft tissue density related to retained fetal pulmonary fluid (Fig. 3–15). This density resolves and is replaced by progressive hyperlucency. On CT, air is in the alveoli, so the interstitial septa and bronchovascular bundles are at the periphery (not center) of the lucency (Fig. 3–16). The airspaces are larger than those in the adjacent normal lung, and pulmonary vessels appear attenuated. The treatment is lobectomy.

Congenital Cystic Adenomatoid Malformation

Congenital cystic adenomatoid malformation (CCAM) is a congenital adenomatoid proliferation that replaces normal alveoli. The majority of cases present either at birth with respiratory distress or are detected prenatally. Most involve only one lobe and, in contrast to congenital lobar emphysema, there is no lobar predilection. Cases of CCAM are divided into one of three types based on how large the cysts appear at imaging or pathologic examination. Type 1 lesions (50%) have one or more large (2 to 10 cm) cysts. Type 2 lesions (40%) have numerous small cysts of uniform size. Type 3 lesions (10%) appear solid on gross inspection and imaging but have microscopic cysts. The classification system has no clinical relevance except that it helps as a reminder that CCAM can have multiple imaging appearances. The imaging appearance reflects the type. CCAM communicate with the bronchial tree at birth and therefore can fill with air within the first hours to days of life. On radiography and CT, a completely cystic (Fig. 3–17) mass, mixed cystic and solid mass (Fig. 3–18), or solid mass is seen, depending on the number and size of cysts and whether the cysts contain air or fluid. Symptomatic CCAMs are managed with surgical resection. The management of asympto-

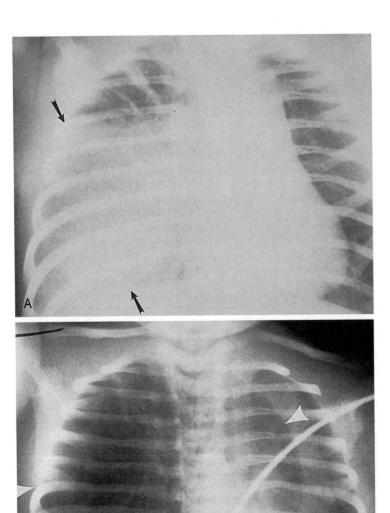

Figure 3–15. Congenital lobar emphysema of the right middle lobe in a female neonate. *A,* Radiograph obtained at 1 day old shows diffuse opacity *(arrows)* and enlargement of right middle lobe. *B,* Radiograph obtained at 12-days old shows hyperlucent and hyperexpanded right middle lobe *(arrowheads)*. Note progressive mediastinal shift. (*A* and *B* from Donnelly LF, Frush DP. Localized lucent chest lesions in neonates: causes and differentiation. AJR Am J Roentgenol 1999; 172:1651–1658.)

Figure 3–16. Congenital lobar emphysema of the right upper lobe in a 1-week-old neonate. *A,* Computed tomographic scan shows hyperlucent lobe with asymmetric attenuation of vascular structures and increased space between interstitial septa. *B,* Photomicrograph of resected lobe shows excessive gas within distended alveoli. (*A* and *B* from Donnelly LF, Frush DP. Localized lucent chest lesions in neonates: causes and differentiation. AJR Am J Roentgenol 1999;172:1651–1658.)

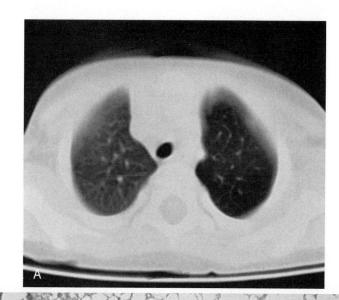

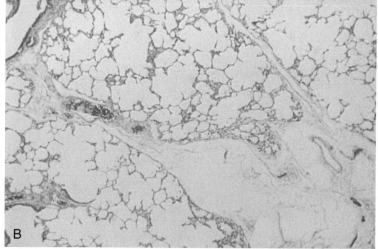

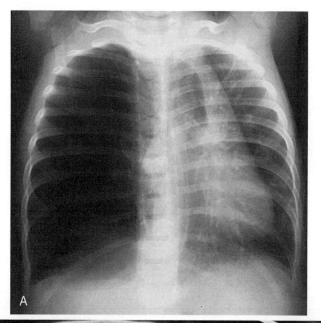

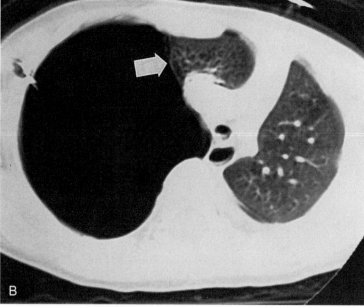

Figure 3–17. Type 1 congenital cystic adenomatoid malformation in a 1-year-old boy. *A,* Chest radiographs shows hyperexpanded, hyperlucent right hemithorax with rightward mediastinal shift. No definite normal lung markings are identified in the right hemithorax. *B,* Computed tomogram shows large, lucent cyst occupying the majority of the right hemithorax and compressing adjacent lung *(arrow).*

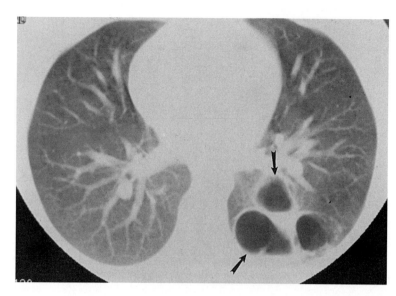

Figure 3–18. Type 1 congenital cystic adenomatoid malformation in a 4-day-old male neonate. Computed tomogram shows multiple large cysts *(arrows)* with associated abnormal soft tissue attenuation within the left lower lobe. (From Donnelly LF, Frush DP. Localized lucent chest lesions in neonates: causes and differentiation. AJR Am J Roentgenol 1999;172:1651–1658.)

matic CCAM is currently somewhat controversial. However, most caregivers advocate elective resection because these lesions have an increased risk of infection and rarely may develop rhabdomyosarcoma.

A scenario that is encountered increasingly consists of a prenatally diagnosed lung mass that becomes less prominent on serial prenatal ultrasonograms and demonstrates only subtle findings or is not detected on a chest radiograph obtained soon after birth. Almost all such lesions are type 2 CCAM and demonstrate abnormalities on CT even in light of a normal chest radiograph (Fig. 3–19).

Persistent Pulmonary Interstitial Emphysema

The more common transient form of PIE was discussed previously. Occasionally, PIE can persist and develop into an expansive, multicystic mass. The air cysts can become large enough to cause mediastinal shift and compromise pulmonary function. The primary therapy for persistent PIE is nonsurgical, including selective intubation of the opposite lung or decubitus positioning. Therefore, differentiation from other air-filled cystic masses that are treated surgically, such as CCAM, is important. CT shows that the air cysts are in the interstitial space by demonstrating that the bronchovascular bundles are positioned within the center of the air cysts and appear as linear or nodular densities in the center of the cysts (Figs. 3–20 and 3–21).

Congenital Diaphragmatic Hernia

Congenital diaphragmatic hernia (CDH) is usually secondary to posterior defects in the diaphragm (Bochdalek hernia). It is more common on the left side (5:1). Most present at birth with severe respiratory distress. The hernia contents may contain stomach, small bowel, colon, or liver. The radiographic appearance depends on the hernia contents and whether there is air within the herniated viscera. On initial radiographs (before air is introduced into the viscera), the appearance may be radiopaque (Fig. 3–22). Later, the herniated viscera contain air, and the hernia will appear as an air-containing cystic mass. Less air-filled viscera in the abdomen than expected and an abnormal position of the support apparatus, such as a nasogastric tube within a herniated stomach, are obvious clues to support the diagnosis (Fig. 3–23). The mortality rate in CDH is related to the degree of pulmonary hypoplasia. Radiographic predictors of a poor prognosis include lack of an aerated ipsilateral lung, low percentage of aerated contralateral lung, and severe mediastinal shift. Treatment includes support for respiratory failure, often with high-frequency ventilation or ECMO, and surgical repair.

Sequestration

Pulmonary sequestration refers to a congenital area of abnormal pulmonary tissue that does not have a normal connection to the bronchial

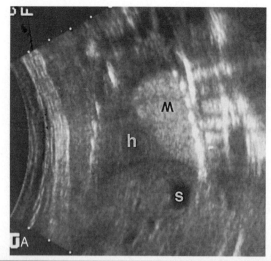

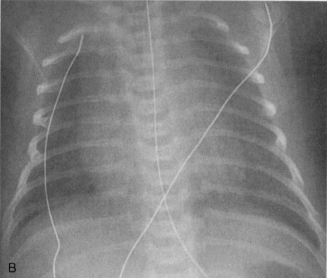

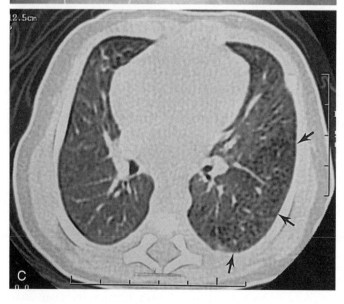

Figure 3–19. Type 2 congenital cystic adenomatoid malformation in female neonate. *A,* Prenatal ultrasonogram obtained at 31 weeks' gestational age and shown in coronal plane demonstrates large echogenic mass (M) occupying entire left hemithorax. H = heart, S = stomach. Follow-up ultrasonograms (not shown) showed a progressive decrease in the size of the mass. *B,* Chest radiograph obtained at 1 day of age shows only minimal, asymmetric ground glass opacity overlying left lower lung. *C,* High-resolution CT performed at 3 days of age shows multiple, small, air-filled cysts confined to the superior segment of left lower lobe *(arrows).* Cysts are homogeneous in size. Distance between septa of cysts is narrower than that of adjacent normal lung. *(A–C* from Donnelly LF, Frush DP. Localized lucent chest lesions in neonates: causes and differentiation. AJR Am J Roentgenol 1999;172:1651–1658.)

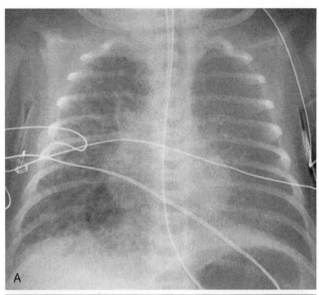

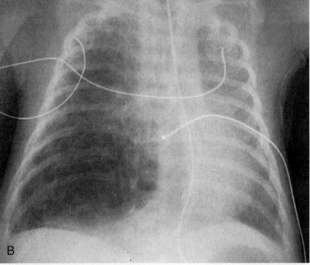

Figure 3–20. Localized persistent pulmonary emphysema requiring surgical resection in male neonate. *A,* Chest radiograph obtained at 4 days of age shows diffuse pulmonary interstitial emphysema throughout right lung. Note endotracheal tube. *B,* Chest radiograph obtained 13 days after that shown in *A* demonstrates the development of multiple expansive cysts throughout what appears to be the entire right lung. Note the resultant mediastinal shift. *C,* Computed tomographic scan obtained 3 days after the radiograph shown in *B* shows cystic airspaces to be confined to right lower lobe. Soft tissue attenuation and linear and nodular densities *(arrows)* in the centers of multiple airspaces are consistent with vascular structures surrounded by air in pulmonary interstitium. Gas surrounding vascular structures documents interstitial location of the abnormal gas. (*A–C* from Donnelly LF, Frush DP. Localized lucent chest lesions in neonates: causes and differentiation. AJR Am J Roentgenol 1999;172:1651–1658.)

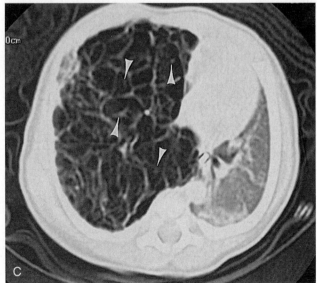

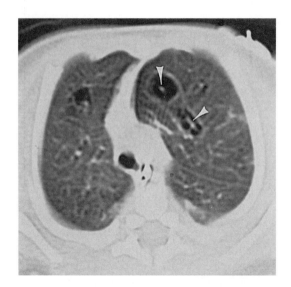

Figure 3–21. Localized persistent pulmonary interstitial emphysema in 9-day-old female neonate. Computed tomogram shows cystic lucencies with soft tissue nodular and linear structures *(arrowheads)* centrally, documenting interstitial location of emphysema. (From Donnelly LF, Frush DP. Localized lucent chest lesions in neonates: causes and differentiation. AJR Am J Roentgenol 1999;172:1651–1658.)

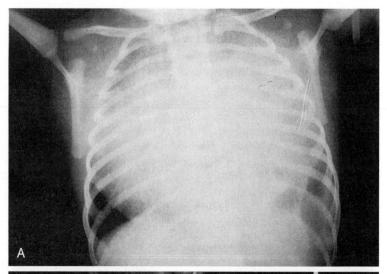

Figure 3–22. Congenital diaphragmatic hernia in a newborn baby boy. *A,* Initial radiograph after birth demonstrates apparent cardiomegaly. *B,* Radiograph obtained later shows aerated bowel within the left hemithorax consistent with congenital diaphragmatic hernia. (*A* and *B* courtesy of Charles A. Gooding, M.D., San Francisco, California.)

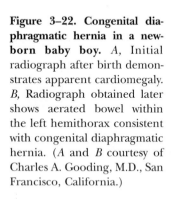

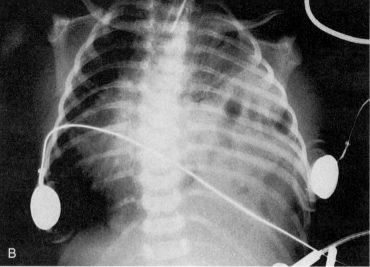

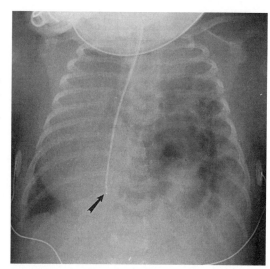

Figure 3–23. Congenital diaphragmatic hernia in a male neonate. Chest radiograph shows cystic lucencies throughout left hemithorax. Note mediastinal shift to right. Left hemidiaphragm is not visualized. The tip of the nasogastric tube *(arrow)* is lodged at the esophageal gastric junction, which is not an uncommon finding in congenital diaphragmatic hernia. (From Donnelly LF, Frush DP. Localized lucent chest lesions in neonates: causes and differentiation. AJR Am J Roentgenol 1999;172:1651–1658.)

tree. The characteristic feature of sequestration is the demonstration of anomalous arterial supply to the abnormal lung via a systemic artery arising from the aorta (Fig. 3–24). All modalities that can demonstrate this abnormal systemic arterial supply—including magnetic resonance imaging (MRI), helical CT, ultrasonography, and arteriography—have been advocated for making the diagnosis of sequestration. I prefer contrast-enhanced helical CT because it visualizes the systemic arterial supply when a sequestration is present (Fig. 3–25) and further characterizes the lung abnormality if a sequestration is not present.

Sequestration most commonly presents with a history of recurrent pneumonia, most commonly in late childhood. Other presentations include a prenatally diagnosed lung mass or respiratory distress in the newborn period. Because sequestrations do not communicate with

Figure 3–24. Sequestration in a 10-month-old girl with a history of recurrent pneumonia. *A,* Chest radiograph shows left lower lobe opacity *(arrow). B,* Obliqued reformat from T1-weighted MR image shows large systemic artery *(arrows)* arising from aorta and ending in lesion.

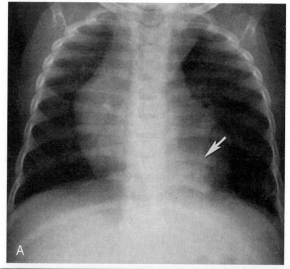

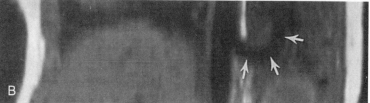

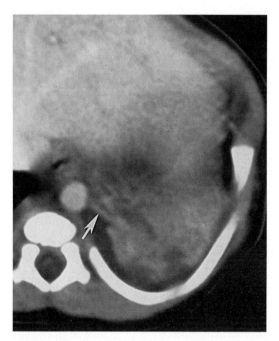

Figure 3–25. Sequestration in a 1-day-old boy with a history of a prenatally diagnosed lung mass. Contrast-enhanced computed tomographic scan shows systemic arterial supply *(arrow)* leading to left lower lobe sequestration.

the bronchial tree unless they become infected, sequestration appears as a radiopaque mass in the neonatal period. After infection has occurred, air may be introduced, and sequestration may appear as a multiloculated cystic mass. The most common location is within the left lower lobe.

There is much discussion concerning differentiation between intralobar and extralobar sequestrations. Extralobar sequestrations have a separate pleural covering, whereas intralobar sequestrations, which are more common, do not. Extralobar sequestrations are associated with other abnormalities in 65% of cases, whereas intralobar sequestrations are not. Differences in venous drainage patterns between intralobar and extralobar sequestrations has been emphasized as the differentiating factor, but such patterns are actually variable with both types. The differentiation between intralobar and extralobar sequestration cannot be made at imaging and does not affect surgical management. Visualization of the supplying systemic artery is the characteristic finding and the documentation that surgeons look for before surgically removing the lesion.

Bronchogenic Cyst

Bronchogenic cysts occur secondary to abnormal budding of the tracheobronchial tree during development and are seen in the lung parenchyma and mediastinum with equal frequency. Like sequestrations, they do not contain air until they become infected and therefore may appear as well-defined soft tissue attenuation or cystic air-fluid–containing masses (Fig. 3–26). They can be large and appear as well-defined cystic structures on imaging (see Fig. 3–26).

Chylothorax

Large pleural effusions can also cause respiratory distress in the newborn. The most common cause is a chylothorax. Most of these children are term and present with respiratory distress during the first several days of life. The cause of the chylothorax usually remains unknown and is possibly related to birth injury of the thoracic duct; most resolve after drainage. If the chylothorax persists, an underlying lymphatic malformation may be present, which may be demonstrated with cross-sectional imaging such as CT or MRI (Fig. 3–27).

PEDIATRIC PNEUMONIA

Roles of Imaging

Respiratory tract infection is the most common cause of illness in children and continues to be a significant cause of morbidity and mortality. Evaluation of suspected community acquired pneumonia is one of the most common indications for imaging in children. Because of the frequency of this scenario, knowledge of the issues concerning the imaging of children with community acquired pneumonia is important. The roles of imaging in these children are multiple: confirmation or exclusion of pneumonia, characterization and prediction of the infectious agent, exclusion of other causes of symptoms, evaluation when the condition fails to resolve, and evaluation of related complications.

Confirmation or Exclusion of Pneumonia

Making the diagnosis of pneumonia, and consequently deciding on treatment and disposi-

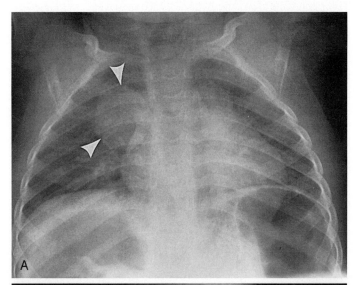

Figure 3–26. Bronchogenic cyst in an 18-month-old boy with wheezing. *A,* Chest radiograph shows well-defined soft tissue attenuation mass *(arrows)* in right upper lobe. *B,* Computed tomogram (at lung windows) shows well-defined mass (m) compressing right upper lobe bronchus and post-obstructive lucency in the posterior segment of the right upper lobe *(arrow). C,* Computed tomogram (at mediastinal windows) shows homogeneous soft tissue attenuation mass (M) with no enhancement.

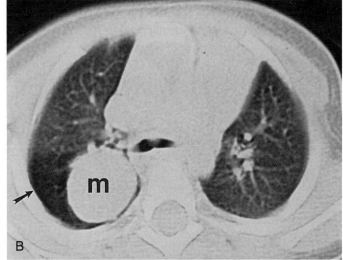

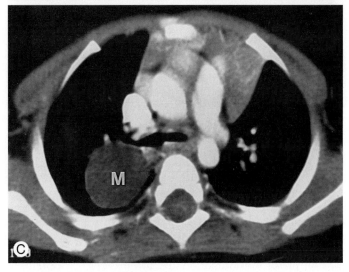

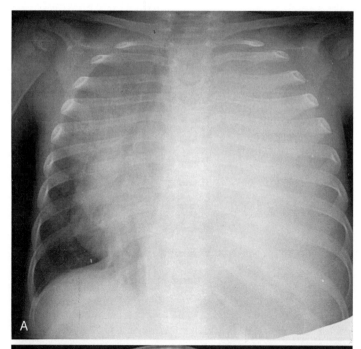

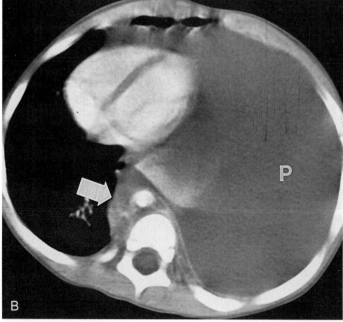

Figure 3–27. Large chylothorax secondary to lymphatic malformation in a 23-month-old boy. *A,* Chest radiograph shows large left pleural effusion with mediastinal shift to the right. *B,* Computed tomographic scan shows large pleural effusion (P), collapsed lung *(arrowhead),* and abnormal soft tissue mass in right paraspinal area, which at surgery was a lymphatic malformation.

tion, is a common but complex and difficult issue. The symptoms and physical findings in children with pneumonia are sometimes non-specific, especially in infants and young children. Many children present with nonrespiratory symptoms such as fever, malaise, irritability, headaches, chest pain, abdominal pain, vomiting, or decreased appetite. Findings on physical examination are also less reliable in children than in adults. Because of the inaccuracy of physical examination, radiography is often requested to evaluate children with suspected pneumonia. Several studies have shown that findings on chest radiography change caregiver's diagnosis and treatment plans (antibiotics, bronchodilators, and patient disposition [admission to hospital versus discharge to home]) in children evaluated for potential pneumonia in a large percentage of cases. In my institution, both a frontal and a lateral film are obtained. It has been shown that obtaining both views increases the negative predictive value of chest radiography for pneumonia. Some findings, such as hyperinflation in an infant, are also much more easily evaluated on the lateral view than on frontal views (Fig. 3–28).

Characterization and Prediction of the Infectious Agent

The historical emphasis of textbooks and articles concerning pneumonia has been on radiographic patterns that suggest a specific infectious agent causing pneumonia, such as staphylococcal or streptococcal pneumonia. However, because of the limited ways in which the lung can respond to inflammation, findings are often not specific. Findings suggestive of a specific diagnosis are uncommonly encountered in the evaluation of the child with suspected community acquired pneumonia. The more general issue in the evaluation of the child with suspected pneumonia is whether the infectious agent is more likely to be bacterial or viral, the pertinent issue being

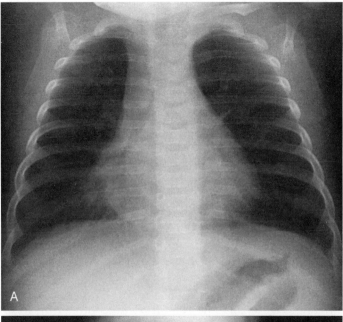

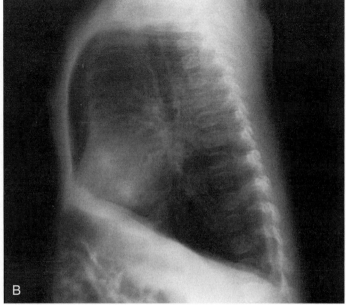

Figure 3–28. Hyperinflation in a 4-month-old boy with viral infection. *A,* Frontal radiograph shows symmetric inflation of lungs to the level of the 10th posterior ribs. Note minimal evidence of hyperinflation. *B,* Lateral radiograph shows marked flattening of hemidiaphragms. Note widened anteroposterior chest diameter and prominent size of retrosternal clear space. The degree of hyperinflation is severe and more easily seen here than in *A.* (*A* and *B* from Donnelly LF. Maximizing the usefulness of imaging in children with community-acquired pneumonia. AJR Am J Roentgenol 1999; 172:505–512.)

whether the patient needs to be given antibiotics. To address this question, it is helpful to review the epidemiology of lower respiratory infections in children, classic radiographic patterns of viral and bacterial pneumonia in children, and what is known about the accuracy of chest radiography in differentiating viral from bacterial infection.

The common etiologic agents causing lower respiratory tract infections in children vary greatly with age. In all age groups, viral infections are much more common than bacterial infections. In preschool-aged infants and children (4 months to 5 years), viruses cause 95% of all lower respiratory tract infections. The epidemiology is much different for school-aged children (6 to 16 years). Although viral agents remain the most common cause of lower respiratory tract infections in school-aged children, the incidence of bacterial infection with *Streptococcus pneumoniae* increases. What is most striking is that *Mycoplasma pneumoniae*, which is an uncommon cause of pneumonia in preschool-aged infants and children, is the cause of approximately 30% of lower respiratory tract infections in school-aged children. Therefore, the odds of a child needing antibiotics for a respiratory tract infection is greatly influenced by age.

Viral infections involve the airways and result in inflammation of the small airways and peribronchial edema. This peribronchial edema appears on radiographs as increased peribronchial opacities that are symmetric, coarse markings radiating from the hila into the lung (Fig. 3–29). The central portions of the lungs appear "dirty" or "busy." It is one of the most subjective findings in radiology. In addition, the combination of bronchial wall edema narrowing the airway lumen and necrotic debris and mucus in the airway lumen leads to small airway occlusion. This results in both hyperinflation and areas of subsegmental atelectasis. Hyperinflation is evident on chest radiographs in children by the presence of hyperlucency, depression of the hemidiaphragm to more than 10 posterior ribs, and an increased anteroposterior chest diameter. Hyperinflation is often much better appreciated on lateral than frontal radiographs in infants and small children (see Fig. 3–28). Subsegmental atelectasis appears as wedge-shaped areas of density that are most common in the lower and middle portions of the lung (Fig. 3–30). There are several anatomic considerations that render small children more predisposed to air trapping and collapse secondary to viral infection than are adults. They include small airway lumen diameter, poorly developed collateral pathways of ventilation, and more abundant mucus production. The misinterpretation of areas of atelectasis as focal opacities suggesting bacterial pneumonia is felt to be one of the more common misinterpretations in pediatric radiology.

In contrast, bacterial pneumonia occurs secondary to inhalation of the infectious agent into the airspaces. There is a resultant progressive development of inflammatory exudate and edema within the acini, resulting in consolidation of the airspaces. On chest radiography, localized airspace consolidation occurs

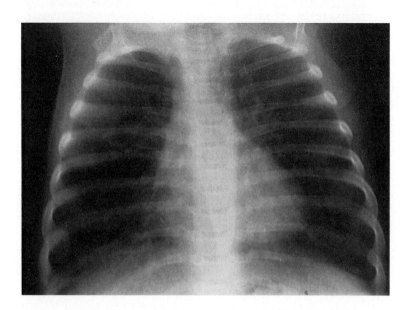

Figure 3–29. Viral illness in a 3-month-old infant girl. Chest radiograph shows increased peribronchial opacities as increased linear markings radiating from the hila.

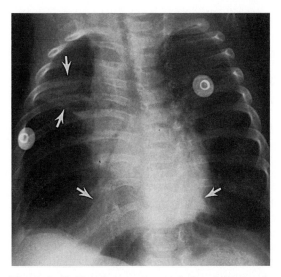

Figure 3–30. Respiratory syncytial virus infection in a 5-month-old girl. Chest radiograph shows increased peribronchial opacities. Note multiple areas of subsegmental atelectasis *(arrows)* to be triangular areas of increased density. Note asymmetric hyperinflation. (From Donnelly LF. Maximizing the usefulness of imaging in children with community-acquired pneumonia. AJR Am J Roentgenol 1999; 172:505–512.)

with air bronchograms. The typical distribution is lobar or segmental, depending on the stage of pneumonia present at the time the radiograph is obtained. Associated pleural effusions are not uncommon. Also, there is a propensity for pneumonia to appear "round" in younger (<8 years) children (Fig. 3–31). It

is most often due to *Streptococcal pneumoniae.* The occurrence of this pattern is thought to be related to poor development of pathways of collateral ventilation. When a round opacity is seen in a child older than 8 years, other pathologic conditions should be suspected.

Do these classic patterns of viral and bacterial infections accurately differentiate which children have bacterial infection and need antibiotics? Studies have shown that these radiographic patterns do have a high negative predictive value (92%) for excluding bacterial pneumonia; however, the positive predictive value is low (30%). In other words, 70% of children who have radiographic findings of bacterial infection actually have viral infection. In regard to the decision about administering antibiotics to children with suspected pneumonia, the goal is to treat all children who have bacterial pneumonia with antibiotics while minimizing the treatment of children with viral illnesses. Therefore, the high negative predictive value of chest radiography for bacterial pneumonia is useful in identifying children who do not need antibiotics.

Exclusion of Other Pathologic Processes

Many of the presenting symptoms in children are nonspecific, and the spectrum of presentation overlaps a number of other pathologic processes involving the chest or other anatomic regions. Therefore, one of the other roles of chest radiography in the evaluation

Figure 3–31. Round pneumonia in 16-month-old boy. Frontal radiograph shows round opacity *(arrows)* overlying the right hilum. Lateral view (not shown) showed opacity to be in superior segment of right lower lobe. (From Donnelly LF. Maximizing the usefulness of imaging in children with community-acquired pneumonia. AJR Am J Roentgenol 1999;172:505–512.)

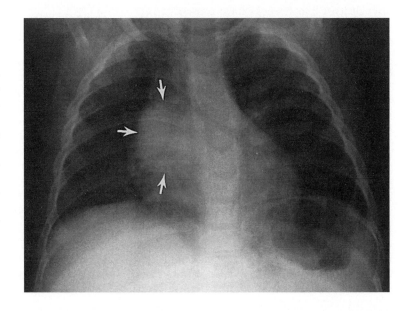

of the child with potential pneumonia is the exclusion of other processes. Two areas that are often "blind spots" for radiologists and may be involved by conditions that mimic pneumonia are the airway and the chest wall. Processes that cause extrinsic compression of the trachea and bronchi can mimic pneumonia, with noisy breathing, lobar collapse, and recurrent infection. Assessment of the diameter of the airway should be stressed as a routine part of evaluating radiographs. Rib abnormalities may be evidence that a lung opacity seen on chest radiography does not represent pneumonia. The presence of rib erosion or asymmetric intercostal spaces helps differentiate neuroblastoma from chest opacity secondary to pneumonia.

Failure to Resolve

In contrast to adults, in whom postobstructive pneumonia secondary to bronchogenic carcinoma is a concern, follow-up radiography to ensure resolution of radiographic findings is not routinely necessary in an otherwise healthy child who has had pneumonia. There is a tendency to obtain follow-up radiographs both too early and too often. Follow-up radiographs should be reserved for children who have persistent or recurrent symptoms and those who have an underlying condition, such as immunodeficiency. The radiographic findings of pneumonia can persist for 2 to 4 weeks, even when the patient is recovering appropriately clinically. When follow-up radiographs are indicated, they should ideally be obtained after at least 2 to 3 weeks have passed.

Causes of failure of suspected pneumonia to resolve include infected developmental lesions, bronchial obstruction, gastroesophageal reflux and aspiration, and underlying systemic disorders. Developmental lung masses that may become infected and present as recurrent or persistent pneumonia include sequestration, bronchogenic cyst, and cystic adenomatoid malformation. These entities have been discussed previously.

Complications of Pneumonia

Evaluation of complications related to pneumonia can be divided into several clinical scenarios: primary evaluation of parapneumonic effusions, evaluation of the child who has persistent or progressive symptoms despite medi-

cal or surgical therapy, and the chronic sequelae of pneumonia.

Primary Evaluation of Parapneumonic Effusions

Parapneumonic effusions occur commonly in patients with bacterial pneumonia. There are multiple therapeutic options available in the management of these effusions, including antibiotic therapy, repeated thoracentesis, chest tube placement, urokinase therapy, and thoracoscopy with surgical débridement. There are great differences in opinion among many pediatric surgeons and pediatric pulmonologists regarding the timing and aggressiveness of the management of parapneumonic effusions. Many investigators advocate antibiotics, drainage tube placement, and thrombolytic therapy. Other investigators advocate early intervention with thoracoscopy and débridement. Traditionally, the aggressiveness of therapy was based on categorizing parapneumonic effusions as empyema or transudative effusion based on needle aspiration and analysis of the pleural fluid. Several imaging modalities have been advocated as helpful in making such decisions. CT findings such as thickening or enhancement of the parietal pleura and thickening or increased attenuation of the extrapleural fat were previously thought to favor empyema over transudative effusion but have been shown to be inaccurate (Fig. 3–32). Ultrasonographic grading of effusions as low grade (anaechoic fluid without internal heterogeneous echogenic structures) or high grade (fibrinopurulent organization demonstrated by the presence of fronds, septations, or loculations) (Fig. 3–33) has been shown to be helpful in identifying which effusions will benefit (high grade) from aggressive drainage. Radiographs obtained with the patient in the decubitus position play a limited role in determining the amount of subpulmonic fluid present and in helping differentiate between pleural fluid and basilar lung opacification.

Evaluation of Persistent or Progressive Symptoms

When children exhibit persistent or progressive symptoms (fever, respiratory distress, sepsis) despite appropriate medical management of pneumonia, there is often an underlying

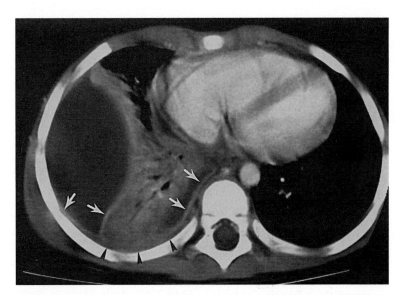

Figure 3–32. Transudative parapneumonic effusion with computed tomographic findings suggestive of empyema in a 5-year-old girl. There is a large elliptical right pleural effusion with mass effect on the adjacent consolidated lung. There is enhancement and thickening of the pleura *(white arrows)* with a "split pleura" sign. The effusion appears loculated. Extrapleural subcostal tissues demonstrate thickening and increased attenuation *(black arrowheads)*. Thoracentesis and chest tube placement yielded transudative pleural fluid. (From Donnelly LF, Klosterman LA. Computed tomographic appearance of parapneumonic effusions in children: findings are not specific for empyema. AJR Am J Roentgenol 1997;169:179–182.)

suppurative complication. Potential suppurative complications include parapneumonic effusions, such as empyema; other inadequately drained effusions or malpositioned chest tubes; parenchymal complications, such as cavitary necrosis or lung abscess; and purulent pericarditis. Although chest radiography is the primary imaging modality used to detect such complications, a significant percentage of these complications are not demonstrated by radiography. In a child with a radiograph that does not contribute to the diagnosis and who has not responded appropriately to therapy, contrast-enhanced CT has been shown to be useful in detecting clinically significant suppurative complications. CT can help differentiate whether the reason for persistent illness is pleural or related to lung parenchyma. Intra-

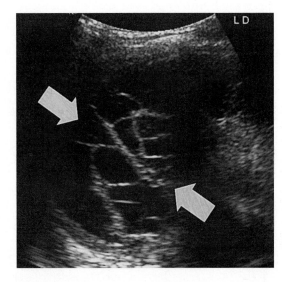

Figure 3–33. Ultrasonography of "high-grade" parapneumonic effusion in a 4-year-old girl. Transverse ultrasonogram shows effusion *(arrows)* with multiple loculations and fronds, which is consistent with fibrinopurulent organization. (From Donnelly LF. Maximizing the usefulness of imaging in children with community-acquired pneumonia. AJR Am J Roentgenol 1999; 172:505–512.)

venous contrast administration is vital to maximize the detection and characterization of both lung parenchyma and pleural complications.

Lung Parenchyma Complications

On contrast-enhanced CT, noncompromised consolidated lung parenchyma diffusely enhances (Fig. 3–34). Large areas of decreased or absent enhancement are indicative of underlying parenchymal ischemia or impending infarction. Suppurative lung parenchymal complications represent a spectrum of abnormalities and include cavitary necrosis, lung abscess, pneumatocele, bronchopleural fistula, and pulmonary gangrene. The name given to the suppurative process depends on several factors, including the severity and distribution, the condition of the adjacent lung parenchyma, and the temporal relationship with disease resolution. Lung abscess represents a dominant focus of suppuration surrounded by well-formed fibrous wall. On contrast-enhanced CT, lung abscesses appear as fluid- or air-filled cavities with definable, enhancing walls (see Fig. 3–34). Typically, there is no evidence of necrosis in the surrounding lung. *Pneumatocele* is a term given to thin-walled cysts seen at imaging and may represent a later or less severe stage of resolving or healing necrosis (Fig. 3–35).

Cavitary necrosis is the most commonly encountered suppurative complication and represents a dominant area of necrosis of a consolidated lobe associated with a variable number of thin-walled cysts. Computed tomographic findings of cavitary necrosis include loss of normal lung architecture, decreased parenchymal enhancement, loss of the lung-pleural margin, and multiple thin-walled cavities containing air or fluid and lacking an enhancing border (Fig. 3–36). Although historically described as a complication most closely associated with staphylococcal pneumonia, cavitary necrosis is currently much more commonly seen as a complication of *S. pneumoniae* infection. The presence of cavitary necrosis is indicative of an intense and prolonged illness. However, unlike in adults in whom the mortality rate of cavitary necrosis is high and early surgical removal of the affected lung has been advocated, the long-term outcome in children with cavitary necrosis is favorable in most cases with medical management alone. In children with cavitary necrosis, follow-up radiographs obtained more than 40 days after the acute illness are most often normal or show only minimal scarring (see Fig. 3–36).

Chronic Pulmonary Complications of Pneumonia

Acute pneumonia can lead to parenchymal damage and long-term sequelae. The most common of these are bronchiectasis and Swyer-James syndrome. *Bronchiectasis* is an enlargement of the diameter of the bronchi related to damage to the bronchial walls. It is best demonstrated on high-resolution CT, when the bronchus is larger in diameter than the adjacent pulmonary artery (Fig. 3–37).

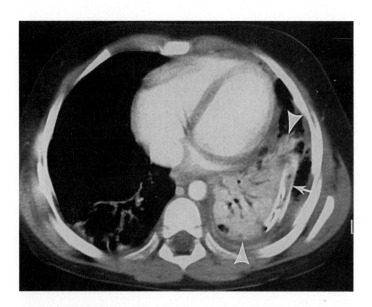

Figure 3–34. Noncompromised, enhancing, consolidated lung in 4-year-old girl with *Streptococcus pneumoniae* pneumonia and previous drainage of a parapneumonic effusion. Contrast-enhanced computed tomogram shows diffuse parenchymal enhancement of consolidated lung *(arrowheads)*. Note left-sided pleural drainage catheter *(arrow)*. (From Donnelly LF. Maximizing the usefulness of imaging in children with community-acquired pneumonia. AJR Am J Roentgenol 1999;172:505–512.)

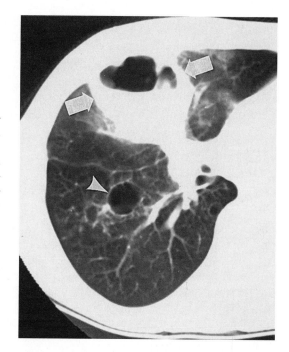

Figure 3–35. Lung abscess and pneumatocele in a 17-year-old boy. Computed tomogram shows cavity in right upper lobe *(arrows)*, which is consistent with abscess. The cavity has a thick, irregular wall and contains an air-fluid level. In contrast, a second air-filled cavity *(arrowhead)* demonstrates a thin wall, consistent with postinflammatory pneumatocele. (From Donnelly LF. Maximizing the usefulness of imaging in children with community-acquired pneumonia. AJR Am J Roentgenol 1999;172:505–512.)

Swyer-James syndrome is characterized by unilateral lung hyperlucency thought to be secondary to a virally induced necrotizing bronchiolitis that leads to an obliterative bronchiolitis. Radiography shows a hyperlucent and enlarged lung with a static lung volume. The number of pulmonary vessels is decreased compared with the normal side.

TUBERCULOSIS

The incidence of tuberculosis in children has been increasing. Children with primary tuberculosis can present with pulmonary consolidation within any lobe. It is often associated with hilar lymphadenopathy or pleural effusion. Therefore, when lung consolidation is seen with associated lymphadenopathy or effusion in a child who is not acutely ill, there should be a high suspicion for tuberculosis. Most of the cases of pulmonary tuberculosis which I have seen have demonstrated unilateral hilar lymphadenopathy alone (Fig. 3–38). Such cases should be considered to be tuberculosis until proven otherwise.

COMMON CHRONIC OR RECURRENT PULMONARY PROBLEMS IN SPECIAL POPULATIONS

In children with certain underlying conditions, the clinical scenarios and differential diagnoses are vastly unlike those seen in the general population. Commonly encountered scenarios include the evaluation of pneumonia in immunocompromised children, acute chest syndrome in sickle cell anemia, and pulmonary complications in cystic fibrosis.

Pneumonia in Immunocompromised Children

Children can be immunocompromised for a variety of reasons, including cancer therapy, bone marrow transplantation, solid organ transplantation, primary immunodeficiency, and acquired immunodeficiency syndrome (AIDS). It is a population that continues to increase. Acute pulmonary processes are a common cause of morbidity and mortality in these patients. As with immunocompetent children, radiography is the primary modality used to confirm or exclude pneumonia. However, because many of the chest radiographs obtained in these children are obtained portably and because of the consequences of missing an infection, CT plays a greater role in evaluating for an acute pulmonary process when chest radiographs do not contribute useful information. I would guess that in many tertiary institutions, the number of chest computed tomographic scans obtained in immunocompromised children outnumber those obtained in immunocompetent children.

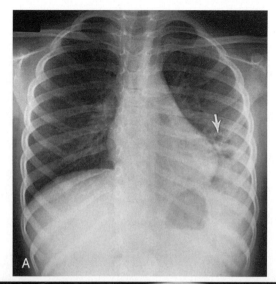

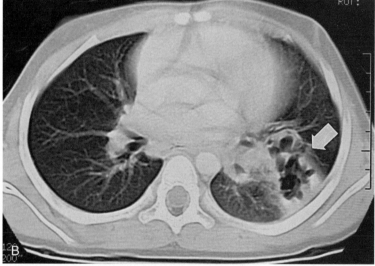

Figure 3–36. Typical course of cavitary necrosis in a 5-year-old boy. *A,* Chest radiograph shows left lower lobe consolidation with cavity *(arrow). B,* Computed tomogram at lung windows shows multiple air-filled cavities *(arrow).*

In contrast to immunocompetent children, in whom the main question is whether a pulmonary process is viral or bacterial, there are many more possible causes of acute pulmonary processes in immunocompromised children. They include alveolar hemorrhage, pulmonary edema, drug reaction, idiopathic pneumonia, lymphoid interstitial pneumonitis, bronchiolitis obliterans, bronchiolitis obliterans with organizing pneumonia, and chronic graft-versus-host disease. The computed tomographic findings in many of these entities are overlapping and nonspecific. A clinical question is often whether there is evidence of fungal infection. The hallmark computed tomographic finding of fungal infection is the presence of nodules (Fig. 3–39). These nodules are often clustered and may exhibit poorly defined margins, cavitation, or a surrounding halo of ground glass opacity. However, many of these findings are also nonspecific. In these cases, CT aids in directing potential interventions, such as bronchoscopy or percutaneous lung biopsy, to high-yield areas.

Acute Chest Syndrome in Sickle Cell Anemia

Children with sickle cell anemia often demonstrate pulmonary opacities on chest radiographs obtained because of fever, chest pain, and hypoxia (Fig. 3–40). There can be an associated increase in cardiomegaly. This clinical scenario is referred to as *acute chest syn-*

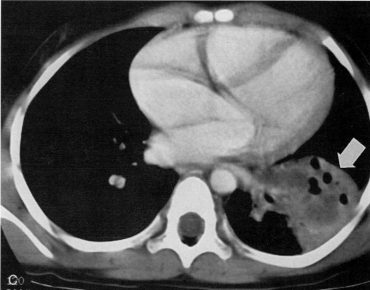

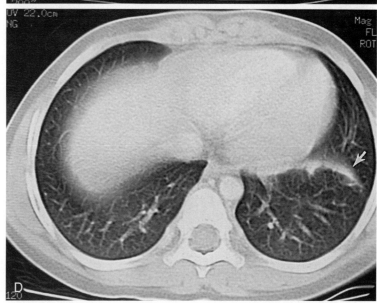

Figure 3–36 *Continued. C,* Computed tomogram at mediastinal windows shows multiple areas of decreased enhancement, air- and fluid-filled cysts, and loss of normal lung architecture *(arrow). D,* Follow-up computed tomograph (CT) performed 3 months later shows resolution of process with only a band of linear scarring *(arrow)* remaining. The lungs are otherwise clear.

drome. Although it is debated whether the cause of such episodes is more often infectious or related to infarction, many believe the lung opacities are related to rib infarction, splinting, and subsequent areas of atelectasis. The children are treated with oxygen, antibiotics, and pain control medication, and the pulmonary opacities are often monitored with radiography.

Cystic Fibrosis

Cystic fibrosis is a genetic disease that most often affects the respiratory tract. Abnormally viscous mucus leads to airway obstruction and infection, which causes bronchitis and bronchiectasis. Children may initially present with recurrent respiratory tract infections. Radiography may be normal in young children but eventually demonstrates hyperinflation, increased peribronchial markings, mucous plugging, and bronchiectasis. The hilar areas are often prominent resulting from a combination of lymphadenopathy secondary to the chronic inflammation and enlarged central pulmonary arteries resulting from the development of pulmonary arterial hypertension. Chest radiography is used to monitor disease and evaluate for complications during acute exacerba-

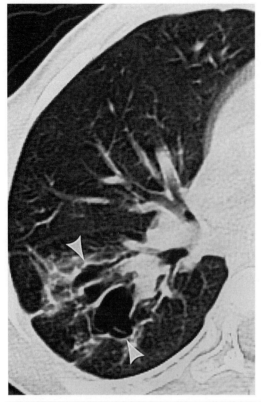

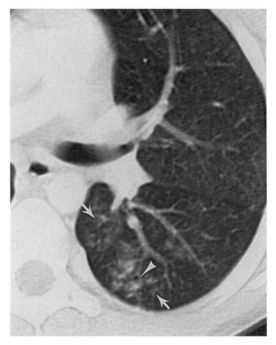

Figure 3–37. Bronchiectasis after pneumonia in an 11-year-old boy. High-resolution CT shows dilated bronchi *(arrowheads)* in right lower lobe.

Figure 3–39. Fungal pneumonia *(Candida)* in a 9-year-old bone marrow transplant recipient. Computed tomogram shows poorly defined nodular densities *(arrows)* in the superior segment of the left lower lobe. There is a small area of cavitation *(arrowhead)*.

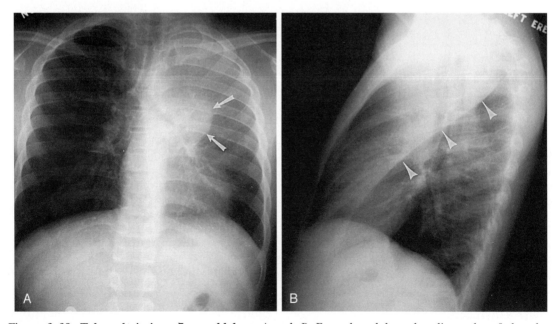

Figure 3–38. Tuberculosis in a 7-year-old boy. *A* and *B,* Frontal and lateral radiographs of the chest demonstrate a left hilar mass *(arrows)* that is consistent with unilateral lymphadenopathy. There is also left upper lobe collapse. Note displaced major fissure on lateral view *(arrowheads)*.

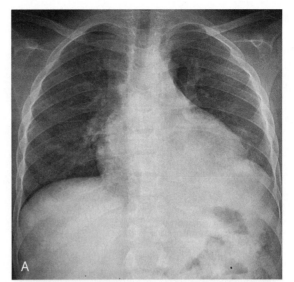

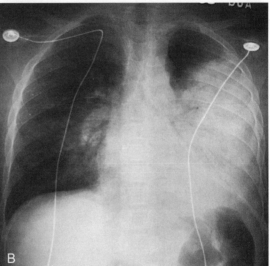

Figure 3–40. Acute chest syndrome in a 6-year-old boy with sickle cell anemia. *A,* Chest radiograph obtained at admission shows low lung volumes and minimal focal opacity within the left lower lobe. *B,* Chest radiograph obtained 1 day later shows consolidation of large portion of left lung. *C,* Chest radiograph obtained 2 days after that shown in *A* reveals complete left lung opacification.

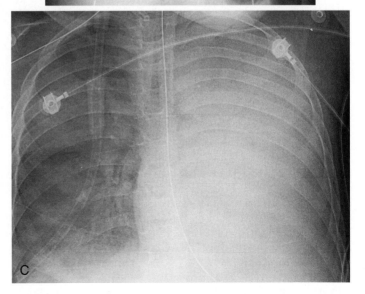

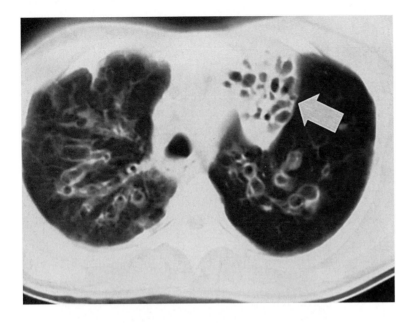

Figure 3–41. Cystic fibrosis in a 20-year-old woman. High-resolution CT shows diffuse bronchiectasis and bronchial wall thickening within the upper lobes. There is cicatricial atelectasis within the left upper lobe *(arrow)*.

tions. Such complications include focal pneumonia, pneumothorax, and pulmonary hemorrhage. Some institutions use high-resolution CT, which more elaborately demonstrates findings such as bronchiectasis and bronchial wall thickening (Fig. 3–41), to monitor the progression of disease.

TRAUMA

Rib Fractures and Lung Contusion

Because there is a greater component of cartilage compared with bone within the chest wall of children, there is more compliance than within the chest wall of adults. Because of this increased compliance, the sequelae of trauma to the pediatric chest are unique in several ways. First, the incidence of rib fractures after high-speed motor vehicle accidents is lower in children than it is in adults. Second, the deceleration forces from high-speed collisions is more apt to be dispersed into the lung, resulting in lung contusion. Children with lung contusions have been shown to have a higher morbidity and mortality rate than those without lung contusions. Although chest CT is not often performed to evaluate for lung contusion, the lower lungs are often seen on CT when it is more commonly performed to evaluate for abdominal trauma. Characteristic findings of lung contusion on CT include non-segmental distribution, posterior location, crescentic shape, and mixed confluent and nodular characteristics (Fig. 3–42). In children with small lung contusions, the compliance of the chest wall can result in a rim of nonopacified lung between the consolidated contusion

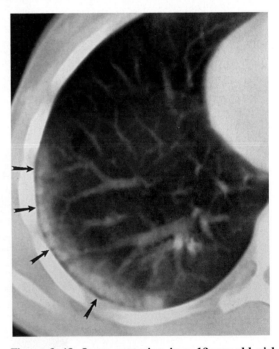

Figure 3–42. Lung contusion in a 12-year-old girl after a motor vehicle accident. Computed tomogram shows characteristic findings of contusion, including posterior location, crescentic shape, nonsegmental distribution, and subpleural sparing *(arrows)*.

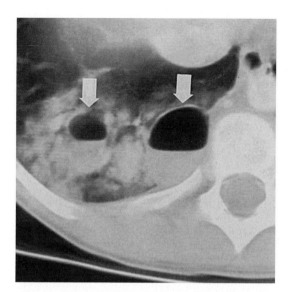

Figure 3–43. Lung laceration in a 10-year-old girl after she fell out of a tree. Computed tomogram shows right lower lobe consolidation with two air- and fluid-filled cavities *(arrows)*.

and the adjacent ribs seen on CT (see Fig. 3–42). This subpleural sparing can be helpful in differentiating lung contusion from other causes of lung opacification. The computed tomographic finding that classifies an opacified area as a lung laceration rather than a lung contusion is the presence of a fluid- or air-filled cyst within the opacified lung (Fig. 3–43).

Finally, the sites of rib fracture are different in children than in adults. Pediatric rib fractures are more likely to be posterior than lateral. As a result of "squeezing" an infant's thorax in child abuse, the posterior ribs can be excessively levered at the costotransverse process articulation, causing posterior fracture at this site. In the appropriate-aged child, these findings are pathognomonic for child abuse.

Mediastinal Injury

The incidence of aortic injury is also much less common in children than in adults. This fact, in combination of the lower incidence of obesity in children than in adults, makes the "uncleared" mediastinum on a chest radiograph after trauma a much more uncommon scenario in children. Otherwise, the use of CT and angiography and the imaging findings of aortic injuries are no different from those in adults.

Hydrocarbon Ingestion

Aspiration of hydrocarbons from ingested gasoline, furniture polish, kerosene, or lighter fluid can cause a combination of chemical pneumonitis and atelectasis secondary to surfactant destruction. Radiographic findings may not manifest for up to 12 hours after ingestion. However, a normal radiograph at 24 hours after suspected ingestion excludes significant aspiration. The lung opacities tend to be in the lung bases (Fig. 3–44) and may

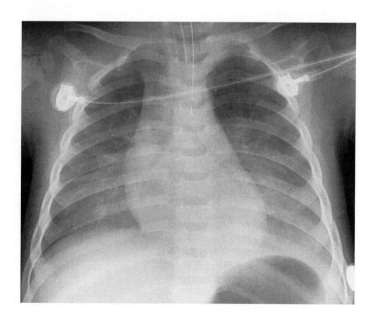

Figure 3–44. Hydrocarbon aspiration in a 1-year-old boy who drank gasoline from an orange juice container on the family's garage floor. Chest radiograph shows bibasilar lung consolidation. The patient is intubated.

persist for weeks after clinical improvement. Pneumatoceles are not uncommon.

MEDIASTINAL MASSES

The mediastinum is the most common location for primary thoracic masses in children. Also, the majority of mediastinal masses occur in children rather than in adults. Like in adults, characterizing the location of the mass as anterior, middle, or posterior mediastinal (Table 3–4) can focus the differential diagnosis of mediastinal masses.

Anterior Mediastinum

By far the most commonly encountered issues in the anterior mediastinum are the normal thymus, mistaken as a mass, and lymphoma. There are a large number of other potential, but much less common, causes of anterior mediastinal masses in children. They include teratoma (and other germ cell tumors), thymoma, and multilocular thymic cysts seen in association with AIDS.

Normal Thymus

One of the most common areas of confusion in the imaging of children is related to differentiating the normal thymus from pathologic processes. This confusion led to "thymic radiation" therapy in the first half of the 20th century and continues to cause diagnostic problems for those who infrequently image children. The appearance of the size and shape of the thymus in children is variable. In children younger than 5 years, and particularly in infants, the thymus can appear very large. The thymus also has a variable configuration.

TABLE 3–4. **Common Mediastinal Masses by Location**

Anterior
  Normal thymus
  Lymphoma
  Teratoma

Middle
  Lymphadenopathy
  Duplication cyst

Posterior
  Neuroblastoma

A number of names have become associated with normal variations in the thymus (Fig. 3–45), including *sail sign, wave sign,* and *notch sign.* Between 5 and 10 years of age, the thymus becomes less prominent radiographically, related to the disproportionate growth of the thymus in relation to growth of the rest of the body. During the second decade of life, the thymus should not be visualized as a discrete anterior mediastinal mass on chest radiography.

Abnormality of the thymus (or anterior mediastinum) is suspected when the thymic silhouette has an abnormal shape or abnormal size for patient age. Displacement of the airway or other structures is suspicious for abnormality. When CT is performed to evaluate suspicious cases, the normal thymus should appear homogeneous in attenuation and typically quadrilateral in shape and may have slightly convex margins. Heterogeneity, calcification, and displacement of the airway or vascular structures indicates an abnormality. True pathologic masses of the thymus are actually rare in children.

"Thymic rebound" is another source of confusion in regard to normal thymic tissue. After a patient has finished chemotherapy for a malignancy, it is normal for the thymus to "grow back" on serial computed tomographic examinations. This interval increase in soft tissue attenuation in the anterior mediastinum should not be considered abnormal when encountered on cross-sectional imaging.

Lymphoma

Lymphoma is the third most common tumor in children, exceeded only by leukemia and brain tumors. It is by far the most common anterior mediastinal mass in children, particularly in older children and teenagers. Therefore, lymphoma is the working diagnosis for newly diagnosed anterior mediastinal masses. Mediastinal lymphoma is often also associated with cervical lymphadenopathy. The most common types of lymphoma to involve the mediastinum include Hodgkin lymphoma and the lymphoblastic type of non-Hodgkin lymphoma. The lesions can appear as discrete lymph nodes or as a conglomerate mass of lymph nodes, most commonly within the anterior mediastinum (Fig. 3–46). Lung involvement, when present, is usually contiguous with mediastinal and hilar disease. Calcifications are rare in untreated lymphoma and when

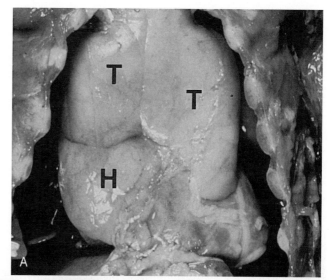

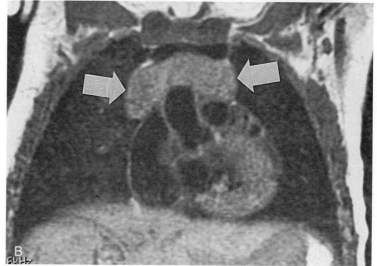

Figure 3–45. Relative large size and variable shape of thymus in infants and young children. *A,* Photograph from autopsy of infant shows frontal view of thymus (T) after thoracotomy. Note prominent size of thymus in relation to heart (H). The thymus is bilobed. In this patient, the left lobe is larger than the right. (Courtesy of Janet L. Strife, M.D., Cincinnati, Ohio). *B,* Coronal, T1-weighted image of 6-month-old boy shows thymus *(arrows)* to be homogeneous in signal and to have convex margins.

present should raise the possibility of other diagnoses, such as teratoma (Fig. 3–47). Most mediastinal masses are initially identified on chest radiography and are then further evaluated with CT, which confirms the presence of an anterior mediastinal mass, evaluates the extent of disease, and evaluates for potential complications. Such complications include airway compression, compressive obstruction of venous structures (superior vena cava, pulmonary veins), and pericardial effusion (see Fig. 3–46). Airway compression is especially important because it may influence decisions concerning general anesthesia and surgical biopsy versus percutaneous biopsy with local anesthesia. If a patient cannot lie recumbent for computed tomographic imaging because of airway compression, the images can often be

obtained with the patient positioned prone because the anterior mediastinal mass "falls away" from the airway.

Middle Mediastinal Masses

Middle mediastinal masses are less common than anterior or posterior mediastinal masses and are most commonly related to either lymphadenopathy or duplication cysts. Lymphadenopathy can be inflammatory, most commonly secondary to granulomatous diseases such as tuberculosis or fungal infection, or neoplastic, secondary to metastatic disease or lymphoma. Duplication cysts can be bronchogenic (Fig. 3–48), enteric, or neurenteric. They appear as well-defined masses that look

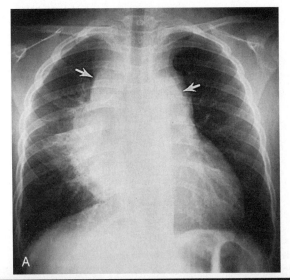

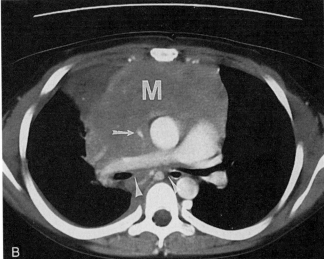

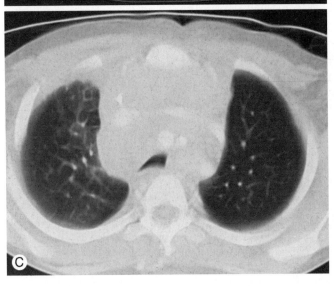

Figure 3–46. Lymphoma in an 11-year-old boy with respiratory distress. *A,* Radiograph shows enlarged superior mediastinum *(arrows)*, enlarged cardiopericardial silhouette, and increased interstitial markings in the right upper lobe. *B,* Computed tomogram shows large anterior mediastinal mass *(M).* The superior vena cava is almost completely obstructed *(arrow).* There is compression of the carina and medial main bronchi *(arrowheads)* from the mass anteriorly. Note that the patient was scanned prone (the opaque line anterior to the patient is the table) because he could not breathe when supine. A pericardial effusion was also present (not shown). *C,* Computed tomogram at lung windows shows increased interstitial markings in the right upper lobe as compared with the left upper lobe secondary to obstruction of the right superior pulmonary vein (not shown).

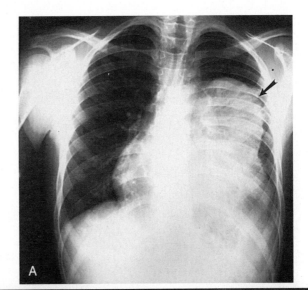

Figure 3–47. Teratoma in an 11-year-old boy. *A,* Chest radiograph shows a leftward anterior mediastinal mass *(arrow)* and marked enlargement of the cardiopericardial silhouette. *B,* Computed tomogram shows the anterior mediastinal mass to contain both fat and calcium attenuation, which is consistent with a teratoma. *C,* Computed tomogram shows large associated pericardial effusion (E).

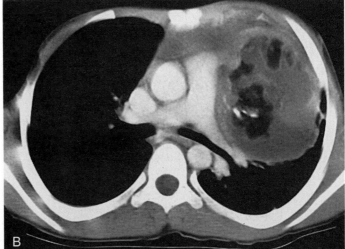

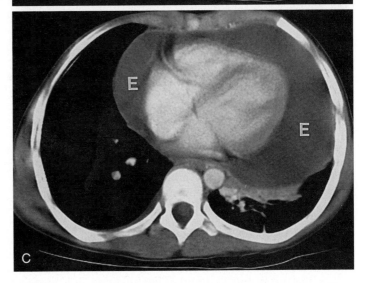

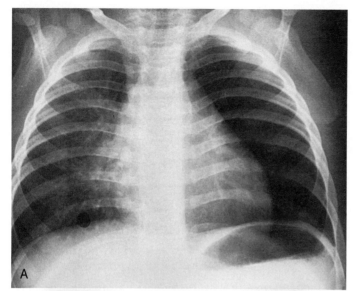

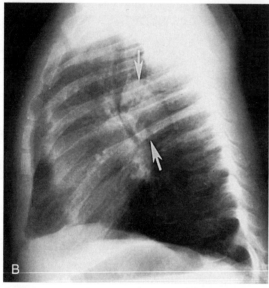

Figure 3–48. Bronchogenic cyst in a 7-month-old girl with wheezing. *A,* Frontal chest radiograph shows asymmetric low attenuation in left hemithorax. *B,* Lateral view shows round soft tissue mass *(arrows)* in middle mediastinum compressing the trachea from a posterior direction.

cystic on cross-sectional imaging. Neurenteric cysts by definition have associated vertebral anomalies (Fig. 3–49). Pathologic processes related to the esophagus can also cause middle mediastinal abnormalities. Chronic foreign bodies can erode from the esophagus and cause a middle mediastinal mass (Fig. 3–50). A dilated esophagus from achalasia or a hiatal hernia may also appear as a middle mediastinal mass on chest radiography.

Posterior Mediastinal Masses

There are a number of causes of posterior mediastinal masses in children. They include neural crest tumors, neurofibromas, lateral meningocele, diskitis, hematoma, and extramedullary hematopoiesis. However, similar to how anterior mediastinal masses in older children are considered to be lymphoma, the working diagnosis for posterior mediastinal masses in young children is neuroblastoma until proved otherwise.

Neuroblastoma

Neurogenic tumors (neuroblastoma, ganglioneuroblastoma, ganglioneuroma) are the most common mediastinal masses of childhood. Neuroblastoma is discussed in detail in the

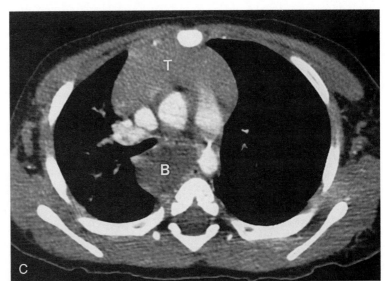

Figure 3–48 *Continued. C,* Computed tomogram shows well-defined, low-attenuation, "cystic"-appearing mass (B) in middle mediastinum compressing the left main bronchus. Note the normal size of the thymus (T) in this 7-month-old girl. *D,* Computed tomogram at lung windows shows hyperlucent left hemithorax. Mass (B) is again noted.

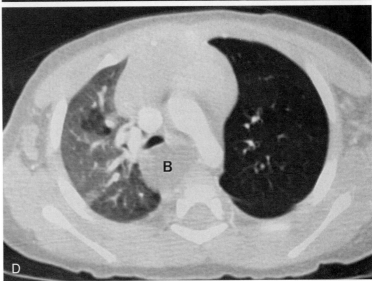

genitourinary chapter of this book. Approximately 15% of neuroblastomas occur in the posterior mediastinum, most before 2 years of age.

Most neuroblastomas are visible on frontal radiographs of the chest as a posterior opacity (Fig. 3–51). In my experience, the soft tissue mass is often poorly visualized on the lateral view. There is often erosion or destruction of the adjacent ribs (see Fig. 3–51). These findings may be subtle; whenever a posterior chest opacity is identified, an effort should be made to look for rib erosion. The neuroforamen may appear enlarged on the lateral view secondary to intraspinal extension of the tumor. Calcification is reported to be visible on chest radiography in up to 25% of cases, although

my experience has shown it to be less frequent. Cross-sectional imaging with CT or MRI confirms the presence of the tumor and evaluates the extent of disease, in particular whether there is intraspinal extension (see Fig. 3–51). Thoracic neuroblastomas have a better prognosis than do abdominal neuroblastomas.

Pediatric Chest Wall Masses

There are a number of malignant processes that can arise in the chest wall of children, including Ewing sarcoma, Askin tumor (primitive neuroectodermal tumor of the chest wall) and, less commonly, other sarcomas, such as osteosarcoma (Fig. 3–52). Most of these le-

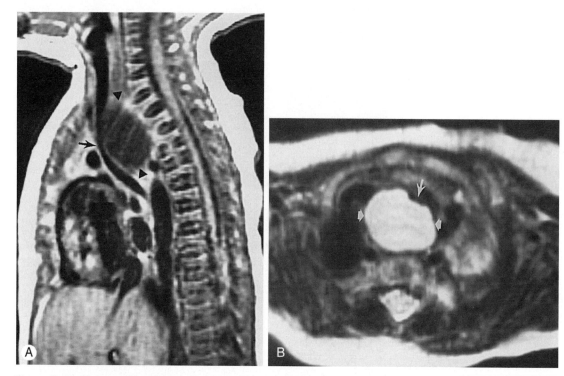

Figure 3–49. Neurenteric cyst in a 2-day-old girl with respiratory distress. *A,* Sagittal T1-weighted MR image shows well-defined retrotracheal mass *(arrowheads)* severely compressing and anteriorly displacing trachea *(arrow)*. Also note multiple segmental vertebral anomalies. *B,* T2-weighted MR image shows displaced trachea *(long arrow)* and mass *(short arrows)* of homogeneously high signal. (*A* and *B* from Donnelly LF, Strife JL, Bisset GS III. The spectrum of extrinsic lower airway compression in children: MR imaging. AJR Am J Roentgenol 1997;168:59–62.)

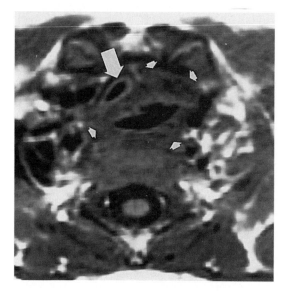

Figure 3–50. Eroded esophageal foreign body (tiddlywink) in 15-month-old boy with chronic stridor. Axial MR image shows anterior displacement and compression of trachea *(large arrow)* secondary to large retrotracheal mass *(small arrows)*. At surgery, low-signal structure in center of mass was found to be a plastic tiddlywink, which had eroded through the anterior wall of the esophagus. (From Donnelly LF, Strife JL, Bisset GS III. The spectrum of extrinsic lower airway compression in children: MR imaging. AJR Am J Roentgenol 1997;168:59–62.)

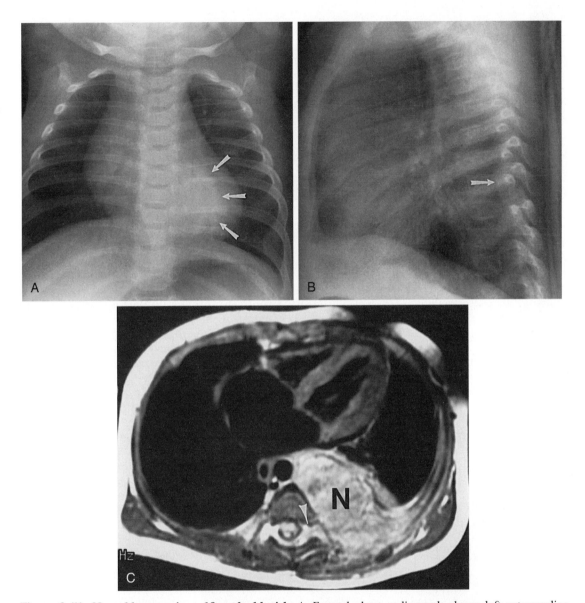

Figure 3–51. Neuroblastoma in a 12-week-old girl. *A,* Frontal chest radiograph shows left retrocardiac density *(arrows)*. There is splaying and thinning (erosion) of the associated left seventh and eighth ribs. *B,* Lateral view shows only minimal pleural thickening *(arrow)*. The opacity is difficult to see on the lateral view. *C,* Axial T2-weighted MR image shows posterior mediastinal mass (N) invading into the posterior chest wall. There is extension of abnormal signal into the left neuroforamina *(arrowhead)*.

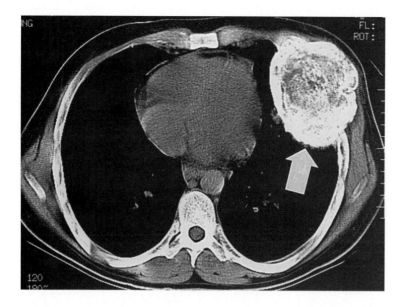

Figure 3–52. Osteosarcoma of the chest wall in a 15-year-old boy. Computed tomogram shows bone attenuation mass *(arrow)* arising from the left anterior chest wall.

sions present with a painful enlargement of the chest wall. Metastatic involvement by neuroblastoma, lymphoma, or leukemia is actually more common than are primary tumors. On imaging, all these malignancies typically appear as nonspecific aggressive lesions: poorly defined margins, bony destruction, and pleural involvement. However, one must consider that up to one third of children have variations in the configuration of the anterior chest wall, including asymmetric findings such as a tilted sternum (Fig. 3–53), prominent convexity of the anterior rib or costal cartilage, prominent asymmetric costal cartilage, parachondral nodules, or mild degrees of pectus excavatum or carinatum. Often, these asymmetric variants

are palpated by the pediatrician, parent, or patient and because of the fear of malignancy, cross-sectional imaging is requested. In a study that reviewed computed tomographic or MR examinations that were performed to evaluate children with suspected chest wall masses, all palpable lesions that were asymptomatic were related to normal anatomic variations. Knowledge of the high frequency of such variations should be communicated to referring physicians and parents when imaging is being contemplated in a child with an asymptomatic chest wall "lump."

Two of the most common abnormalities of chest wall configuration are pectus excavatum and pectus carinatum. Although the majority

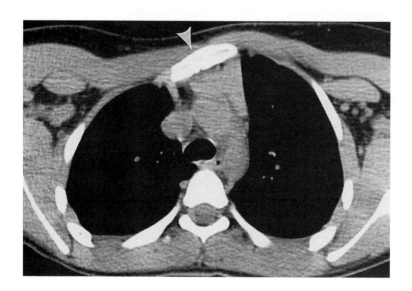

Figure 3–53. Tilted sternum in a 12-year-old girl. Computed tomographic image shows the sternum *(arrowhead)* to be tilted with respect to the horizontal right-to-left axis of the body. The left margin of the sternum is more anterior than the right. This asymmetry was palpated on physical examination and imaged to rule out a chest wall mass.

of problems due to these deformities are cosmetic, pectus deformities can cause chest pain, fatigability, dyspnea on exertion, palpitations, and restrictive lung disease. When the deformities are severe, surgical repair is often performed. Although the diagnosis is made visually and does not involve imaging, cross-sectional imaging with CT or MRI has been useful in demonstrating the anatomy of severe deformities and in evaluating for complications after surgical repair.

Suggested Reading

Condon VR. Pneumonia in children. J Thorac Imaging 1991;6:31–44.

Donnelly LF. Maximizing the usefulness of imaging in children with community-acquired pneumonia. AJR Am J Roentgenol 1999;172:505–512.

Donnelly LF, Frush DP. Localized lucent chest lesions in neonates: causes and differentiation. AJR Am J Roentgenol 1999;172:1651–1658.

Donnelly LF, Frush DP. Abnormalities of the chest wall in pediatric patients. AJR Am J Roentgenol 1999;173:1595–1601.

Donnelly LF, Frush DP, Foss JN, et al. Anterior chest wall: frequency of anatomic variations in children. Radiology 1999;212:837–840.

Donnelly LF, Klosterman LA. CT appearance of parapneumonic effusions in children: findings are not specific for empyema. AJR Am J Roentgenol 1997;169:179–182.

Donnelly LF, Klosterman LA. Pneumonia in children: decreased parenchymal contrast enhancement—CT sign of intense illness and impending cavitary necrosis. Radiology 1997;205:817–820.

Donnelly LF, Klosterman LA. Subpleural sparing: a CT finding of lung contusion in children. Radiology 1997;204:385–387.

Donnelly LF, Klosterman LA. Cavitary necrosis complicating pneumonia in children: sequential findings on chest radiography. AJR Am J Roentgenol 1998;171:253–256.

Donnelly LF, Klosterman LA. The yield of CT of children who have complicated pneumonia and noncontributory chest radiography. AJR Am J Roentgenol 1998;170:1627–1631.

Donnelly LF, Strife JL, Bisset GS III. The spectrum of extrinsic lower airway compression in children: MR imaging. AJR Am J Roentgenol 1997;168:59–62.

Donnelly LF, Taylor CNR, Emery KH, Brody AS. Asymptomatic, palpable, anterior chest wall lesions in children: is cross-sectional imaging necessary? Radiology 1997;202:829–831.

Griscom NT, Wohl MB, Kirkpatrick JA. Lower respiratory infections: how infants differ from adults. Radiol Clin North Am 1978;16:367–387.

Griscom NT. Respiratory problems of early life now allowing survival into adulthood: concepts for radiologists. AJR Am J Roentgenol 1992;158:1–8.

Merton DF. Diagnostic imaging of mediastinal masses in children. AJR Am J Roentgenol 1992;158:825–832.

Singleton EB. Radiologic consideration of intensive care in the premature infant. Radiology 1981;140:291–300.

Swischuk KE, John SD. Immature lung problems: can our nomenclature be more specific? AJR Am J Roentgenol 1996;166:917–918.

Heart

APPROACH TO THE CHEST RADIOGRAPH IN CONGENITAL HEART DISEASE

Many radiologists dread evaluating radiographs in children with potential congenital heart disease. This most likely stems from a combination of factors, including minimal exposure to cases of congenital heart disease as well as a lack of an organized approach. When evaluating a chest radiograph in a patient with potential congenital heart disease, it is important to evaluate the following findings: pulmonary vascularity, heart size, situs, and the position of the aortic arch.

Pulmonary Vascularity

The most important radiographic finding needed to generate the appropriate differential diagnosis of congenital heart disease is pulmonary vascularity. Unfortunately, it is probably also the most difficult. Pulmonary vascularity can be normal or it can demonstrate increased pulmonary arterial flow, increased pulmonary venous flow, or decreased pulmonary flow. In cases of increased pulmonary arterial flow, the pulmonary arteries will seem too prominent both in size and in the number of visualized pulmonary arterial structures (Fig. 4–1). One helpful rule is that if the right interlobar pulmonary artery is larger in diameter than the trachea, one should consider that increased pulmonary arterial flow is present. The prominent vascular structures seen in increased pulmonary arterial flow are distinct with well-defined borders. With increased pulmonary venous flow, the pulmonary vascular structures appear prominent in size and distribution but are very indistinct

and poorly defined (Fig. 4–2). In many cases (e.g., left-to-right shunts), there is both increased pulmonary arterial flow from left-to-right shunting and increased pulmonary venous flow from congestive heart failure. If I see that any of the pulmonary arteries in a particular patient appear well defined, I will consider at least a component of increased pulmonary arterial flow to be present. In decreased pulmonary arterial flow, there is a paucity of visualized arterial structures throughout the lung (Fig. 4–3). It can at times be difficult to differentiate increased pulmonary arterial flow from the increased peribronchial markings seen with viral pneumonia (see Fig. 3–29).

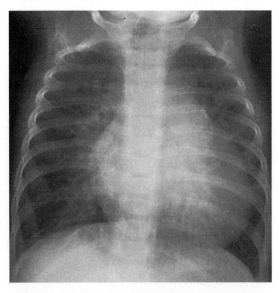

Figure 4–1. Increased pulmonary arterial flow in a 2-week-old boy with a ventricular septal defect. Note the prominent but distinct pulmonary vascular markings.

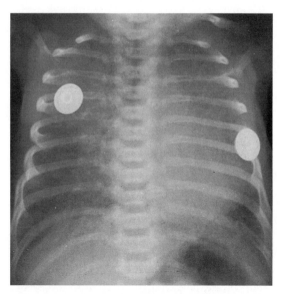

Figure 4–2. Increased pulmonary venous flow in a 9-day-old girl with congestive heart failure secondary to myocarditis. Note the prominent and indistinct pulmonary vascularity.

Heart Size

The cardiac size may be normal or enlarged. In older children and adults, there may be findings that suggest specific chamber enlargement. However, in infants in whom films are often obtained anteroposteriorly and who have a large thymus, specific chamber enlargement may be difficult to ascertain. In these infants, the lateral view often offers more in-

sight into whether cardiomegaly is present or absent than does the frontal view (Fig. 4–4). On the lateral view, if the posterior aspect of the cardiac silhouette extends over the vertebral bodies, cardiomegaly should be considered present. The *cardiac axis* is the name given to the configuration of the apex of the heart in regard to whether it points superiorly or inferiorly. If the cardiac apex is oriented superiorly, right-sided cardiac enlargement is suggested (Fig. 4–5), and if the cardiac access or apex is oriented inferiorly, left-sided cardiac enlargement is suggested.

Situs

The important structures to identify when evaluating situs are the cardiac apex, stomach bubble, and position of the liver. When the cardiac apex and gastric bubble appear on the same side, left or right, there is a much lower incidence of congenital heart disease than when the cardiac apex is on the side opposite the gastric bubble. When there is such discordance between the cardiac apex and the gastric bubble, there is a nearly 100% incidence of congenital heart disease.

Polysplenia and asplenia are syndromes in which there is bilateral left (polysplenia) or right (asplenia) sidedness. Asplenia is associated with complex, cyanotic congenital heart disease. Patients are susceptible to infections with encapsulated bacteria because of the lack of a spleen. Other findings include malrota-

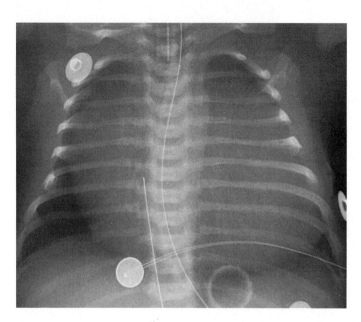

Figure 4–3. Decreased pulmonary venous flow in a newborn boy with pulmonary atresia and an intact ventricular septum. Note the lack of pulmonary markings and associated massive cardiomegaly.

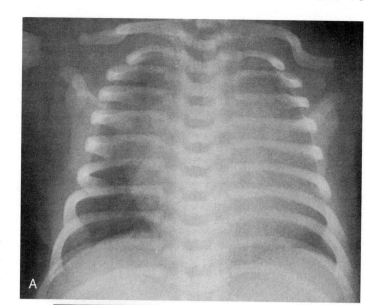

Figure 4–4. Exaggerated size of cardiothymic silhouette on anteroposterior (AP) frontal radiograph in a newborn. *A,* Frontal radiograph shows the cardiothymic silhouette to extend nearly across the entire chest. *B,* Lateral radiograph shows the posterior border of the heart to be normally positioned. There is no cardiomegaly present. The findings on the frontal radiograph are secondary to AP, lordotic technique. (*A* and *B* from Donnelly LF, Gelfand KJ, Schwartz DC, Strife JL. The wall to wall heart: differential diagnosis for massively large cardiothymic silhouette in newborns. Appl Radiol 1997;26:23–28.)

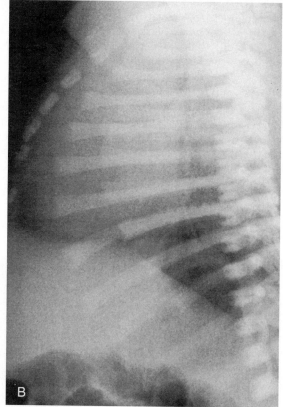

tion, microgastria, and a midline gallbladder. Radiographic findings include a midline liver, bilateral right-sided–appearing bronchi, decreased pulmonary arterial flow, azygous continuation of the inferior vena cava (IVC), and other findings that reflect the specific type of cyanotic heart disease (Fig. 4–6).

Polysplenia is typically associated with less complex acyanotic heart disease, usually left-to-right shunts. Other associations include azygos continuation of the IVC, a bilateral superior vena cava (SVC), malrotation, and lack of a gallbladder. Radiographic findings include absence of the IVC shadow, a prominent azygous vein, a midline liver, and increased pulmonary arterial flow.

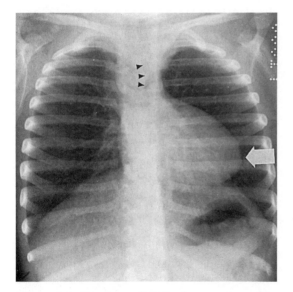

Figure 4–5. Tetralogy of Fallot in a newborn boy. Chest radiograph demonstrates an upturned cardiac apex *(arrow)* consistent with right-sided cardiac enlargement. There is a right-sided aortic arch. The trachea deviates leftward, rather than the normal rightward direction, and there is an indentation on the right border of the trachea *(arrowheads)*, rather than on the normal left. There is decreased pulmonary arterial flow.

Position of the Aortic Arch

The identification of a right-sided aortic arch is also a red flag for the presence of congenital heart disease. When evaluating the position of the aortic arch, identification of the aortic knob is possible in most adults and older children, which makes it obvious which side the aortic arch is on. However, in infants, the aortic knob often is not identified. In such cases, secondary findings for the presence of the aortic arch must be used. Such findings include position of the descending aorta, tracheal displacement, and tracheal indentation. In a normal left-sided aortic arch, the trachea is displaced slightly toward the right as it moves inferiorly. Also in such cases, there is an indentation on the left border of the trachea as visualized on the frontal view of the chest. If the trachea deviates slightly leftward as it moves inferiorly, or if there is a soft tissue indentation on the right border of the trachea, a right-sided aortic arch should be suspected (see Fig. 4–5).

CATEGORIZATION OF CONGENITAL HEART DISEASE

Once the preceding radiographic features have been identified, it is much easier to identify the category and appropriate differential diagnosis in congenital heart disease. It is important to note, however, that many of the classic features described for particular types of congenital heart disease were established when there was no surgical therapy and patients lived beyond the neonatal period without treatment. Because most cases of congenital heart disease are often identified either in

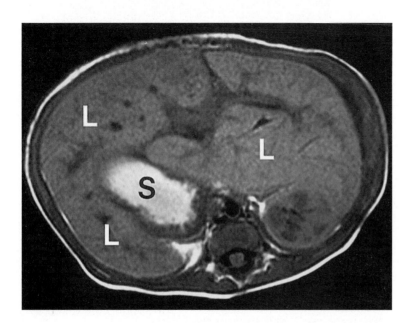

Figure 4–6. Asplenia and midline liver in a neonate with biliary atresia. The liver (L) is midline, extending from the right to left upper abdomen. The stomach (S) is on the right. There is azygous continuation of the inferior vena cava (IVC), with no intrahepatic IVC identified. There is no spleen in the left upper quadrant.

utero with ultrasonography or within the first days of life, and because many types of congenital heart disease are treated during the first week of life with surgery, many of these classic radiographic appearances are no longer seen. In the neonate, increased pulmonary resistance is present physiologically, and the findings of increased pulmonary arterial flow often are not present radiographically. In addition, the classic cardiac configurations described with many of these disease entities do not appear until several weeks of life. Finally, to learn about congenital heart disease, we study the isolated types of congenital heart lesions. This is an oversimplification because many of these abnormalities often occur simultaneously (complex congenital heart disease).

However, radiographic diagnosis of congenital heart disease remains important. In many neonates, chest radiographs obtained in the intensive care unit may be the first suggestion of the presence of congenital heart disease. Two of the major features when categorizing congenital heart disease appropriately include (1) whether the patient is cyanotic or not and (2) whether the pulmonary arterial flow is decreased or increased (Table 4–1). Once

TABLE 4–1. **Categorization of Congenital Heart Disease**

Cyanosis

Decreased flow
  Normal heart size
    Tetralogy of Fallot
  Giant heart size
    Ebstein anomaly
    Pulmonary atresia with intact ventricular septum

Increased flow
  Truncus arteriosus
  Total anomalous pulmonary venous return

Variable flow
  D-Transposition of the great arteries
  Tricuspid atresia

Pink

Increased pulmonary arterial flow
  Left-to-right shunt (VSD, ASD, AVC, PDA)

Increased pulmonary venous flow
  CHF in the newborn

Normal pulmonary flow
  Obstructive lesions
    Coarctation of the aorta
    Aortic stenosis
    Pulmonary artery stenosis
  After surgery

VSD = Ventricular septal defect; ASD = atrial septal defect; AVC = atrioventricular canal; PDA = patent ductus arteriosus; CHF = congestive heart failure.

these two major features are identified, other radiographic findings help to limit the differential diagnosis.

Cyanosis, Decreased Pulmonary Arterial Flow, and Mild Cardiomegaly

In any patient who is cyanotic and demonstrates decreased pulmonary arterial flow on chest radiography, the differential diagnosis can be further limited by whether there is mild or massive cardiomegaly. When the heart size is normal or there is only mild cardiomegaly, the differential diagnosis includes tetralogy of Fallot or pulmonary atresia with an associated ventricular septal defect (VSD). These two entities are essentially different spectrums of the same disease.

Tetralogy of Fallot

Tetralogy of Fallot is the most common type of cyanotic congenital heart disease in children. There are four classic anatomic components of tetralogy of Fallot, which include (1) right ventricular outflow tract obstruction, (2) VSD, (3) overriding aorta, and (4) right ventricular hypertrophy. Radiographic features include a normal-sized to slightly enlarged cardiac silhouette, with uplifting of the ventricular apex (a superiorly oriented cardiac access) secondary to right ventricular hypertrophy (see Fig. 4–5). The main pulmonary artery segment is concave because of the small associated pulmonary arteries. The combination of the deficient main pulmonary artery and upturned cardiac apex makes the configuration of the cardiac silhouette appear boot-shaped. The pulmonary vascularity is decreased. In tetralogy of Fallot, the central pulmonary arteries may be confluent or not confluent. Because this is often difficult to evaluate with echocardiography, magnetic resonance imaging (MRI) can be used to evaluate the status of the pulmonary arteries in patients with tetralogy of Fallot (Fig. 4–7). Pulmonary atresia with a VSD is considered to be the most severe form of tetralogy of Fallot. It is synonymous with pseudotruncus or truncus arteriosus, type 4 because of the larger bronchial arteries arising from the aorta and supplying the lungs.

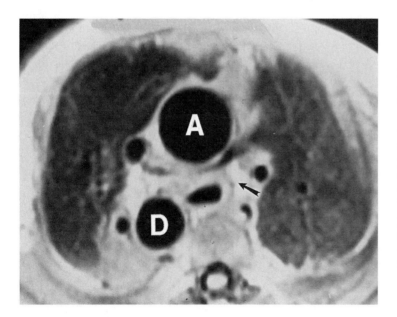

Figure 4–7. Tetralogy of Fallot in a 2-month-old boy. Axial T1-weighted magnetic resonance (MR) image, obtained to evaluate the confluence of the pulmonary arteries, demonstrates no main pulmonary artery. The arrow denotes the expected location of the main pulmonary artery. There is no confluence of the pulmonary arteries. Note the right-sided aortic arch. A = ascending aorta; D = descending aorta.

Cyanosis, Decreased Pulmonary Arterial Flow, and Massive Cardiomegaly

In patients who are cyanotic and demonstrate decreased pulmonary flow but have massive cardiomegaly, the first two entities that should be considered are Ebstein anomaly and pulmonary atresia with an intact septum. In these conditions, the degree of cardiomegaly may be massive—the most massive cardiomegaly seen on radiography. The right atrium can dilate immensely, rather like a balloon; when massive cardiomegaly is encountered, causes that may lead to marked enlargement of the right atrium should be considered.

Ebstein Anomaly

In Ebstein anomaly there is redundancy of the tricuspid valve, which is displaced into the right ventricle, causing atrialization of part of the right ventricle. There is functional obstruction at the level of the tricuspid valve that results in massive dilatation of the right atrium

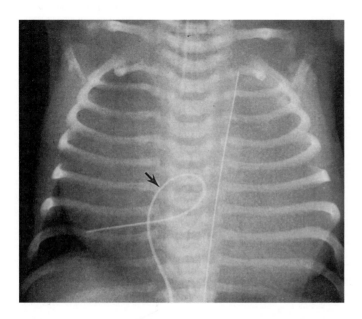

Figure 4–8. Ebstein anomaly in a newborn. There is massive cardiomegaly and decreased pulmonary arterial flow. Note the umbilical venous catheter *(arrow)* curled in the right atrium. (From Donnelly LF, Gelfand KJ, Schwartz DC, Strife JL. The wall to wall heart: differential diagnosis for massively large cardiothymic silhouette in newborns. Appl Radiol 1997;26:23–28.)

and the atrialized portion of the right ventricle. When the anomaly is severe, infants present with severe cyanosis. On radiography, there is massive cardiomegaly and decreased pulmonary arterial flow (Fig. 4–8).

Pulmonary Atresia with Intact Ventricular Septum

Unlike pulmonary atresia with a VSD (severe tetralogy of Fallot), in patients with pulmonary atresia and an intact septum, there is no forward flow from the right side of the heart, leading to massive dilatation of the right atrium and, to a lesser degree, the right ventricle. Such patients present with marked cyanosis in infancy. The radiographic appearance may be identical to that of Ebstein anomaly (Fig. 4–9; see also Fig. 4–3). Note that there are many other abnormalities that may cause the appearance of a massive cardiopericardial silhouette on the chest radiograph of a new-

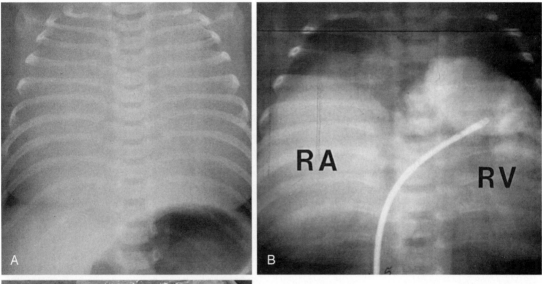

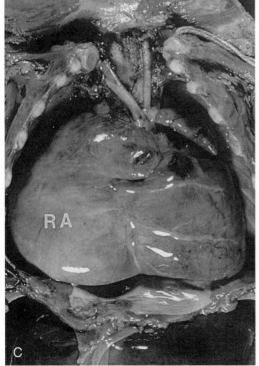

Figure 4–9. Pulmonary atresia with intact ventricular septum in a newborn. *A,* Radiograph shows massive cardiomegaly filling the entire chest. *B,* Contrast injection of right ventricle shows massive dilatation of right atrium (RA) and right ventricle (RV). *C,* Postmortem photograph after thoracotomy shows massively dilated right atrium (RA). (*A–C* from Donnelly LF, Gelfand KJ, Schwartz DC, Strife JL. The wall to wall heart: differential diagnosis for massively large cardiothymic silhouette in newborns. Appl Radiol 1997;26:23–28.)

born. They include cardiac tumors such as rhabdomyoma (Fig. 4–10), noncardiac mediastinal masses, congenital diaphragmatic hernia before aeration of the herniated valve, and peripheral arteriovenous fistulas with associated high-output failure (Fig. 4–11). However, when massive cardiomegaly is encountered in the presence of decreased pulmonary flow, Ebstein anomaly and pulmonary atresia with an intact septum should be the primary considerations.

Cyanosis and Increased Flow

Patients who are cyanotic and have increased pulmonary arterial flow have add-mixture lesions. In infancy, the two entities that should be considered first are truncus arteriosus and total anomalous pulmonary venous return (TAPVR).

Truncus Arteriosus

In truncus arteriosus, the primitive truncus arteriosus fails to divide into an aorta and pulmonary artery. Therefore, one single vessel arises from the heart and gives rise to the coronary, systemic, and pulmonary circulations. There is always an associated VSD. The types of truncus arteriosus are classified based on how the pulmonary arteries arise from the primitive truncus. It is an uncommon lesion and usually presents with cyanosis early in infancy.

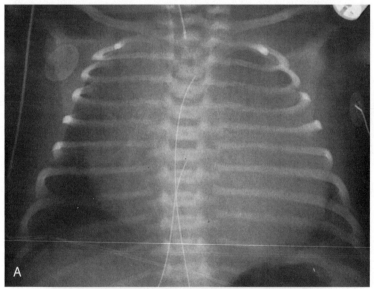

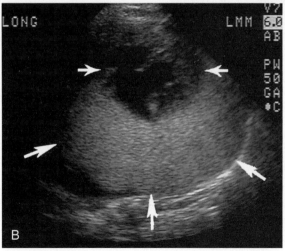

Figure 4–10. Cardiac rhabdomyoma with massive cardiomegaly mimicking Ebstein anomaly on radiography. *A,* Frontal radiograph demonstrates apparent massive cardiomegaly. *B,* Substernal longitudinal ultrasonogram demonstrates large infiltrative mass *(large arrows)* arising from and surrounding the heart *(small arrows).* (*A* and *B* from Donnelly LF, Gelfand KJ, Schwartz DC, Strife JL. The wall to wall heart: differential diagnosis for massively large cardiothymic silhouette in newborns. Appl Radiol 1997; 26:23–28.)

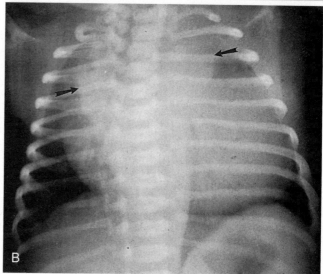

Figure 4–11. Marked enlargement of the cardiac silhouette secondary to peripheral arteriovenous shunting in a neonate with a scalp hemangioma. *A*, Photograph shows large scalp hemangioma. *B*, Chest radiograph shows marked enlargement of the cardiac silhouette. Note the enlargement of the superior mediastinum *(arrows)* secondary to increased flow in the vessels to and from the head. (*A* and *B* from Donnelly LF, Gelfand KJ, Schwartz DC, Strife JL. The wall to wall heart: differential diagnosis for massively large cardiothymic silhouette in newborns. Appl Radiol 1997;26:23–28.)

On chest radiography, there is increased pulmonary arterial flow. A right aortic arch is present in one third of patients. When a right aortic arch is identified in the presence of increased pulmonary arterial flow, the diagnosis is highly suggestive (Fig. 4–12). There is usually moderate cardiomegaly as well as superimposed pulmonary venous congestion.

Total Anomalous Pulmonary Venous Return

In TAPVR, the pulmonary venous return does not connect to the left atrium but connects to the systemic venous structures such as the SVC, right atrium, or portal vein. TAPVR can be divided into subtypes that include supracardiac, cardiac, or infracardiac. Supracardiac is the most common form; the pulmonary veins converge and form a left vertical vein that runs superiorly and connects to the innominate vein. With infracardiac TAPVR, the returning veins penetrate the diaphragm and connect to the IVC below the level of diaphragm. These veins may become obstructed, and the patient may present with a pattern of pulmonary edema on chest radiography (Fig. 4–13). Supracardiac TAPVR classically demonstrates a "snowman" appearance. The dilated left vertical vein and dilated SVC form the superior portion of the snowman (Fig. 4–14). This classic appearance does not develop until later in life and currently is not seen often because these lesions are fixed during infancy.

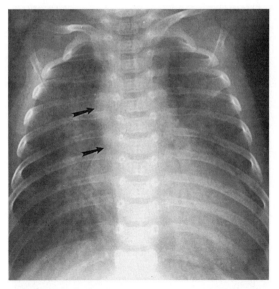

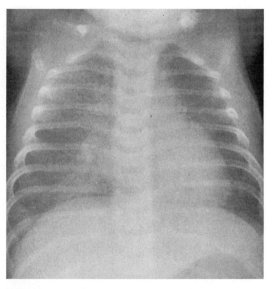

Figure 4–12. Truncus arteriosus in a 5-day-old boy. Chest radiograph shows increased pulmonary arterial flow, cardiomegaly, and a right-sided aortic arch *(arrows)*. Note the indentation on the right wall of the trachea and the leftward course of the trachea from a superior to inferior direction, secondary to the right aortic arch.

Figure 4–13. Total anomalous pulmonary venous return, infracardiac type, with venous obstruction in a newborn. Chest radiograph demonstrates diffuse pulmonary opacity with indistinctness of the pulmonary vascularity.

Cyanosis and Variable Pulmonary Arterial Flow

Both D-transposition of the great arteries and tricuspid atresia can present with variable flow, depending on the anatomy associated with the lesion as well as the age of the patient.

D-*Transposition of the Great Arteries*

D-Transposition of the great arteries (D-TGA) is the most common congenital heart disease presenting with cyanosis during the first 24 hours of life. With this abnormality, the aorta and pulmonary arteries are transposed. The ascending aorta arises from the right ventricle,

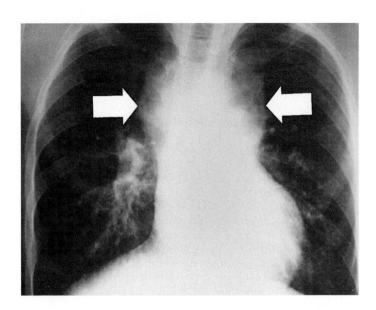

Figure 4–14. Total anomalous pulmonary venous return, supracardiac type, in an older child. Chest radiograph shows "snowman" appearance of mediastinum. There is enlargement of the superior mediastinum *(arrows)* secondary to dilated left vertical vein and superior vena cava. There is also increased pulmonary arterial flow.

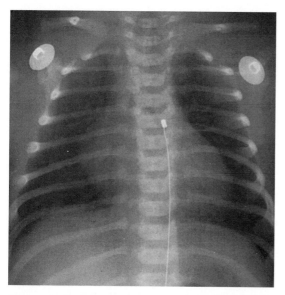

Figure 4–15. D-Transposition of the great arteries (D-TGA) in a newborn boy. Chest radiograph shows normal pulmonary vascularity. The classically described findings of D-TGA, such as increased pulmonary arterial flow and an egg-on-a-string appearance of the mediastinum, are absent.

and the pulmonary artery arises from the left ventricle. Therefore, blood flow runs in two parallel circuits, systemic and pulmonary. Survival depends on communication between these two circles via a patent foramen ovale, atrial septal defect (ASD), VSD, or a patent ductus arteriosus (PDA). Historically, D-TGA

was categorized as a cardiac lesion associated with increased pulmonary arterial flow. However, in areas with well-developed health care systems, pulmonary arterial switch procedures are performed during the first week of life, and increased pulmonary flow, which occurs in older children with transposition, is rarely seen now. The most common radiographic appearance of a newborn with D-TGA is a normal chest radiograph (Fig. 4–15). Classically described radiographic findings include narrowing of the superior mediastinum resulting from decreased thymic tissue and abnormal relationships of the great vessels and, as previously mentioned, increased pulmonary arterial flow. The appearance of the mediastinum has been likened to an "egg on a string."

Tricuspid Atresia

In tricuspid atresia, the classic description is that the right atrium greatly increases in size, leading to marked cardiomegaly associated with decreased pulmonary flow. However, in my experience, this classic appearance is seen in the minority of patients. The radiograph can vary greatly in cases of tricuspid atresia, making radiographic diagnosis a humbling experience (Fig. 4–16).

Pink with Increased Pulmonary Arterial Flow

Children who are acyanotic and demonstrate increased pulmonary arterial flow on chest ra-

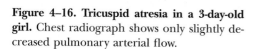

Figure 4–16. Tricuspid atresia in a 3-day-old girl. Chest radiograph shows only slightly decreased pulmonary arterial flow.

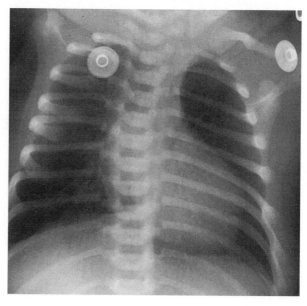

diography have a left-to-right shunt. Potential shunts include ASD, VSD, PDA, atrial ventricular canal (AVC), partial anomalous pulmonary venous return, and aortopulmonary window. Which cardiac chambers are enlarged are often a clue as to which type of shunt is present. In ASD, the right atrium and right ventricle are enlarged. In VSD, the right ventricle, left atrium, and left ventricle are enlarged. In PDA, the left atrium, left ventricle, and aorta are enlarged. However, as previously mentioned, determining chamber enlargement is next to impossible in infants. Perhaps a more practical way to predict which type of shunt is present is based on age at presentation. Patients with very large shunts present in infancy. Typically these are VSDs or AVCs. ASDs more typically present later in childhood or in early adulthood. The most common population to have a PDA is premature infants. AVCs often occur in patients with Down syndrome.

On chest radiography, neonates with left-to-right shunts demonstrate increased pulmonary arterial flow, a variable amount of associated increased pulmonary venous flow (pulmonary edema), and cardiomegaly (see Fig. 4–1). It is common for infants with large left-to-right shunts to also have marked hyperinflation on chest radiography (Fig. 4–17). This is thought to be secondary to air trapping from the peribronchial edema. Therefore, the presence of marked hyperinflation should not dissuade one from the diagnosis of a left-to-right shunt.

Pink (or Dusky) with Increased Pulmonary Venous Flow

A noncyanotic patient with increased pulmonary venous flow is essentially a patient with congestive heart failure. In the neonate, the differential diagnosis of congestive heart failure is extensive and somewhat different from that seen in older children and adults. In my experience, residents have more difficulty with a reasonable differential diagnosis of congestive heart failure in the newborn than with any other differential diagnosis in pediatric radiology. An easy way to approach the differential diagnosis is to consider two large categories of disease. The first category is that of

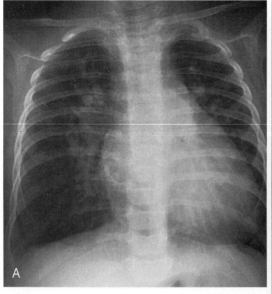
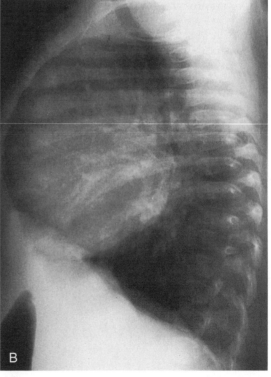

Figure 4–17. Ventricular septal defect in a 3-month-old boy. *A,* Frontal radiograph demonstrates cardiomegaly and increased pulmonary arterial flow. *B,* Lateral radiograph demonstrates marked hyperinflation, which is commonly seen in infants with large left-to-right shunts. Cardiomegaly is again present.

anatomic left-sided obstruction (Table 4–2). Anything that obstructs the left side of the heart can cause congestive heart failure. By working proximally starting at the level of the aorta, one is less likely to forget any of the likely candidates. In the aorta, both coarctation of the aorta and critical aortic stenosis can cause left-sided obstruction. Anything that causes the left ventricle to be dysfunctional also can cause left-sided cardiac obstruction. The list of possibilities is long and includes cardiomyopathy (see Fig. 4–2), glycogen storage disease, anomalous origin of the left coronary artery with associated cardiac ischemia (Fig. 4–18), maternal diabetes, and hypoplastic left heart syndrome. Within the region of the left atrium, both mitral valve stenosis and cor triatriatum can cause left-sided heart failure. *Cor triatriatum* is defined as the presence of a membrane dividing the left atrium into two separate chambers. The membrane has a pin-like hole centrally as the only route for forward blood flow and causes relative obstruction. Pulmonary venous atresia can also cause left-sided heart failure. Of the previously mentioned list of entities, the most commonly encountered include hypoplastic left heart syndrome and coarctation of the aorta.

The second large category of entities that can result in left-sided heart failure include systemic causes such as anemia and polycythemia, sepsis, high-output failure from a peripheral arterial venous malformation, or birth asphyxia (shock myocardium).

TABLE 4–2. **Differential Diagnosis for Congestive Heart Failure in the Newborn**

Anatomic

Coarctation
Aortic stenosis
Left ventricular dysfunction
  Anomalous origin of the left coronary artery
  Myocarditis
  Shock myocardium (birth asphyxia)
  Glycogen storage disease
  Infant of diabetic mother
Hypoplastic left heart
Mitral stenosis
Cor triatriatum
Pulmonary venous atresia-stenosis

Systemic

Anemia-polycythemia
Hypoglycemia, hyperglycemia
Hypothyroidism, hyperthyroidism
Sepsis
Peripheral arteriovenous malformation
  Vein of Galen malformation
  Hepatic hemangioendothelioma

Pink with Normal Pulmonary Arterial Flow

The three main categories of congenital heart disease that are associated with acyanosis and normal pulmonary arterial flow include obstructive lesions, extrinsic airway compression, and patients who have previously had surgery for congenital heart disease and have had the increased or decreased pulmonary arterial flow corrected. Extrinsic airway compression was discussed in Chapter 2.

Obstructive Lesions

Obstructive lesions of the great arteries include aortic stenosis, pulmonic stenosis, and coarctation of the aorta. These lesions can present subtle findings on chest radiography. When a scenario suggests congenital heart disease and the initial impression is that the chest radiograph is normal, a second glance for subtle mediastinal contour abnormalities may prove fruitful.

Aortic Stenosis

Aortic stenosis may be secondary to a bicuspid aortic valve or previous rheumatic disease. With aortic valve stenosis, there may be dilatation of the ascending aorta secondary to the "jet" effect through the stenotic valve (Fig. 4–19). The ascending aorta should never be identified in a normal child by radiography alone. If the righthand border of the ascending aorta is visualized, a dilated aorta should be suspected (Fig. 4–20). In addition to aortic stenosis, other causes of a dilated ascending aorta include aneurysm secondary to disorders such as Marfan syndrome. Other supportive signs of aortic stenosis include findings of left ventricular enlargement secondary to hypertrophy.

Pulmonic Stenosis

In pulmonary valve stenosis, there may be dilatation of the main pulmonary artery secondary to the jet effect. On chest radiography, this appears as a prominent main pulmonary artery segment (Fig. 4–21). Aortic stenosis can also be supravalvular in location. Williams syndrome (Fig. 4–22) is associated with supraval-

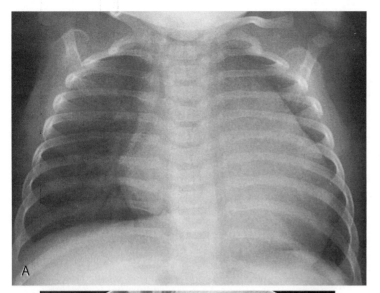

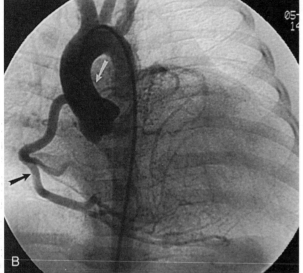

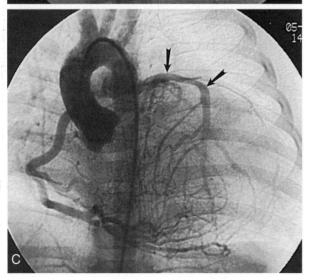

Figure 4–18. Anomalous origin of the left coronary artery with congestive heart failure secondary to left ventricular ischemia in a newborn girl. *A,* Chest radiograph shows cardiomegaly and prominent and indistinct pulmonary vascularity. *B,* Early image from aortogram shows contrast in right coronary artery *(black arrow)* but no visualized origin of the left coronary artery *(white arrow). C,* Delayed image from aortogram shows reconstitution of left coronary artery *(arrows)* from collaterals from right coronary artery. The left coronary artery arises from the pulmonary artery.

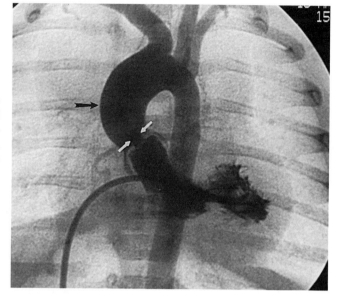

Figure 4–19. Aortic stenosis with poststenotic dilatation in a child with a bicuspid aortic valve. Left ventriculogram shows dilated ascending aorta with the rightward border of the ascending aorta *(black arrow)* protruding well to the right of the spine. A jet of contrast *(white arrows)* can be seen extending from the stenotic valve.

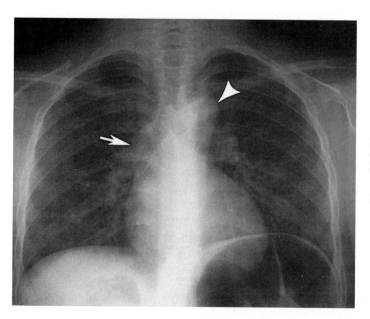

Figure 4–20. Aortic stenosis in a 10-year-old boy. Chest radiograph shows visualization of the ascending aorta *(arrows)* and prominence of the aortic knob *(arrowhead).*

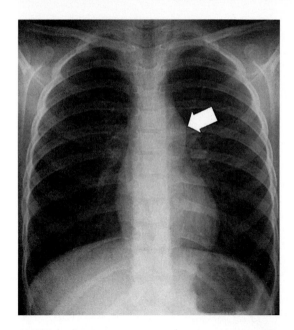

Figure 4–21. Pulmonic stenosis in a 7-year-old girl. There is slight prominence of the main pulmonary artery *(arrow)*.

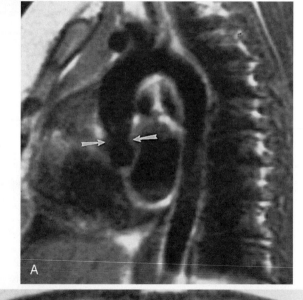

Figure 4–22. Supravalvular aortic stenosis and pulmonic stenosis in a 10-year-old boy with Williams syndrome. *A,* Obliqued sagittal MR image shows narrowing *(arrows)* of the ascending aorta just above the aortic valve. There is poststenotic dilatation. *B,* Axial, T1-weighted MRI shows diffuse narrowing of the main (p) and proximal right and left pulmonary arteries *(arrowheads).*

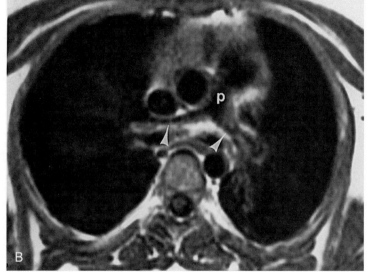

vular stenosis, peripheral pulmonary artery stenosis, and other symptoms, including mental retardation.

Coarctation of the Aorta

Coarctation is defined as a congenital narrowing of the aorta. This narrowing can be either diffuse or localized. The localized type, which is usually positioned juxtaductal, is more common. A typical location of the localized type of coarctation is just beyond the left subclavian artery in the vicinity of the level of the ductus arteriosus. The clinical presentation is determined by the severity of the narrowing. Severe narrowing presents in infancy with congestive heart failure. Less severe narrowing may present later in childhood with upper extremity hypertension. On chest radiography, the appearance of the lefthand border of the superior mediastinum has been likened to an inverse 3 in coarctation (Fig. 4–23). The superior portion of the inverse 3 is caused by the prestenotic dilatation of the aorta above the coarctation. The middle or narrow part of the 3 is caused by the coarctation itself, and the inferior part of the 3 is caused by the poststenotic, dilated portion of the descending aorta. Rib notching may be present secondary to erosion by dilated intracostal arteries (see Fig. 4–23) and most commonly occurs at the level of the fourth through eighth ribs. Coarctation of the aorta has an increased association with bicuspid aortic valve, and such patients

can present later in life with resultant aortic stenosis (Fig. 4–24). In coarctation, MRI can be used for diagnosis, presurgical planning (site, length, severity, relationship to left subclavian artery, and extent of collateralization) (Fig. 4–25), and postsurgical follow-up in the evaluation of restenosis, aneurysm, or left ventricular hypertrophy.

Abnormalities of Conotruncal Rotation

A number of types of congenital heart disease can result from abnormalities of conotruncal rotation. Because there is often confusion concerning this group of diseases, I will discuss how they arise from abnormal rotation of the conotruncus. The primitive truncus is an anterior midline structure during fetal development. Normally, it divides into the aorta and the pulmonary artery, which rotate 150 degrees in a clockwise direction (Fig. 4–26). As a result, the pulmonary artery ends up anterior and to the left of the aorta. Abnormal division or rotation of this primitive truncus may result in a number of diseases, including D-TGA, L-transposition of the great arteries (L-DGA), truncus arteriosus, double-outlet right ventricle, or situs inversus. The anatomic relationship between the aorta and the pulmonary artery as viewed in cross-section at the level of the semilunar valves is characteristic of these abnormalities. With truncus arteriosus, there is a failure of division of the primitive truncus

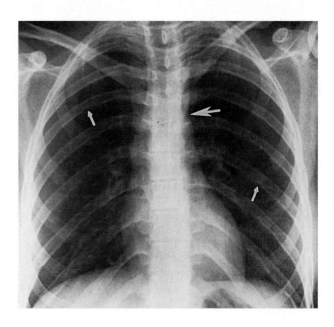

Figure 4–23. Coarctation of the aorta in a 12-year-old girl. Chest radiograph shows reverse 3 appearance of the left superior mediastinal border (arrow denotes middle indentation between dilated prestenotic and poststenotic portions) and rib notching *(small arrows).*

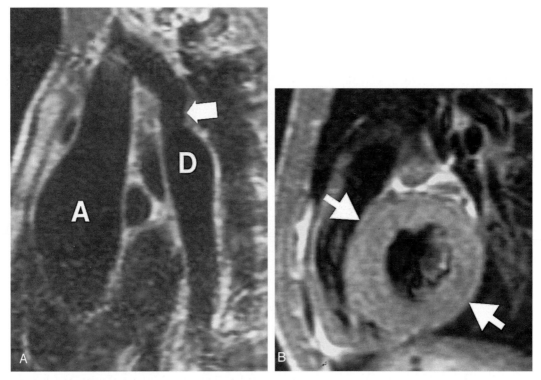

Figure 4–24. Eighteen-year-old boy with history of previous coarctation repair as an infant who presented with increasing shortness of breath on exertion. *A,* Oblique, sagittal T1-weighted MR image shows dilatation of the ascending aorta (A). There is dilatation of the descending aorta (D) just beyond the previous coarctation repair. However, the level of the previous coarctation *(arrow)* is not significantly narrower than the descending aorta beyond the level of poststenotic dilatation (meaning the stenosis is not significant). *B,* Oblique, sagittal T1-weighted MR image shows marked hypertrophy of the left ventricular walls *(arrows).* The combination of the dilatation of the ascending aorta and left ventricular hypertrophy are consistent with aortic stenosis secondary to bicuspid aortic valve.

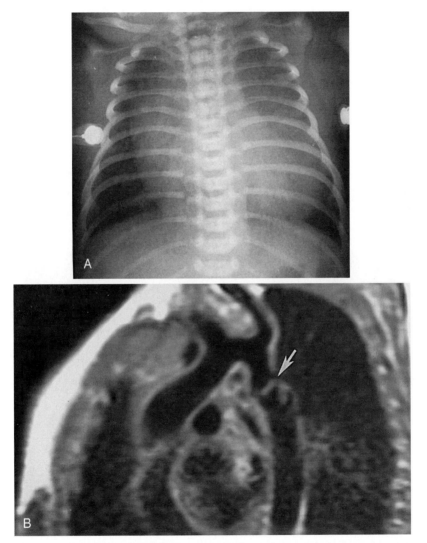

Figure 4–25. Coarctation of the aorta leading to congestive heart failure in a newborn. *A,* Chest radiograph shows cardiomegaly and increased pulmonary venous flow, an edematous pattern. *B,* Oblique, sagittal T1-weighted MR image shows focal, web-like coarctation *(arrow)* in a juxtaductal location.

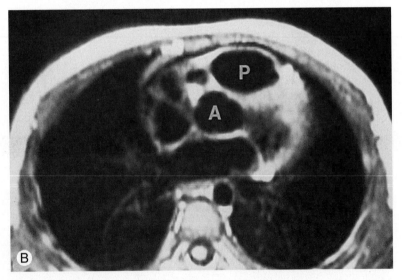

Figure 4–26. Conotruncal rotation. *A,* Diagram shows relationship of the great arteries at the level of semilunar valves as depicted by axial cross-sectional MR imaging. During embryologic development, the primitive truncus is an anterior midline structure. With normal development, the primitive truncus divides into the aorta and the pulmonary artery, which then rotate 150 degrees counterclockwise. The pulmonary artery then lies anterior and leftward of the aorta. Variations in this rotation are characteristic of various conotruncal abnormalities. PT = primitive truncus; A = aorta; P = pulmonary artery; DORV = double-outlet right ventricle; TGA = transposition of the great arteries. *B,* Normal conotruncal position on axial, T1-weighted MR image. The pulmonary artery (P) is anterior and leftward of the aorta (A). (*A* from Donnelly LF, Higgins CB. MR imaging of conotruncal abnormalities. AJR Am J Roentgenol 1996;166:925–928.)

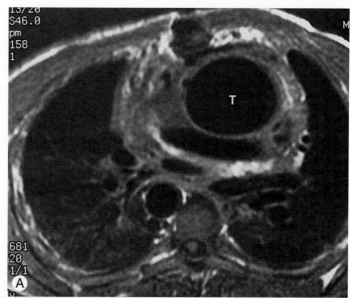

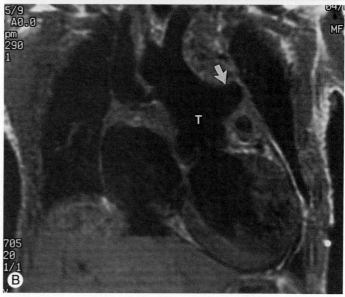

Figure 4–27. Truncus arteriosus is shown on T1-weighted MR image. *A,* Axial image shows a large single vessel; the truncus (T) arises from base of heart. *B,* Coronal image shows left pulmonary artery *(arrow)* arising from ascending aorta. (*A* and *B* from Donnelly LF, Higgins CB. MR imaging of conotruncal abnormalities. AJR Am J Roentgentol 1996;166:925–928.)

into a separate aorta and pulmonary artery. Therefore, a single large vessel gives rise to the coronary, systemic, and pulmonary arterial circulation (Fig. 4–27). Truncus arteriosus was discussed earlier.

In L-TGA, or congenitally corrected transposition of the great arteries, the ventricles and arterial ventricular valves are inverted so that there is both atrioventricular and ventriculoarterial discordance. Therefore, the morphologic right ventricle is in the position of, and serves as, the anatomic left ventricle. L-TGA is often associated with complex congenital heart disease but may occur as an isolated lesion. With L-TGA, there is 30-degree clock-

wise rotation of the primitive truncus, resulting in the aorta being anterior and leftward compared with the pulmonary artery (see Fig. 4–26).

In contrast, with D-TGA, or complete transposition of the great arteries, there is ventricular–great vessel discordance, with the aorta arising from the right ventricle and the pulmonary artery arising from the left ventricle. With D-TGA, there is 30-degree clockwise rotation of the primitive truncus, resulting in the aorta being rightward and anterior to the pulmonary artery (Fig. 4–28).

With double-outlet right ventricle, more than half of the great arteries arise from the

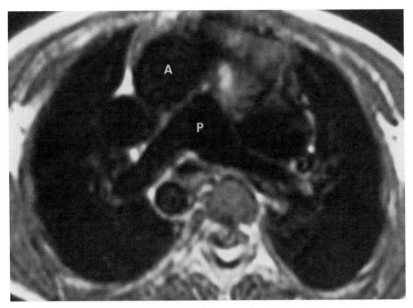

Figure 4–28. D-Transposition of the great vessels is shown on T1-weighted axial MR image. The aorta (A) is anterior and rightward in relationship to the pulmonary artery (P). (From Donnelly LF, Higgins CB. MR imaging of conotruncal abnormalities. AJR Am J Roentgenol 1996;166:925–928.)

morphologic right ventricle. The only outlet for the left ventricle is a VSD. This lesion is often associated with other complex congenital heart disease. With double-outlet right ventricle, there is 45-degree counterclockwise rotation of the primitive truncus, resulting in the aorta and pulmonary artery being side by side, with the aorta on the right (see Fig. 4–26).

In situs inversus, the rotation of the aorta and pulmonary artery can be completely opposite that of normal (see Fig. 4–26).

SURGERY FOR CONGENITAL HEART DISEASE

In order to understand the radiographic or MRI or computed tomographic appearance of patients who have undergone surgery for congenital heart disease, a knowledge of the types of procedures performed is required. Table 4–3 lists the name, flow alteration, and indications for commonly performed cardiac procedures.

MAGNETIC RESONANCE IMAGING FOR EVALUATING CONGENITAL HEART DISEASE

With the continuous technologic advances in MRI, helical CT, and echocardiography, there

is a constant redefining of the role of MRI in cardiac imaging. To put things in perspective, at the Children's Hospital Medical Center in Cincinnati, Ohio, which is fairly well known for pediatric cardiac MR imaging, there are more than 200 echocardiograms performed for every MRI of the chest. At most institutions, MRI is used in cases when echocardiography cannot provide all the necessary information. General indications for MRI are listed in Table 4–4. The use of MRI in the evaluation of aortic anomalies includes evaluation of coarctation (see Figs. 4–24 and 4–25), supravalvular aortic stenosis (see Fig. 4–22), aneurysm (Fig. 4–29), dissection, or vascular rings. In the evaluation of the pulmonary arteries, MRI is often used to determine the confluence of the pulmonary arteries in tetralogy of Fallot and pulmonary atresia (see Fig. 4–7). Pulmonary vein stenosis or atresia or cor triatriatum can also be imaged with MRI. In the patient who has had previous surgery for congenital heart disease, MRI can be useful in the evaluation of stenoses, thromboses, aneurysm formation, or hematoma surrounding shunts. In the evaluation of congenital heart disease with MRI, the primary information is anatomic and is obtained on T1-weighted images in multiple planes. Functional information can also be obtained through a combination of cine MRI, MR spectroscopy, and gradient echo imaging.

TABLE 4–3. **Common Surgical Procedures for Congenital Heart Disease**

Procedure	Indication	Connection
Fontan	Tricuspid atresia Single ventricle Hypoplastic right ventricle Complex CHD	RA-to-PA conduit or anastomosis
Glenn	Tricuspid atresia Hypoplastic RV Pulmonary atresia	SVC-to-right PA anastomosis (bidirectional provides flow to both pulmonary arteries)
Rastelli	Pulmonary atresia	RV-to-PA conduit
Mustard-Senning (intraatrial baffle)	D-Transposition of the great arteries	Atrial rerouting of venous blood flow
Arterial switch procedure (Jatene)	D-Transposition of the great arteries	Switch of aorta and PA with reanastomosis of coronary arteries
Norwood	Hypoplastic right ventricle	*First stage:* use of main PA as ascending aorta, enlargement of aortic arch, systemic shunt to distal PA *Second stage:* modified Fontan
Blalock-Taussig shunt	Palliative shunt for obstruction of pulmonary blood flow (TOF, pulmonary atresia, tricuspid atresia)	Subclavian artery-to-PA graft
Waterston-Cooley	Palliative shunt for obstruction of pulmonary blood flow	Ascending aorta-to-right PA anastomosis
Potts	Palliative shunt for obstruction of pulmonary blood flow	Descending aorta-to-right PA anastomosis
PA banding	Left-to-right shunting	Band around main PA

RA = right atrium; PA = pulmonary artery; CHD = congestive heart failure; SVC = superior vena cava; RV = right ventricle; TOF = tetralogy of Fallot.

ACQUIRED HEART DISEASE

In addition to congenital heart disease, there are multiple types of acquired heart disease that can occur during childhood. Many, such as cardiomyopathy and rheumatic heart disease, have overlapping features with adult disease. One of the unique types of acquired heart disease that can occur in children is Kawasaki disease.

Kawasaki Disease

Kawasaki disease (mucocutaneous lymph node syndrome) is an inflammatory disease of un-

TABLE 4–4. **General Uses of Magnetic Resonance Imaging in the Evaluation of Congenital Heart Disease**

Aortic abnormalities
Vascular ring
Pulmonary vein abnormalities
Pulmonary artery abnormalities
Cardiac masses
Complex congenital heart disease
Postoperative complications

known cause. Characteristic findings include fever, rash, conjunctivitis, erythema of the lips and oral cavity, and cervical lymphadenopathy. There is an associated generalized vasculitis. Cardiac involvement includes acute myocarditis, which can lead to congestive heart failure (Fig. 4–30). Delayed cardiac complications include the development of coronary artery aneurysms as well as coronary artery stenoses. Chest radiographs can show findings of congestive heart failure when the myocarditis is severe. Rarely the coronary artery calcifications can calcify. Gallbladder hydrops, as seen on ultrasonography, has also been described as a finding. However, this is not included as one of the criteria in making the diagnosis, and ultrasonography of the upper abdomen is rarely useful. Treatment is with gamma globulin.

Cardiac Masses

There are a number of causes of cardiac masses in children. The majority present during the newborn period. The most common type of congenital heart mass is rhabdomyoma (Fig. 4–31). This lesion is most often seen in

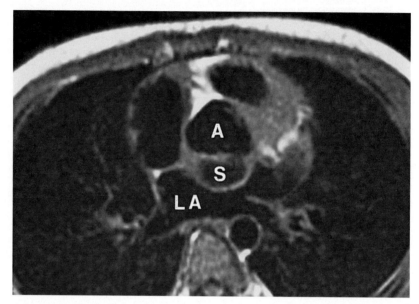

Figure 4–29. Sinus of Valsalva aneurysm in a 6-year-old boy who presented with embolic, ischemic myositis. Axial, T1-weighted image shows an abnormal vascular structure (S), the aneurysm, situated between the ascending aorta (A) and the left atrium (LA).

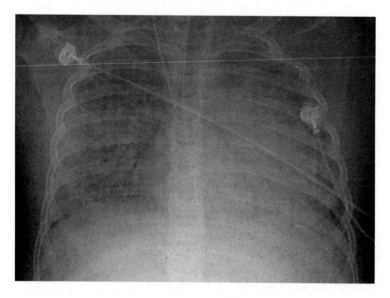

Figure 4–30. Kawasaki disease in a 5-year-old child resulting in acute myocarditis. Chest radiograph shows diffuse lung opacity secondary to congestive heart failure.

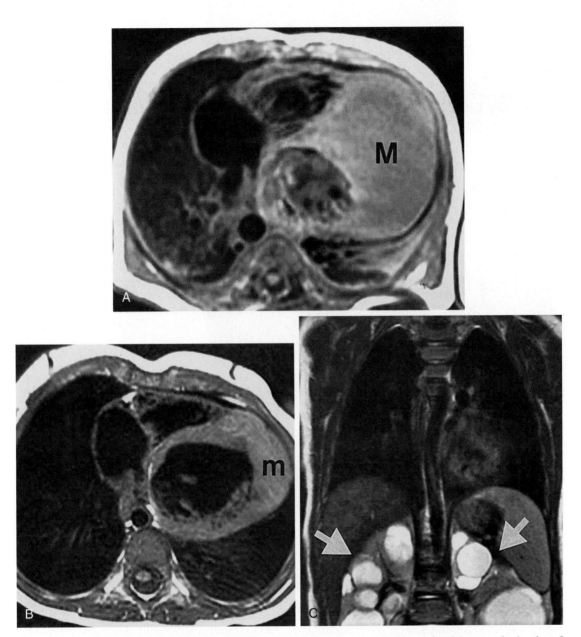

Figure 4–31. Rhabdomyoma in a girl with tuberous sclerosis. *A,* Axial, T1-weighted image obtained at 2 days of life shows large mass (M) arising from the myocardium of the left and right ventricle, splaying the intraventricular septum. *B,* Axial, T1-weighted image obtained at 2 years of age shows interval decrease in size of mass (m). *C,* Coronal, T2-weighted image obtained at the same time as that in *B* shows multiple cysts in kidneys *(arrows).*

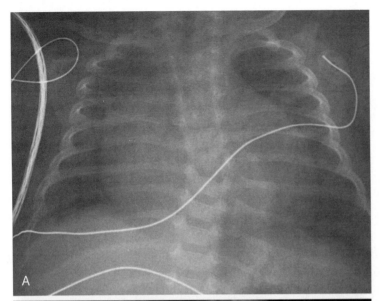

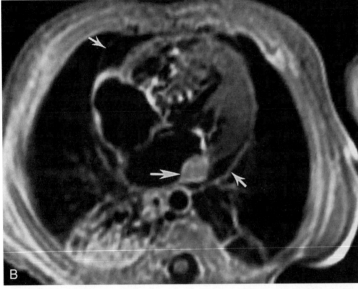

Figure 4–32. Left atrial hemangioendothelioma causing pericardial effusion in a newborn boy. *A,* Chest radiograph shows enlargement of the cardiopericardial silhouette. There is also a segmental vertebral anomaly present. *B,* Axial, T1-weighted MR image after injection of gadolinium shows well-defined enhancing mass *(large arrow)* arising from the lateral wall of the left atrium. There is low signal *(small arrows)* in the pericardial sac consistent with residual air after pericardiocentesis.

patients with tuberous sclerosis. Rhabdomyomas typically involute over time and are usually treated conservatively (see Fig. 4–31). Other potential cardiac masses include angiosarcoma, fibroma, teratoma, and hemangioma. The most common cause of cardiac tumor associated with pericardial effusion is hemangioma (Fig. 4–32). These cases are often initially diagnosed on in utero or postnatal ultrasonography and then further characterized with MR imaging.

Suggested Readings

Coussement AM, Gooding CA. Objective radiographic assessment of pulmonary vascularity in children. Radiology 1973;109:649–654.

Donnelly LF, Gelfand KJ, Schwartz DC, Strife JL. The wall to wall heart: differential diagnosis for massively large cardiothymic silhouette in newborns. Appl Radiol 1997;26:23–28.

Donnelly LF, Higgins CB. MR imaging of conotruncal abnormalities AJR Am J Roentgenol 1996;166:925–928.

Fellows KE, Weinberg PM, Baffa JM, Hoffman EA. Evaluation of congenital heart disease with MR imaging: current and coming attractions. 1992;159:925–931.

Strife JS, Sze RW. Radiographic evaluation of the neonate with congenital heart disease. Radiol Clin North Am 1999;37:1093–1107.

Swischuk LE, Stansberry SD. Pulmonary vascularity in pediatric heart disease. J Thorac Imaging 1989;4:1–6.

Winer-Muram HT, Tonkin IL. The spectrum of heterotaxic syndromes. Radiol Clin North Am 1989;27:1147–1170.

Chapter

5

Gastrointestinal Tract

NEONATAL GASTROINTESTINAL TRACT

Necrotizing Enterocolitis

Necrotizing enterocolitis (NEC) is a disease primarily of premature infants in the intensive care unit. It can less commonly be seen in older infants under extreme stress, such as after cardiac surgery. It is an idiopathic enterocolitis that is most likely related to some combination of infection and ischemia and most commonly affects the ileum and ascending colon. It most commonly presents during the first or second week of life with abdominal distention, feeding intolerance, increased aspirates from the nasogastric tube, or sepsis. When NEC is suspected, infants are given nothing orally,

are treated with antibiotics, and are monitored with serial abdominal radiographs (anteroposterior [AP] and supine, and a free air view: cross-table lateral or left lateral decubitus).

Radiographic findings range from normal to suggestive to diagnostic. Suggestive findings include focal dilatation of bowel (especially within the right lower quadrant) or featureless, "unfolded"-appearing small bowel loops with separation of bowel loops, suggesting bowel wall thickening (Fig. 5–1). An unchanging bowel gas pattern over serial films is worrisome. The most definitive finding of NEC is the presence of pneumatosis (gas in the bowel wall) (Fig. 5–2). Pneumatosis appears as multiple bubble-like or curvilinear lucencies overlying the bowel. It can be similar to the appear-

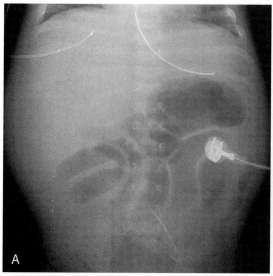
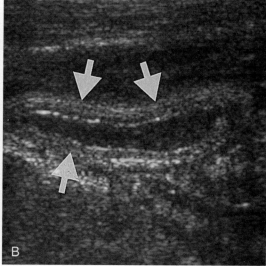

Figure 5–1. Necrotizing enterocolitis in a 2-month-old premature infant. *A,* Radiography shows featureless, "unfolded"-appearing small bowel loops, with separation of bowel loops suggestive of bowel wall thickening. The bowel gas pattern was unchanging over many days. *B,* Ultrasonography shows bowel wall thickening *(arrows)* of small bowel loops within the right lower quadrant.

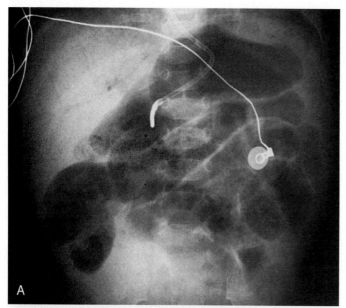

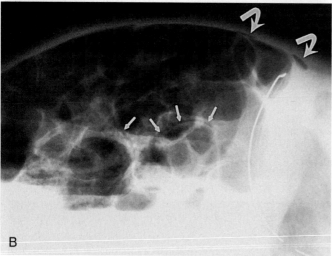

Figure 5–2. Necrotizing enterocolitis in a newborn infant. *A*, Frontal radiograph shows portal venous gas as branching lucencies overlying the liver. There are also bubble-like lucencies, which may indicate pneumatosis overlying multiple dilated bowel loops. *B*, Cross-table lateral radiograph a day later shows curvilinear lucencies *(arrows)*, which are diagnostic of pneumatosis. There are two triangular areas of lucency *(curved arrows)* anteriorly, which are consistent with free intraperitoneal gas.

ance of stool. However, such stool patterns are uncommon in sick, premature neonates in the intensive care unit. Portal venous gas can occur (see Fig. 5–2). It appears as branching linear lucencies overlying the liver. Free intraperitoneal air is considered the only radiographic finding seen in NEC that is an absolute indication for surgery. Otherwise, the decision to perform surgery is made based on a combination of clinical and radiographic findings. Free air may be seen as triangles of anterior lucency on cross-table lateral radiographs, as overall increased lucency on supine radiographs (see Fig. 5–2), or as visualization of both sides of the bowel wall (Rigler sign); free air may also outline intraperitoneal structures such as the falciform ligament (football sign) (Fig. 5–3).

In NEC when the abdomen is distended but relatively gasless, ultrasonography can be helpful. The ultrasonographic identification of thickened bowel loops (see Fig. 5–1) with increased or absent color Doppler flow is suggestive of inflamed or infarcted bowel. Large amounts of free fluid is also a poor prognostic finding.

A delayed complication seen in survivors of NEC is bowel stricture. These strictures most commonly involve the descending colon.

High Intestinal Obstruction in Neonates

Neonates with suspected intestinal obstruction can be divided into those with suspected upper

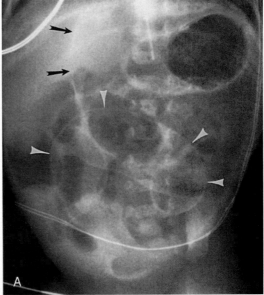

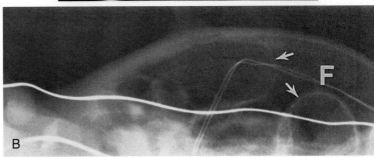

Figure 5–3. Necrotizing entero-colitis in a newborn premature infant. *A,* Frontal radiograph shows multiple findings of free intraperitoneal air. There is increased lucency overlying the liver, outlining the falciform ligament (football sign) *(arrows).* Both internal and external walls of the bowel (the Rigler sign) *(arrowheads)* are seen. *B,* Cross-table lateral view confirms free intraperitoneal gas as a large anterior area of lucency (F) outlining bowel wall *(arrows).*

gastrointestinal (GI) obstruction and those with lower intestinal obstruction on the basis of clinical symptoms and radiographic findings. Infants with high intestinal obstruction present predominantly with vomiting. Radiographs may show distention involving the stomach, duodenum, or jejunum, or a combination of these organs, depending on the level of obstruction. The number of distended small bowel loops is much less than seen with distal bowel obstruction. The most common causes of upper GI tract obstruction in neonates include duodenal atresia or stenosis, duodenal web, annular pancreas, midgut volvulus or obstruction by Ladd bands, or jejunal atresia (Table 5–1).

Duodenal Atresia, Duodenal Stenosis, Duodenal Web, and Annular Pancreas

Duodenal atresia, duodenal stenosis, duodenal web, and annular pancreas are a spectrum of similar abnormalities. All cause either complete or partial duodenal obstruction and usually present at birth or within the first couple days of life. Often, components of more than one diagnosis are present. For example, many cases of duodenal atresia have a component of annular pancreas, and annular pancreas almost never occurs without a component of intrinsic duodenal stenosis.

TABLE 5–1. **Common Causes of Intestinal Obstruction in Neonates**

High
Midgut volvulus-malrotation
Duodenal atresia-stenosis
Duodenal web
Annular pancreas
Jejunal atresia

Low
Hirschsprung disease
Meconium plug syndrome (small left colon syndrome)
Ileal atresia
Meconium ileus
Anal atresia-anorectal malformations

The duodenum is the most common site of intestinal atresia. Duodenal atresia and duodenal stenosis almost always occur in the region of the ampula of Vater. Approximately 30% of cases of duodenal atresia are associated with Down syndrome. Additional associations include other intestinal atresias, biliary abnormalities, congenital heart disease, and VATER (vertebral defects, imperforate anus, tracheoesophageal fistula, and radial and renal dysplasia) associations. On radiographs, neonates with duodenal atresia typically demonstrate a dilated stomach and proximal duodenum with no gas distal to the proximal duodenum. The two dilated structures are referred to as a *double-bubble* sign (Fig. 5–4). In the appropriate clinical setting, a double bubble is diagnostic of duodenal atresia, and additional imaging with an upper gastrointestinal (UGI) series is unnecessary. The question that often arises is, How do we know that this is not an acute obstruction from a midgut volvulus, a surgical

emergency? Dilatation of the duodenal bulb is seen only with chronic causes of obstruction. There is not enough time for the bulb to become dilated with acute obstruction from causes such as midgut volvulus. If the diagnosis is not clear, a UGI series can be performed to document the cause of obstruction. With duodenal stenosis, the double bubble is seen in association with the presence of distal bowel gas (Fig. 5–5).

Duodenal web is another cause of congenital duodenal obstruction. Typically, a web consists of an obstructing membrane (Fig. 5–6), with a pin-sized hole in its center being the only lumen. The web may "stretch" downstream, forming a windsock configuration seen on the UGI series. Because the obstruction is not complete, these patients may present later in life than do those with atresia.

Malrotation and Midgut Volvulus

The possibility of midgut volvulus is one of the few true emergencies in pediatric GI imaging. A delay in the diagnosis of midgut volvulus can result in ischemic necrosis of large portions of the bowel or in death (Fig. 5–7). With normal embryonic rotation, both the duodenojejunal and ileocolic portions of the bowel rotate 270 degrees around the axis of the superior mesenteric artery. An understanding of the embryogenesis is often emphasized, but an understanding of the result is more important. With normal rotation, the duodenojejunal junction is positioned in the left upper quadrant and the cecum is positioned in the right lower quadrant. This results in a long, fixed base that keeps the mesentery from twisting. If the duodenojejunal and ileocecal junctions are not in their normal positions, the base of the small bowel mesentery may be short and predispose the small bowel to twisting—the development of midgut volvulus. In addition to midgut volvulus, malrotation can be associated with duodenal obstruction from Ladd bands (abnormal fibrous peritoneal bands) and periduodenal hernias.

In patients with malrotation, midgut volvulus may happen at any age; however, most present during the first month of life with bilious vomiting. In a child with bilious vomiting, demonstration of findings of malrotation on UGI series, with or without findings of midgut volvulus, is considered a surgical emergency. The diagnosis of malrotation is made on UGI series by determining that the duode-

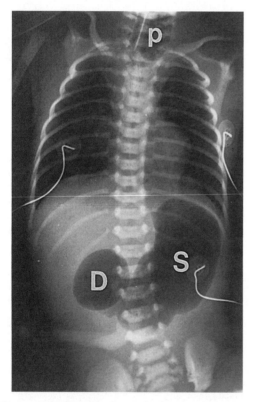

Figure 5–4. Duodenal atresia in association with esophageal atresia and distal tracheoesophageal fistula in a newborn infant. Radiograph shows air-filled, dilated stomach (S) and duodenal bulb (D) giving the appearance of a double bubble. There is also air in a distended pharyngeal pouch (P).

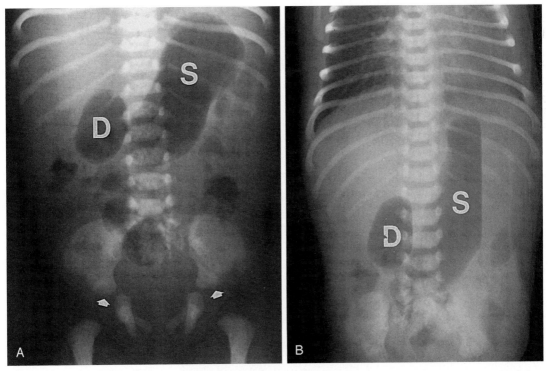

Figure 5–5. Duodenal stenosis in a newborn infant with Down syndrome. Frontal *(A)* and left lateral decubitus *(B)* radiographs show double bubble with air-filled distended stomach (S) and duodenal bulb (D). There is distal gas present, which is consistent with stenosis rather than complete atresia. There are other radiographic findings associated with Down syndrome. Cardiomegaly and increased pulmonary arterial flow seen on *B* are consistent with an arteriovenous (AV) canal. The pelvis demonstrates decreased acetabular angles *(A; arrows)* and an associated "Mickey Mouse" appearance.

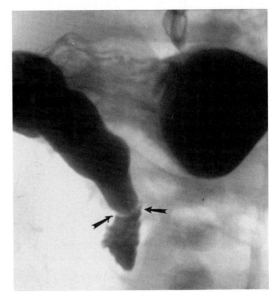

Figure 5–6. Duodenal web in an infant with vomiting. Oblique upper gastrointestinal view shows web-like diaphragm *(arrows)* traversing the duodenum with dilatation of more proximal duodenum. There was a marked delay in passage of contrast into more distal bowel.

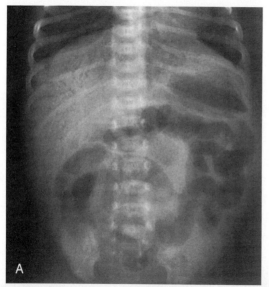

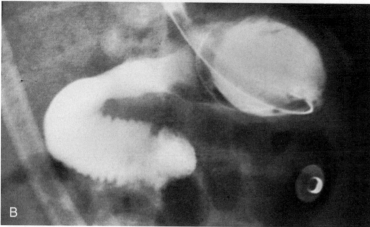

Figure 5–7. Midgut volvulus with resultant bowel necrosis in a 2-week-old infant. *A*, Radiography shows multiple dilated bowel loops and portal venous gas, which are seen as tubular lucencies overlying the liver. *B*, Emergency contrast study shows complete obstruction of the duodenum, which is consistent with volvulus.

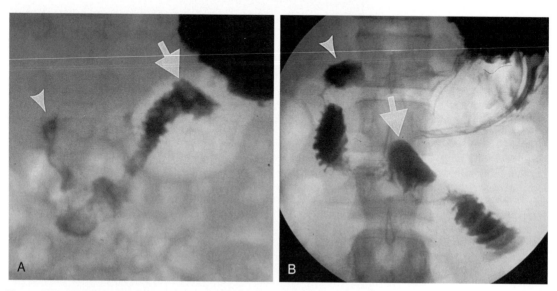

Figure 5–8. Position of the duodenojejunal junction (ligament of Treitz). *A*, Normal position. The duodenojejunal junction *(arrow)* is to the left of the spine and as far superior as the duodenal bulb *(arrowhead)*. *B*, Abnormal position, consistent with malrotation. The duodenojejunal junction *(arrow)* is to the right of the left border of the spine and inferior to the duodenal bulb *(arrowhead)*.

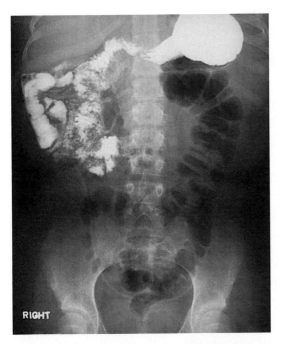

Figure 5–9. Malrotation. The duodenum courses rightward and never crosses the spine. The opacified proximal small bowel is in the right upper quadrant. The unopacified colon is in the left side of the abdomen.

nojejunal junction (ligament of Treitz) is abnormally positioned. The duodenojejunal junction is considered normal when it meets the following two criteria: (1) it is to the left of the spine and (2) it is at the same level as or more superior to the duodenal bulb. It is important to evaluate the position of the duodenojejunal junction during the first pass of contrast through the duodenum and jejunum (see further on) (Fig. 5–8).

In many cases of malrotation, the findings are grossly obvious: The duodenum will course rightward, rather than leftward, and never cross the spine (Fig. 5–9). However, when performing UGI series in children, there are many cases that do not meet the criteria for normal but are very close. It is probably inappropriate to send all these patients to the operating room. I have come to consider the two criteria for normalcy as guidelines rather than rules. In borderline cases (not as high as the bulb, not quite to the right of the spine), I follow the contrast through the small bowel. If the jejunum is in the left upper quadrant and the ileum and cecum are in the right lower quadrant, the patient is probably not at risk for midgut volvulus. Also, the duodenojejunal junction is a mobile structure in children and

can "factiously" be moved into an abnormal position by space-occupying lesions such as a mass (Fig. 5–10) or distended bowel loops. In addition, the presence of a nasojejunal tube may alter the apparent position of the duodenojejunal junction. With midgut volvulus, the duodenum and jejunum appear on UGI series as a corkscrew (Fig. 5–11) or as duodenal obstruction (see Fig. 5–7).

Malrotation or midgut volvulus may also be encountered on cross-sectional imaging studies, such as computed tomography (CT) or ultrasonography, when these studies are ordered to evaluate abdominal pain or vomiting. This is particularly true in older children in whom malrotation is not suspected as the cause of acute abdominal symptoms. On cross-sectional imaging, the bowel may be seen in a swirling pattern around the superior mesenteric vessels (see Fig. 5–11). In addition, the superior mesenteric vein, which is normally to the right of the superior mesenteric artery, is more often to the left of the superior mesenteric artery in patients with malrotation (see Fig. 5–11). However, this is neither sensitive nor specific.

Performing an Upper Gastrointestinal Series in Infants

Perhaps, this is an appropriate place to discuss how to perform a UGI series in infants. First, there are various ways to accomplish a UGI series in an infant, and many pediatric radiologists disagree about the details. The following is how I perform the procedure. I prefer to have the infant secured to an octagon board (immobilization device). This allows me to concentrate on the examination rather than on keeping the child from wiggling or getting hurt, to get images in the appropriate positions rapidly, and to minimize the radiation dose. Some radiologists prefer to administer barium orally and some prefer to use a nasogastric tube. When the child is willing and able to drink, I administer the contrast medium orally, usually by bottle. Contrary to adults, in whom many images of the stomach and duodenum are obtained to exclude ulcers and cancer, few images are needed in a normal infant UGI series. The most important task is to document the position of the duodenojejunal junction.

I start with the child feeding in the supine position because they typically are more likely to suck in this position. Once they begin drinking, I obtain an AP image of the esophagus and turn the patient to a lateral, right side

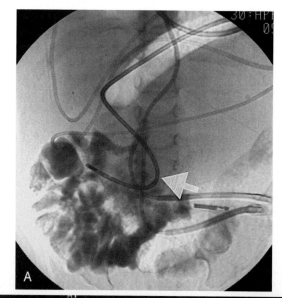

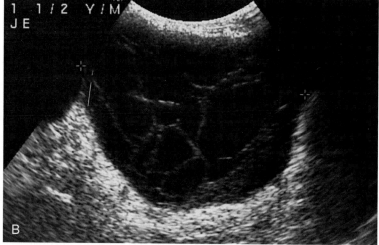

Figure 5–10. Displacement of the duodenojejunal junction by extrinsic compression in a 1-year-old boy with a ventriculoperitoneal shunt and a nasojejunal feeding tube placed because of vomiting. *A,* Fluoroscopic image after placement of nasojejunal tube *(arrowheads)* demonstrates that the location of the duodenojejunal junction *(arrow)* is inferior to the duodenal bulb. *B,* Ultrasonography, performed because of the findings on fluoroscopy, demonstrates a large pseudocyst within the left upper quadrant at the tip of the ventriculoperitoneal shunt. The pseudocyst is causing mass effect, displacing the duodenojejunal junction. Shunt malfunction, rather than gastrointesintal problems, was the cause of the patient's vomiting.

down position. I then obtain a lateral view of the esophagus and wait for contrast to pool in the antrum. When contrast passes through the pylorus and begins to fill the first and second portions of the duodenum, I obtain a lateral view documenting that the pylorus appears normal and that the duodenum courses posteriorly. This is the crucial point in the examination. The infant is then quickly turned supine and an image obtained as contrast courses into the duodenum and proximal jejunum. If the infant is turned supine too early and not enough contrast is in the duodenum, contrast will not pass leftward over the spine. One can always turn the child back to a right side–down position and get more contrast into the duodenum. If the child is turned supine too late (the worst case scenario), contrast will have passed into more distal loops of jejunum and obscure visualization of the position of the duodenojejunal junction. Appropriate timing comes with experience. The next image that I obtain is an oblique view with the left side down, which produces an image of the air-filled antrum and bulb. Finally, I obtain either a fluoroscopic spot view or overhead radiograph once more contrast has passed into the jejunum to document nondilatation of the jejunum and show that there is no gastroesophageal reflux. Therefore, a normal UGI series in an infant should consist of only six images.

Low Intestinal Obstruction in Neonates

Neonates who fail to pass meconium are not uncommon and are considered to have a distal

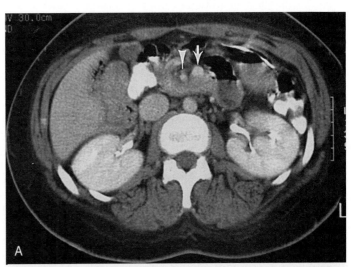

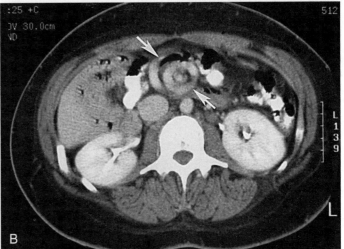

Figure 5–11. Malrotation presenting with intermittent abdominal pain secondary to midgut volvulus in a 17-year-old girl. *A,* Computed tomographic image of the upper abdomen shows inversion of normal relationship between superior mesenteric artery *(arrowhead)* and vein *(arrow),* with the vein situated to the left of the artery. *B,* More caudal image shows characteristic swirling pattern of bowel loops *(arrows)* twisting around the axis of the mesenteric vessels, which is consistent with volvulus. *C,* Upper gastrointestinal series demonstrates an abnormal course of the duodenum and jejunum, resulting in the "corkscrew" appearance of volvulus. (From Zarewych ZM, Donnelly LF, Frush DP, Bisset GS III. Imaging of pediatric mesenteric abnormalities. Pediatr Radiol 1999;29:711–719.)

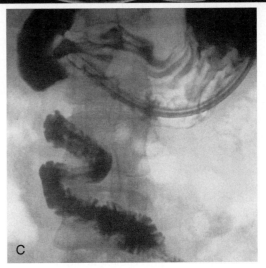

obstructive process. On radiographs of the abdomen, dilatation of multiple loops of bowel is consistent with a distal obstructive process (Figs. 5–12 and 5–13). The only proximal bowel process that may be associated with multiple dilated loops of bowel is midgut volvulus, when the bowel dilates secondary to ischemia or infarction. These infants, however, are very ill. The neonate with multiple dilated loops of bowel on radiography, abdominal distention, and failure to pass adequate amounts of meconium and is otherwise well on physical examination does not have midgut volvulus as a cause of bowel dilatation and should be evaluated with a contrast enema, rather than a UGI series. In a patient without anal atresia on physical examination, the diagnosis is likely to be one of four entities (see Table 5–1). Two of these entities involve the colon (Hirschsprung disease and meconium plug syndrome) and two involve the ileum (ileal atresia and meconium ileus).

Neonatal contrast enemas are typically performed with dilute, ionic, water-soluble agents and a non–balloon tip catheter of appropriate size. Barium typically is not used because it can exacerbate the evacuation of meconium plugs or meconium ileus, whereas, water-soluble enemas can be therapeutic. If a microcolon (a narrow-caliber colon resulting from disuse) is identified on the enema, the cause is likely to be secondary to ileal pathology (see Fig. 5–12). If contrast is refluxed into collapsed terminal ileum and the noncontrast filled, more proximal bowel loops are disproportionately dilated, the diagnosis is likely ileal atresia. If the terminal ileum is distended, with multiple filling defects, the diagnosis is meconium ileus (see Fig. 5–12).

Meconium ileus is secondary to obstruction of the distal ileum resulting from accumulation of abnormally tenacious meconium. It occurs almost exclusively in patients with cystic fibrosis and is the presenting finding of cystic fibrosis in about 10% of patients. It may be complicated by perforation, bowel volvulus, or peritonitis. Plain radiographs show findings of distal obstruction (see Fig. 5–12). There may be associated bubble-like lucencies, secondary to the accumulated meconium, or calcification

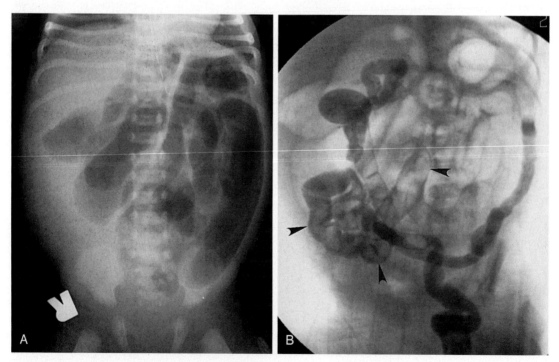

Figure 5–12. Meconium ileus in a newborn infant with abdominal distention and failure to pass meconium. It was confirmed that the infant had cystic fibrosis. *A,* Radiograph shows dilatation of multiple loops of bowel and no definite colonic gas, findings that are consistent with a distal obstruction. *B,* Contrast enema demonstrates small-caliber microcolon and multiple tubular filling defects *(arrowheads)* within dilated distal ileum, consistent with meconium ileus. The more proximal, unopacified small bowel loops are disproportionately dilated, which is consistent with obstruction.

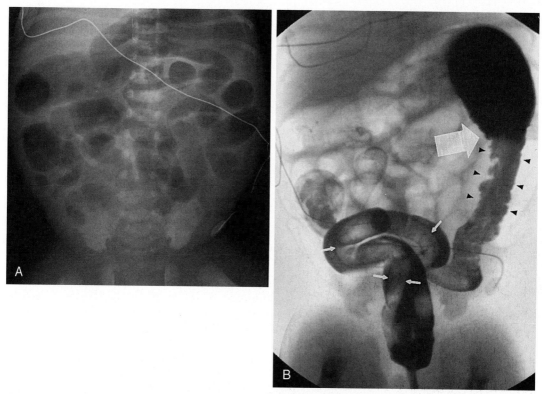

Figure 5–13. Hirschsprung disease in a newborn with abdominal distention and failure to pass meconium. *A*, Radiograph shows dilatation of multiple loops of bowel and no definite colonic gas, findings that are consistent with a distal obstruction. *B*, Contrast enema demonstrates multiple filling defects *(small arrows)* within the colon, which is consistent with meconium plugs. There is a transition zone *(large arrow)* from the dilated proximal colon to the narrower distal colon. The mucosa of the descending colon demonstrates a saw-toothed appearance *(arrowheads)*.

when perforation is present. Serial, water-soluble enemas are often used in an attempt to remove the obstruction nonsurgically. There is much debate regarding the optimal contrast agent to use for such serial therapeutic enemas.

On contrast enemas for neonatal distal obstruction, if the proximal colon is distended and not a microcolon, the cause of distal obstruction is likely colonic, secondary to Hirschsprung disease or meconium plug syndrome.

Hirschsprung Disease

Hirschsprung disease is related to the absence of the ganglion cells that innervate the colon. The deinnervated colon spasms and causes a functional obstruction. Therefore, the affected portions of colon are small in caliber, and the more proximal, normally innervated colon is dilated secondary to the obstruction. The affected colon involves the rectum and a variable

amount of more proximal colon. There are no skip lesions. Most patients with Hirschsprung disease present in the neonatal period with failure to pass meconium (see Fig. 5–13). However, patients can present later in life with problems related to constipation. Hirschsprung disease is much more common in boys than in girls and is associated with Down syndrome in 5% of cases.

When enema series are being performed to evaluate for possible Hirshsprung disease, it is essential to obtain early filling views, collimated to include the rectum and sigmoid colon, in both the lateral and the frontal positions. Findings of Hirschsprung disease include a transition zone from an abnormally small rectum and distal colon to a dilated, normally innervated proximal colon (see Fig. 5–13). In a normal patient, the rectum will have the largest luminal diameter of the left-sided colon. When the rectum alone is involved by Hirschsprung disease, the sigmoid colon will be larger than the rectum (Fig. 5–

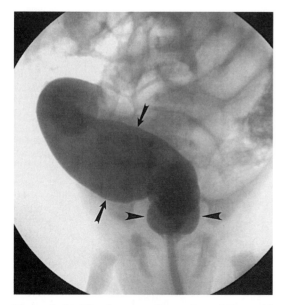

Figure 5–14. Hirschsprung disease in an infant with constipation. Frontal image demonstrates that the diameter of the rectum *(arrowheads)* is smaller than the diameter of the sigmoid colon *(arrows)*, which is an abnormal rectosigmoid ratio.

14). This is referred to as an *abnormal rectosigmoid ratio.* Other less common findings include fasciculations or saw-toothed irregularity of the deinnervated segment (see Fig. 5–13). If the entire colon is involved by Hirschsprung disease, it may appear small in caliber and may mimic a microcolon. Patients with Hirschsprung disease may present with associated colitis. Therefore, in patients who are suspected to have Hirschsprung disease and are ill, contrast enemas should be avoided.

Definitive diagnosis is obtained by rectal biopsy, and patients are treated by surgical resection of the deinnervated segment.

Meconium Plug Syndrome

Meconium plug syndrome, also referred to as *functional immaturity of the colon* or *small left colon syndrome,* is a common cause of distal neonatal obstruction. It is the most frequently encountered diagnosis in neonates who fail to pass meconium. It is thought to be related to functional immaturity of the ganglion cells. As with Hirschsprung disease, the distal colon does not have normal motility, and a functional obstruction results. Unlike Hirschsprung disease, it is a temporary phenomenon and resolves. Although most neonates with me-

conium plug syndrome are otherwise normal and have no abnormal associations, there is an increased incidence in patients who are infants of diabetic mothers or mothers who receive magnesium sulfate for eclampsia. In neonates with meconium plug syndrome, there is always the concern of underlying Hischsprung disease, and at many centers, all neonates who have findings of meconium plug syndrome undergo a rectal biopsy. In contrast to meconium ileus, there is not a significant relationship between meconium plug syndrome and cystic fibrosis.

Infants with meconium plug syndrome present with failure to pass meconium. On contrast enemas, multiple filling defects (meconium plugs) (Fig. 5–15) are seen within the colon. There is not a microcolon. The ascending and transverse colon may be more dilated than the descending colon (small left colon syndrome) (see Fig. 5–15), although these findings are variable. The rectum tends to be normal in luminal diameter, as compared with infants with Hirschsprung disease. During or shortly after the enema, plugs of meconium are often passed. The enema is

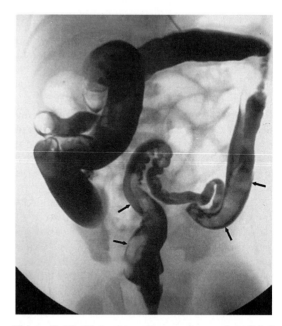

Figure 5–15. Meconium plug syndrome (small left colon syndrome) in a newborn infant born of a diabetic mother. Contrast enema demonstrates multiple filling defects *(arrows)* within the colon, which is consistent with meconium plugs. The left colon is small in caliber. Rectal biopsy, performed to exclude Hirschsprung disease, demonstrated normal ganglion cells.

often therapeutic, with symptoms of obstruction often resolving within hours after enema administration.

Esophageal Atresia and Tracheoesophageal Fistula

With esophageal atresia, the esophagus is atretic for a variable length, usually at the junction of the proximal and middle thirds of the esophagus. Esophageal atresia can occur in the presence or absence of a tracheoesophageal fistula. The most common type is that of esophageal atresia with a fistulous communication between the distal esophageal segment and the trachea. Much less commonly, the fistula can connect the proximal, or both the proximal and distal esophageal segments, to the trachea. In addition, rarely, tracheoesophageal fistulas can occur in the absence of esophageal atresia, the so-called H-type fistula.

Esophageal atresia presents at birth and is usually encountered by the radiologist after there is failure to pass an orogastric tube. Radiographic findings include a distended air-filled pharyngeal pouch, with or without an indwelling tube. If there is no abdominal bowel gas, there is no associated tracheoesophageal fistula, and if there is distal bowel gas,

there is probably a distal fistula (see Fig. 5–4). Further imaging, such as a UGI series, is rarely needed. Because the surgery for esophageal atresia is performed through a thoracotomy contralateral to the aortic arch, it is important to determine the side of the arch. Often, echocardiography is used.

Esophageal atresia is associated with other congenital anomalies. The acronym VACTERL is used: *v*ertebral anomalies, *a*nal atresia, *c*ardiac anomalies, *t*racheoesophageal fistula, *re*nal anomalies, and *l*imb (radial array) anomalies. Chest radiographs in such patients should be scrutinized for vertebral or cardiac anomalies.

Children with an H-type fistula present with coughing or choking during feeding or with recurrent pneumonia. Often a UGI series is requested to exclude an H-type fistula. Some authors advocate that such examination be performed prone with a tube positioned in the esophagus to fully distend the esophagus and maximize potential visualization of the fistula. Others state that this offers no advantage over routine oral administration of contrast via a bottle.

Complications after repair of esophageal atresia include recurrent fistula and esophageal leak during the immediate postoperative period (Fig. 5–16). A large extrapleural fluid

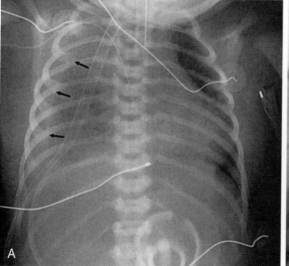 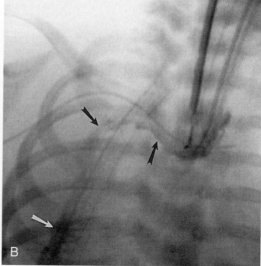

Figure 5–16. Leaking from anastomotic site after repair of esophageal atresia from an extrapleural approach in a 10-day-old boy. *A*, Radiograph 2 days after surgery shows extrapleural effusion *(arrows)* and adjacent extrapleural drains. *B*, Water-soluble contrast injection of the esophagus shows extraluminal extravasation of contrast *(arrows)* in communication with extrapleural space along drainage catheters. (From Donnelly LF, Frush DP, Bisset GS III. The appearance and significance of extrapleural fluid after esophageal atresia repair. AJR Am J Roentgenol 1999;172:231–233.)

collection seen on chest radiographs is highly suggestive of a leak. Long-term problems include esophageal stricture, esophageal dysmotility, and gastroesophageal reflux.

Abnormalities of the Anterior Abdominal Wall

The closure of the anterior abdominal wall occurs during fetal life, and failure of proper closure may result in a number of abnormalities, the most common of which are omphalocele, gastroschisis, and cloacal exstrophy. Omphalocele results from failure of fusion of the lateral folds. It is a midline defect in which the herniated abdominal contents (bowel or liver, or both) are covered by a sac of peritoneum (Fig. 5–17). Up to two thirds of patients with omphalocele have associated congenital anomalies, most commonly cardiac anomalies. In contrast, the defect in gastroschisis is lateral to midline, typically there are no associated abnormalities, and the herniated content (usually just bowel) is not covered by a membrane. The lack of a covering membrane in gastroschisis exposes the bowel to the amniotic fluid, and this is toxic to the bowel. These patients often have severe dysmotility problems and often present with multiple episodes of pseudoobstruction. Cloacal exstrophy is a

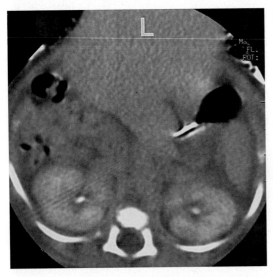

Figure 5–17. Omphalocele demonstrated on computed tomography (CT) (obtained for other reasons) in an 8-day-old boy. CT shows midline abdominal defect, with the liver (L) in an external position.

severe malformation in which there is bladder exstrophy, omphalocele, and epispadias. There is associated diastasis of the pubic bones and spinal dysraphism.

VOMITING INFANT

The referral of an infant for a UGI series to "rule out reflux" is a common event. Typically, such infants are referred to radiology because of excessive "spitting up" or vomiting. There are a number of significant causes for excessive vomiting in infants, including hypertrophic pyloric stenosis, gastroesophageal reflux, congenital stenosis, lactobeazor, and possibly midgut volvulus. The problem for pediatricians is that spitting up (regurgitation) after feedings is a common, normal event. The degree of such spitting up is also variable. I often tell the parents of patients the story of my two children. If you look back through our family photo albums, there are no pictures of my first-born daughter when she was younger than 1 year in which she is not wearing a bib. This is because she spit up constantly and excessively. My wife and I did not think much of it at the time, and it eventually resolved. My second-born son never spit up and does not have a bib on in any photographs. Both children are now relatively normal. How do pediatricians differentiate prominent but normal regurgitation from vomiting secondary to obstruction or pathologic amounts of gastroesophageal reflux? Associated problems such as failure to gain weight, failure to thrive, or respiratory symptoms suggest pathology. This difficult question often results in the performance of a UGI series. Although such UGI studies are often ordered to "rule out reflux," they are actually performed to exclude an anatomic reason for excessive reflux, rather than to exclude reflux itself. Although it is appropriate to document the presence and anatomic extent of gastroesophageal reflux when it occurs, it is not necessary to do maneuvers to provoke reflux. A UGI series in an infant can be performed in a manner similar to the technique previously described for neonates.

HYPERTROPHIC PYLORIC STENOSIS

Hypertrophic pyloric stenosis is a common, idiopathic thickening of the muscle of the pylorus that results in a progressive gastric outlet obstruction. It usually occurs in otherwise healthy infants (1 week to 3 months) who typically present with projectile, bile-free emesis. It is much more common in males (5:1 ratio). On physical examination, the hypertrophied pylorus can be palpated as an olive-sized mass in the right upper quadrant. It is suggested that palpation of an "olive" with the appropriate clinical symptoms is diagnostic and that such infants do not need confirmatory imaging studies. However, in my experience as a pediatric radiologist, I do not know of a single child who has gone to the operating room without some type of imaging study. It should be noted that imaging to confirm or exclude hypertrophic pyloric stenosis is not a medical emergency, and in the middle of the night such a request can usually wait.

On radiographs, children with hypertrophic pyloric stenosis may show gastric distention, peristaltic waves (caterpillar sign), and mottled retained gastric contents. There is continuous debate as to which is the best test to perform in the child suspected of having hypertrophic pyloric stenosis: ultrasonography or a UGI series. There are advocates for both. Ultrasonography directly visualizes the pyloric muscle and does not use radiation but does not typically exclude other diagnoses such as midgut volvulus. A UGI series excludes other, more serious causes of pathology, but the findings of a UGI series infer rather than directly visualize the hypertrophied muscle. The following guidelines may be helpful in making such decisions. If hypertrophic pyloric stenosis is highly suspected on clinical grounds and the purpose of the study is to confirm the diagnosis, I start with ultrasonography. If the symptoms or patient age are not classic, a UGI series may be better to both evaluate for hypertrophic pyloric stenosis and exclude other pathologic conditions.

On ultrasonography, the diagnosis of hypertrophic pyloric stenosis is often obvious and is made on gestalt appearance (Fig. 5–18). The pylorus is located near the gallbladder, so an easy technique is to find the gallbladder and turn obliquely sagittal to the body in an attempt to visualize the pylorus longitudinally. The hypertrophied muscle is hypoechoic, and the central mucosa is hyperechoic (see Fig. 5–18). The pylorus is not seen to open during real-time evaluation. There are measurement criteria that vary slightly from source to

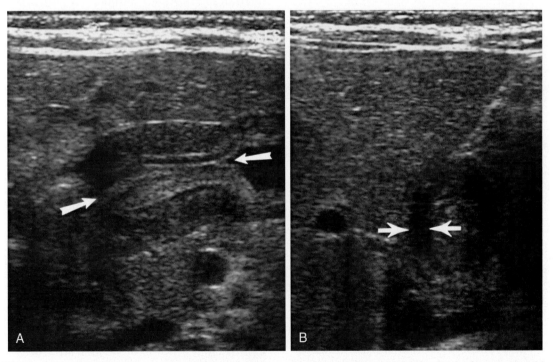

Figure 5–18. Hypertrophic pyloric stenosis seen on ultrasonography. *A*, Longitudinal ultrasonographic image demonstrating findings of hypertrophic pyloric stenosis. The hypertrophied pyloric muscle is hypoechoic, and the mucosa is echogenic. The length of the pylorus *(arrows)* is 20 mm. *B*, Transverse ultrasonographic image shows pyloric thickness *(arrows)* to be 5 mm.

source. The pyloric muscle thickness (diameter of a single muscular wall on a transverse image) should normally be less than 3 mm (Fig. 5–19). The length (longitudinal diameter) should not exceed 15 mm. Another good rule of thumb is that if an inexperienced ultrasonographer or resident scans the child and easily finds the pylorus, it is probably abnormal. A normal pylorus is much harder to image than an abnormal pylorus.

On the UGI series, there is delayed gastric emptying. When some contrast does pass into the duodenum, the pylorus appears elongated with a narrow pyloric channel (string sign). The lumen may be puckered into more than one apparent lumen (double-track sign). The pylorus indents the contrast-filled antrum (shoulder sign) or base of the duodenal bulb (mushroom sign), and the entrance to the pylorus may be beak-shaped (beak sign) (Fig. 5–20). After the diagnosis is made, excess barium should be removed from the stomach by nasogastric tube to avoid the risk of aspiration.

INTESTINAL OBSTRUCTION IN CHILDREN

As in adults, the key finding of bowel obstruction on radiography is the presence of dispro-

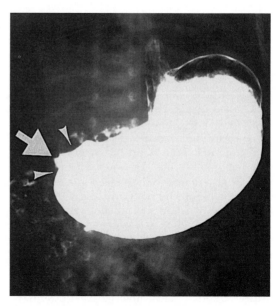

Figure 5–20. Hypertrophic pyloric stenosis on an upper gastrointestinal view. Image shows distention of the stomach and delayed gastric emptying. The entrance of the pylorus *(arrow)* has a beak-like configuration, with shoulder-type impressions of the pylorus on the antral walls *(arrowheads)*.

portionately dilated proximal small bowel compared with a less dilated, more distal small bowel or colon. In contrast to adults, however, it may be difficult to differentiate small bowel from colon in infants and small children, because of a lack of well-defined haustra and valvulae conniventes. The addition of a prone view to the standard two-view abdominal series (supine and upright, cross-table lateral, or left decubitus) can be helpful when differentiation of small from large bowel is difficult. On the prone view, gas moves into the more posterior structures of the colon—the ascending and descending colon and rectum. On supine views, the colonic gas lies in the more anterior structures—the transverse and sigmoid colon. The position of gas on the combination of these two views is often helpful in identifying gas to be in the colon rather than in dilated small bowel. Demonstration of the presence or absence of gas in the ascending colon can be of particular help when evaluating for potential ileocolic intussusception.

The most common causes of bowel obstruction in children beyond infancy are listed in Table 5–2. The pneumonic "take AAIIMM" against small bowel obstruction, championed by Donald R. Kirks, M.D., is helpful in recalling this list when under pressure. Each letter

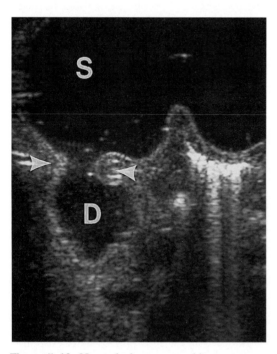

Figure 5–19. Normal ultrasonographic appearance of the pylorus. The pylorus *(arrowheads)* is open connecting the stomach (S) and duodenum (D) and is only 5 mm in length.

TABLE 5–2. **Common Causes of Intestinal Obstruction in Older Children: Take AAIIMM**

Adhesions
Appendicitis
Intussusception
Incarcerated inguinal hernia
Malrotation with volvulus
Meckel diverticulum

in AIM represents two diagnoses. Appendicitis, intussusception, and Meckel diverticulum are discussed in more detail in the following sections.

Appendicitis

Appendicitis is the most common reason for abdominal surgery in children. Obstruction of the appendiceal lumen results in distention of the appendix, superimposed infection, ischemia, and eventually perforation. In older children with nonperforated appendicitis, the classic symptoms include pain that begins in the periumbilical region and migrates to the right lower quadrant, tenderness over the McBurney point, and a combination of anorexia, nausea, vomiting, diarrhea, and fever. Patients with classic symptoms are typically taken to the operating room with outimaging. However, the clinical presentation is nonspecific in up to one third of patients. This is particularly true in young patients whose diagnosis is often delayed and who have a higher rate of perforation. It is in these patients with nonspecific presentations in whom imaging plays a role. The goals of imaging include decreasing the rate of negative results on laparotomy, increasing the rapidity of diagnosis to reduce the rate of perforation, and to identify alternative diagnoses.

Radiographs demonstrate an appendicolith in 5 to 10% of patients (Fig. 5–21). Other findings may include air-fluid levels within the right lower quadrant, splinting, and loss of the psoas margin. With perforated appendicitis, there may be findings of small bowel obstruction, right lower quadrant extraluminal gas, and displacement of bowel loops from the right lower quadrant (see Fig. 5–21). Free intraperitoneal gas is extremely uncommon secondary to appendicitis.

There is much debate over appropriate imaging algorithms for suspected appendicitis. Some advocate ultrasonography as the primary diagnostic test and others advocate CT. Some have advocated primary use of ultrasonography, with CT performed in questionable cases. Others claim that the low negative predictive value of a negative ultrasonographic examination renders ultrasonography essentially useless in the diagnosis of appendicitis. There is also debate over the technical factors on how to perform CT: intravenous contrast, oral contrast, rectal contrast, or noncontrast studies. Imaging algorithms for appendicitis will continue to vary among institutions. However, several factors may be helpful in making such decisions. Ultrasonography is much more useful in patients of thin body habitus and in girls than in fat individuals and in boys. In girls—in whom ovarian causes of right lower quadrant pain such as hemorrhage, cyst, or torsion are not uncommon, ultrasonography may be the first test of choice. Features that may favor the use of CT include cases in which perforated appendicitis is highly suspected, evaluation for abscess, postoperative evaluation, and obesity.

The technique for ultrasonographic evaluation of appendicitis is graded compression of the right lower quadrant using a high-frequency transducer. Findings include a shadowing, echogenic appendicolith (Fig. 5–22), a noncompressible blind-ending tubular structure that measures greater than 6 mm in diam-

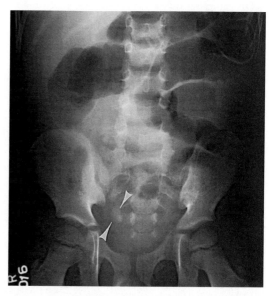

Figure 5–21. Perforated appendicitis in an 8-year-old girl. Radiography shows appendicolith *(arrowheads)*, displacement of bowel loops out of right lower quadrant, and findings of small bowel obstruction.

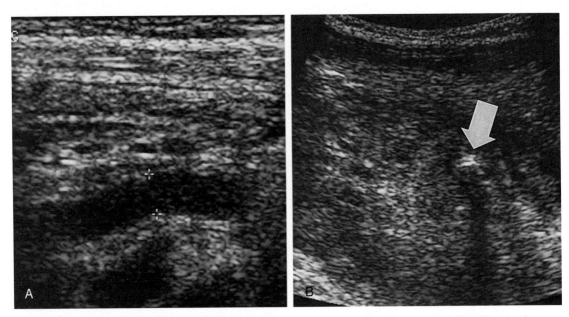

Figure 5–22. Nonperforated appendicitis demonstrated by ultrasonography. *A,* Longitudinal image demonstrates noncompressible, blind-ending tube that measures 8 mm in diameter. *B,* Image at base of appendix shows shadowing, echogenic appendicolith *(arrow).*

eter (see Fig. 5–22), or right lower quadrant fluid, phlegmon, or abscess. Computed tomographic findings include identification of an appendicolith, a distended appendix, periappendiceal soft tissue stranding (Fig. 5–23), and wall thickening of the cecum or terminal ileum. In perforated appendicitis, findings of small bowel obstruction may be present, and inflammatory fluid collections may be seen in

the right lower quadrant (Fig. 5–24) or in the pelvic cul-de-sac.

Intussusception

Intussusception occurs when forward peristalsis results in invagination of the more proximal bowel (the intussusceptum) into the lumen of the more distal bowel (the intussus-

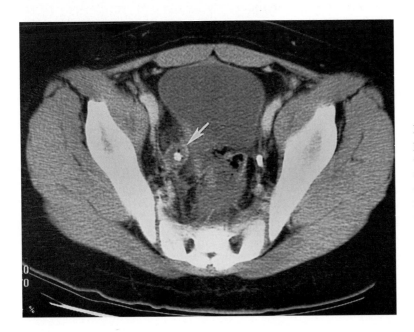

Figure 5–23. Nonperforated appendicitis on CT in a 13-year-old boy. CT shows a distended appendix *(arrow)* containing a calcified appendicolith. There is soft tissue stranding in the periappendiceal fat.

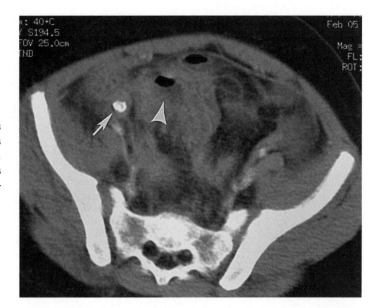

Figure 5–24. Perforated appendicitis on CT in a 7-year-old boy. CT shows a calcified appendicolith *(arrow)* in the right lower quadrant. There is an adjacent inflammatory fluid collection *(arrowhead)* and phlegmon.

cipiens) in a telescope-like manner. Intussusception is ileocolic in more than 90% of cases. The other cases are typically ileum-ileum or ileo-ileocolic. Intussusception can be divided into two categories: idiopathic and pathologic. The pathologic variety occurs secondary to a pathologic lead point and accounts for approximately 10% of cases. Lead points include the Meckel diverticulum, lymphoma, inspissated feces (cystic fibrosis), or bowel wall hemorrhage (Henoch-Schönlein purpura). The age of presentation is related to the cause of the lead point.

In children, most (90%) of cases of intussusception are idiopathic. They are thought to be related to lymphoid hypertrophy in the terminal ileum secondary to viral disease. Most of these cases are ileocolic intussusception. It is more common during the winter and spring months, when more viral illness occurs, and occurs more commonly in girls than in boys. The typical age for presentation is between 3 months and 1 year, with almost all cases of idiopathic intussusception occurring before 3 years of age. Presenting symptoms include crampy abdominal pain, bloody (currant jelly) stools, vomiting, or a palpable right-sided abdominal mass.

Radiographs are rarely completely normal in cases of intussusception. Findings include a paucity of gas within the right abdomen, nonvisualization of an air-filled cecum or ascending colon, the meniscus of a soft tissue mass typically within the ascending colon or hepatic flexure, and small bowel obstruction

(Fig. 5–25). Because the key to identifying or excluding the diagnosis is related to seeing or not seeing gas in the ascending colon, left side–down decubitus and prone–positioned radiographs are helpful. If air-fluid levels are identified within the distal colon, intussusception is unlikely, and viral gastroenteritis is the more likely cause of the patient's symptoms. Ultrasonography has also been advocated as useful in confirming and excluding the presence of ileocolic intussusception. On ultrasonography, the intussusception appears as a mass with alternating rings of hyper- and hypoechogenicity (Fig. 5–26). In the transverse plane, the mass has been likened to a donut, and in the longitudinal plane it has been said to resemble a pseudokidney. When encountered on CT, ileocolic intussusception appears as a mass in the cecum or ascending colon, with alternating rings of low and high attenuation (see Fig. 5–26).

Imaging-Guided Reduction of Intussusception

There are several methods of increasing the pressure within the colon in an attempt to invert the intussusception into a normal position using imaging guidance. They include air insufflation with fluoroscopic guidance, contrast enema with fluoroscopic guidance, and hydrostatic reduction with ultrasonographic guidance. Such methods are the primary therapy for intussusception, with surgery reserved for cases in which imaging-guided reduction

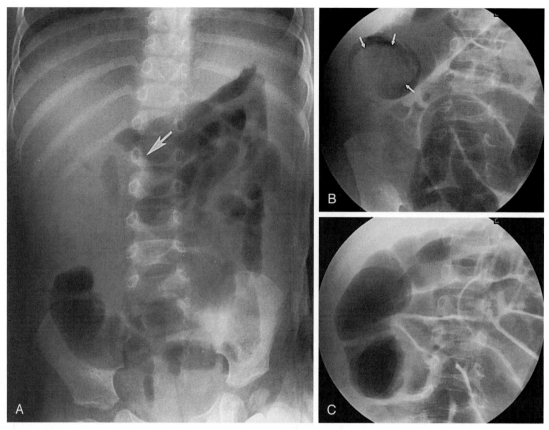

Figure 5–25. Intussusception in a 10-month-old child with crampy abdominal pain and bloody stools. *A,* Radiograph obtained with the patient in the left lateral decubitus position demonstrates nonvisualization of gas within the ascending colon or cecum and a soft tissue meniscus *(arrow)* overlying the hepatic flexure, suggesting a mass. *B,* Fluoroscopic image obtained during air enema procedure demonstrates soft tissue mass *(arrows)* in descending colon. *C,* Fluoroscopic image obtained after reduction of the intussusception demonstrates resolution of the soft tissue mass and reflux of air into the small bowel.

fails. Which method is used varies among institutions. At my institution, air reduction is used. This will be described here.

Contraindications for attempting pressure reduction of an intussusception include peritonitis on physical examination or pneumoperitoneum on radiography. The following guidelines use used for preparing a patient for attempted reduction: adequate hydration with intravenous fluids if needed, a working intravenous (IV) line, abdominal examination by an experienced physician, and consultation with the pediatric surgery service. The surgery service must at least know that the reduction is going to be attempted, and someone from the service preferably should have examined the patient. For air reduction, the patient is immobilized and a Shiels intussusception air reduction system (Custom Medical Products, Mainville, OH) is used. A key to success is generating an adequate rectal seal so that ade-

quate colonic pressures can be obtained without leakage of air from the rectum. Pressure generated within the colon should not exceed 120 mm Hg. With air insufflation, the intussusception is encountered as a mass. The reducing intussusception moves retrograde to the level of the ileocecal valve. Criteria for successful reduction include resolution of the soft tissue mass and free reflux of gas into the small bowel (see Fig. 5–25). Success rates are approximately 80 to 90%. The risk of perforation is less than 0.5%. The risk of recurrent intussusception is 5 to 10%, with most occurring within the first 72 hours after the reduction.

Meckel Diverticulum

The omphalomesenteric duct is a fetal structure that connects the umbilical cord to the

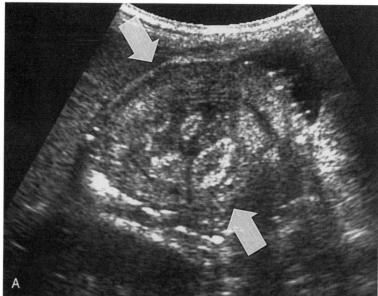

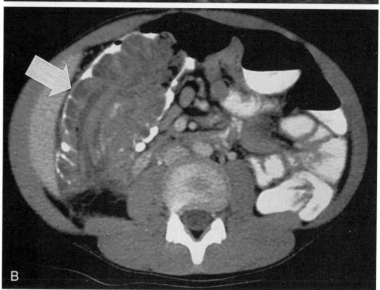

Figure 5–26. Appearance of intussusception on ultrasonography and CT. *A*, Ultrasonography shows mass *(arrows)* of alternating hyperechogenic and hypoechogenic rings. *B*, CT shows mass *(arrow)* within the hepatic flexure of colon. It is surrounded by intraluminal enteric contrast. The mass demonstrates alternating rings of variable density.

portion of the gut that becomes the ileum. Any or all of the structure can persist abnormally into postnatal life, resulting in cysts, sinuses, or fistulas from umbilicus to ileum. Most commonly, the portion adjacent to the ileal end persists and results in a *Meckel diverticulum,* which can cause symptoms secondary to bleeding, focal inflammation, perforation, or intussusception. Bleeding is the most common complication and occurs secondary to the presence of ectopic gastric mucosa. Although most Meckel diverticula do not contain gastric mucosa, almost all of those associated with bleeding do. The imaging modality of choice to detect Meckel diverticulum is nuclear scin-

tigraphy with pertechnetate 99m, which accumulates in gastric mucosa. Such studies demonstrate a foci of increased activity within the right lower quadrant of the abdomen (Fig. 5–27). Meckel diverticula are difficult to visualize on other studies such as CT or small bowel follow-through.

Gastrointestinal Duplication Cysts

Gastrointestinal duplication cysts are congenital lesions that are typically round, attached to the gastrointestinal tract, and do not communicate with the gastrointestinal lumen. The

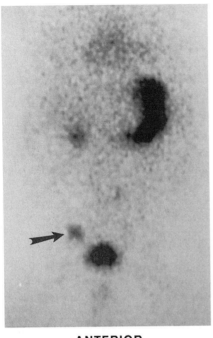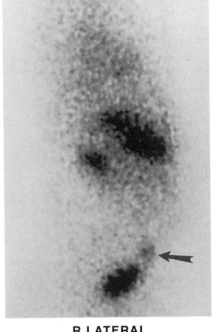

ANTERIOR   **30 MIN**   **R LATERAL**

Figure 5–27. Meckel diverticulum shown on pertechnetate 99m images. Anterior and right lateral views demonstrate abnormal increased activity *(arrows)* within the anterior right lower quadrant. There is normal activity seen within the stomach, right kidney, and bladder.

most common locations are the terminal ileum and distal esophagus. Presentation can be related to a palpable mass, compression of adjacent anatomic structures, bowel obstruction, or ulceration and perforation. Most present during the first year of life. Duplication cysts have a typical ultrasonographic appearance: a cystic mass with a "bowel wall signature." The wall of the cyst demonstrates alternating hypoechoic and more hyperechoic layers, which correlate with the mucosal (hyperechoic) and muscular layers (hypoechoic) (Fig. 5–28). Much less commonly, duplications can appear tubular, rather than round, and

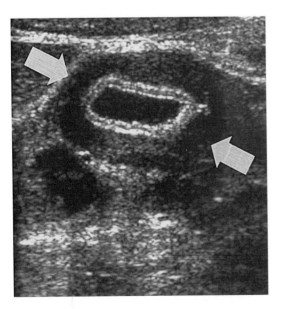

Figure 5–28. Gastric duplication cyst demonstrated on ultrasonography. The structure appears as a cystic lesion *(arrows)* with "bowel wall signature" of alternating hyperechoic and hypoechoic rings.

can communicate with the gastrointestinal lumen.

DISORDERS OF THE PEDIATRIC ESOPHAGUS

Two disorders that may be encountered by radiologists within the esophagi of children include esophageal foreign bodies and esophageal strictures.

The majority of foreign bodies swallowed by children pass through the gastrointestinal tract without complication. If the initial series of radiographs demonstrates that the foreign body lies within the stomach or more distally in the gastrointestinal tract, follow-up films are not indicated unless the child develops obstructive symptoms or peritonitis. However, foreign bodies may lodge within the esophagus. The most common site of esophageal foreign bodies, and also the least likely area from which foreign bodies will spontaneously pass, is the proximal esophagus at the thoracic inlet. Because most infants with esophageal foreign bodies are initially asymptomatic, when ingestions are witnessed, radiographs should be obtained, regardless of whether symptoms are present, to confirm that the object has passed into the stomach. The most common foreign body to lodge in the esophagus is a coin (Fig. 5–29). Such coins may be removed from the esophagus by using a Foley balloon catheter and fluoroscopic guidance (see Fig. 5–29). The catheter is inserted via the nose, and the balloon is blown up in the esophagus beyond the level of the coin. The catheter is pulled retrograde, moving the coin into the oropharynx. Chronic esophageal foreign bodies may result in complications such as tracheoesophageal fistula (Fig. 5–30). They may also cause an inflammatory mass that leads to compression of the trachea. Such foreign bodies may present with respiratory, rather than gastrointestinal, symptoms. Lodged esophageal foreign bodies may also reveal an underlying pathologic condition that caused the foreign body not to pass, such as a stricture (Fig. 5–31) or vascular ring.

Esophageal strictures can occur secondary to a number of causes in children, including ingestion of a corrosive agent, previous esophageal atresia repair (see Fig. 5–31), epidermolysis bullosa, or gastroesophageal reflux. Such strictures are often dilated using balloon catheters and fluoroscopic guidance.

ABNORMALITIES OF THE PEDIATRIC MESENTERY

The mesentery does not have easily recognizable boundaries on imaging. Localization of an abnormality to the mesentery can therefore

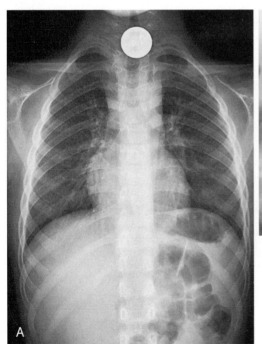

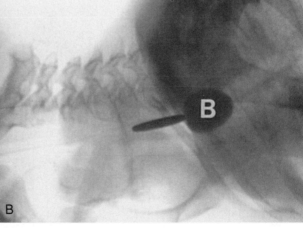

Figure 5–29. Quarter lodged within the esophagus at the thoracic inlet in a 7-year-old boy. *A,* Radiograph shows coin at thoracic inlet. *B,* Fluoroscopic image during Foley catheter removal of the coin demonstrates the contrast-filled balloon (B) distal to the quarter. The catheter is pulled retrograde, moving the coin into the mouth. Removal was successful.

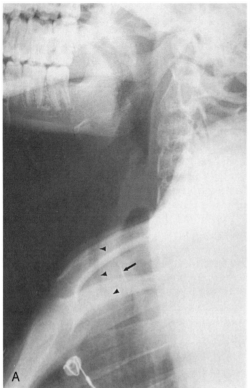

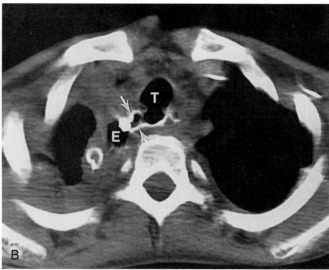

Figure 5–30. Chronic esophageal foreign body resulting in extraluminal migration and tracheoesophageal fistula in a 15-year-old mentally retarded girl. *A*, Radiograph demonstrates marked thickening of the tracheoesophageal interface with compression of the posterior aspect of the trachea *(arrowheads)*. There is a radiopaque liner structure *(arrow)* within the soft tissues consistent with a foreign body. *B*, Computed tomographic scan obtained later after foreign body removal demonstrates contrast that was injected into indwelling esophageal tube to communicate directly between trachea (T) and esophagus (E) through fistula *(arrows)*.

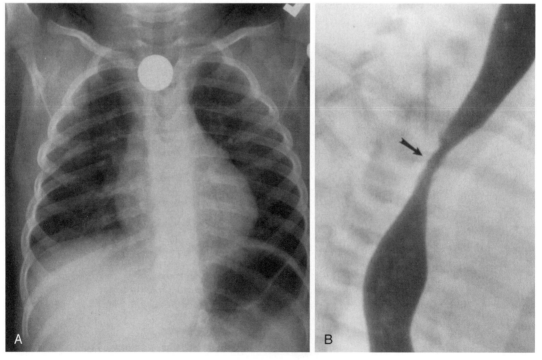

Figure 5–31. Lodged coin unmasking esophageal stricture in a 2-year-old boy with history of previous esophageal atresia repair. *A*, Chest radiograph shows coin lodged in upper esophagus. *B*, Esophagram demonstrates stricture *(arrow)* in region of previous surgery.

be difficult. The relative paucity of mesenteric fat seen in the pediatric population can make detection and localization of processes in the mesentery even more difficult than in adults in whom fat is typically abundant. The following criteria are helpful in localizing a process to the mesentery in children: (1) partial or complete envelopment of the superior mesenteric artery or vein, (2) peripheral displacement of jejunal or ileal bowel loops, or (3) extension of the process from a superocentral to an inferoperipheral position in a cone-like manner. Disorders are divided into the specific patterns of involvement that can readily be identified by imaging: developmental abnormalities of mesenteric rotation, diffuse mesen-

teric processes, focal mesenteric masses, and multifocal mesenteric masses. Abnormalities of mesenteric rotation have previously been discussed.

Processes that can involve the mesentery diffusely include edema, hemorrhage, and inflammation. Characteristic findings of a diffuse mesenteric process include replacement of mesenteric fat with soft tissue attenuation, with resultant loss of vascular definition (Fig. 5–32). Focal masses within the mesentery in the pediatric population can be secondary to lymphoma, mesenteric cysts, desmoid tumors, teratomas, and lipomas. Mesenteric cysts, also known as lymphatic malformations, are developmental anomalies in which focal lymphatic

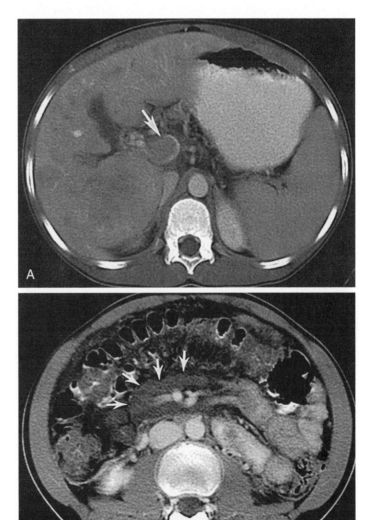

Figure 5–32. Mesenteric edema resulting from portal vein obstruction by tumor thrombus in a 12-year-old boy with hepatocellular carcinoma. *A*, Computed tomographic image shows nearly complete portal vein occlusion by tumor thrombus *(arrow)*. Irregular liver contour with heterogeneous enhancement is due to diffuse, multifocal tumor involvement. *B*, At the level of the mesenteric vessels, increased attenuation within the mesentery *(arrows)* represents edema secondary to portal vein obstruction. The mesenteric location of the edema is determined by the envelopment of the superior mesenteric artery and vein by the edema. (From Zarewych ZM, Donnelly LF, Frush DP, Bisset GS III. Imaging of pediatric mesenteric abnormalities. Pediatr Radiol 1999; 29:711–719.)

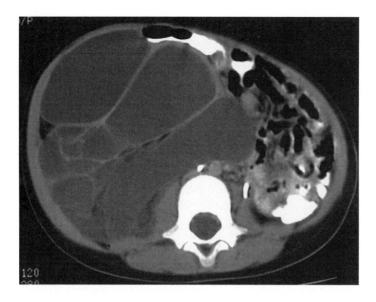

Figure 5–33. Cystic lymphatic malformation in a 3-year-old girl. CT demonstrates a large, multiseptated focal mass displacing bowel loops leftward. (From Zarewych ZM, Donnelly LF, Frush DP, Bisset GS III. Imaging of pediatric mesenteric abnormalities. Pediatr Radiol 1999; 29:711–719.)

channels fail to establish connections with the central lymphatic system. Lymphatic malformations are often multiseptated and quite large (Fig. 5–33).

Multifocal mesenteric masses most commonly represent lymphadenopathy. On imaging studies such as CT, mesenteric lymph nodes are considered abnormal if they are greater than 5 mm in diameter. Mesenteric lymphadenopathy can be a manifestation of either a malignant neoplastic or inflammatory process. Malignant entities include lymphoma, lymphoproliferative disorder, and metastatic disease. Lymphomatous involvement of the mesentery is usually by non-Hodgkin disease and usually involves both the mesentery and retroperitoneum (Fig. 5–34). Most cases of non-Hodgkin lymphoma that involve the abdomen demonstrate lymphadenopathy rather than parenchymal masses. Mesenteric lymphadenopathy can also be due to infectious causes such as tuberculosis, cat scratch disease, or fungal infection. Central low attenuation with peripheral enhancement favors an inflammatory cause over a neoplastic one. This appearance has been described as characteristic of tuberculosis and is present in up to 60% of cases (Fig. 5–35). With tuberculosis, it has

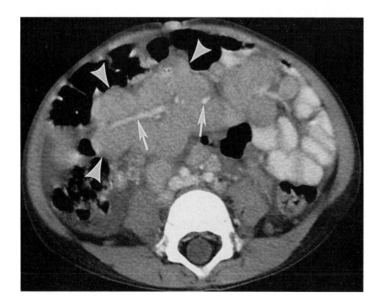

Figure 5–34. Non-Hodgkin lymphoma in a 3-year-old boy. CT shows large, multifocal mesenteric *(arrowheads)* and retroperitoneal adenopathy. Note encasement of mesenteric vessels *(arrows)*. (From Zarewych ZM, Donnelly LF, Frush DP, Bisset GS III. Imaging of pediatric mesenteric abnormalities. Pediatr Radiol 1999; 29:711–719.)

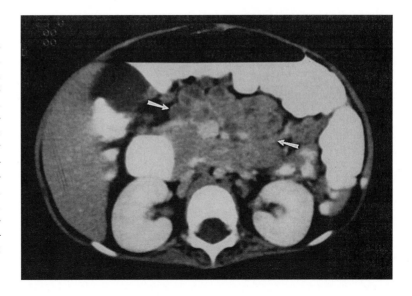

Figure 5–35. Tuberculosis in a 16-year-old girl. Computed tomographic image through the superior mesentery shows a conglomeration of matted lymph nodes *(arrows)* surrounding the mesenteric vessels. There are several areas of central low attenuation, which are characteristic of tuberculous lymphadenopathy. (From Zarewych ZM, Donnelly LF, Frush DP, Bisset GS III. Imaging of pediatric mesenteric abnormalities. Pediatr Radiol 1999;29: 711–719.)

been suggested that the mesenteric adenopathy is often more pronounced relative to the degree of retroperitoneal adenopathy.

Mesenteric Adenitis

Mesenteric adenitis is a clinical entity that is related to benign inflammation of the mesenteric lymph nodes, sometimes associated with enteritis. Patients present with nausea, vomiting, diarrhea, right lower quadrant abdominal pain and tenderness, fever, and leukocytosis. Because of the marked overlap in clinical symptoms, differentiation between appendicitis and mesenteric adenitis can be extremely difficult, if not impossible, on a clinical basis. The diagnosis is often made at laparotomy and nontherapeutic appendectomy. On CT, there is enlarged and clustered lymphadenopathy in the bowel mesenteries, just anterior to the right psoas muscle (78% of cases) and in the small bowel mesentery (56% of cases) (Fig. 5–36). There may also be associated ileal wall thickening (33% of cases) or inflammatory changes in the mesentery (see Fig. 5–36). The presence of diffuse mesenteric lymph nodes and absence of findings of appendicitis suggest mesenteric adenitis as the cause of right lower quadrant pain.

NEONATAL JAUNDICE

Some degree of "physiologic jaundice" or hyperbilirubinemia is common in neonates and is related to physiologic destruction of red blood cells in the polycythemic newborn. Jaundice that persists beyond 4 weeks of age is due to biliary atresia or neonatal hepatitis in 90% of cases.

Biliary Atresia Versus Neonatal Hepatitis

It is important to identify children with biliary atresia. These infants benefit from early surgical intervention (before 3 months of age). In contradistinction, it is essential to avoid unnecessary laparotomies in patients with neonatal hepatitis. Because the two entities have similar clinical, laboratory, and pathologic findings, diagnostic imaging plays an important role in differentiating these two entities. In biliary atresia, there is congenital obstruction of the biliary system, with bile duct proliferation intrahepatically and focal or total absence of the extrahepatic bile ducts. Cirrhosis ultimately develops unless there is corrective surgery. There is an association with the abdominal heterotaxia syndromes, such as polysplenia, and with trisomy 18.

Ultrasonography is also the initial imaging procedure in neonates with jaundice. It can exclude the presence of choledocal cysts or dilatation of the bile duct system from other causes of obstruction. Absence of a visualized gallbladder is suggestive of biliary atresia. However, 20% of patients with biliary atresia have a small or, rarely, normal gallbladder. The finding of a normal or enlarged gallbladder is supportive of the diagnosis of neonatal hepatitis. The hepatic parenchyma and intrahepatic

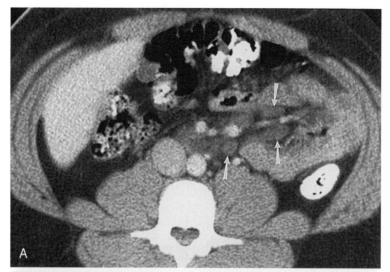

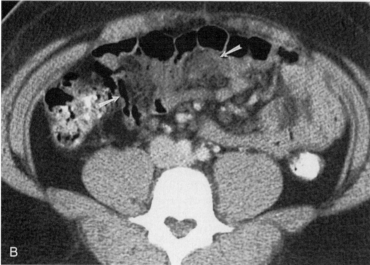

Figure 5–36. Mesenteric adenitis in a 16-year-old boy with right lower quadrant pain. *A,* CT shows multiple lymph nodes in the mesentery *(arrows)* adjacent to the mesenteric vessels and centrally located in relationship to adjacent bowel. *B,* More inferior computed tomographic image shows soft tissue stranding *(arrows)* within the mesenteric fat as well as more lymphadenopathy. (From Zarewych ZM, Donnelly LF, Frush DP, Bisset GS III. Imaging of pediatric mesenteric abnormalities. Pediatr Radiol 1999;29:711–719.)

bile ducts usually appear normal in patients with neonatal hepatitis and in those with biliary atresia. Hepatobiliary scintigraphy with technetium 99m iminodiacetate (IDA) derivatives can be one of the most reliable ways to differentiate between neonatal hepatitis and biliary atresia. The radiopharmaceutical agent is usually administered after pretreatment with oral phenobarbital. Normally, radiopharmaceutical uptake and clearance by hepatocytes exceeds cardiac blood pool tracer activity and radiotracer is normally visualized within the biliary tree and intestines by 15 minutes after administration. The classically described scintigraphic appearance of neonatal hepatitis includes delayed uptake of radiotracer by hepatic sites, slow clearance of blood pool radiotracer, but eventual radiotracer excretion into the intestines. In biliary atresia, radiotracer uptake and clearance by hepatocytes are

adequate, with prominent low activity identified but tracer never reaches the GI tract, even on 24-hour delayed imaging (Fig. 5–37).

Choledocal Cyst

Choledocal cyst is defined as a local dilatation of the biliary duct system and is categorized into types based on anatomic distribution of dilatation. Types include localized dilatation of the common bile duct below the cystic duct, dilatation of the common bile and hepatic ducts, localized cystic diverticula of the common bile duct, dilatation of the distal intramedullary portion of the common bile duct (choledococele), and multiple cystic dilatations involving both the intra- and extrahepatic bile duct radicals (Caroli disease). Choledocal cysts are uncommon and the cause is unknown. Choledocal cysts most commonly

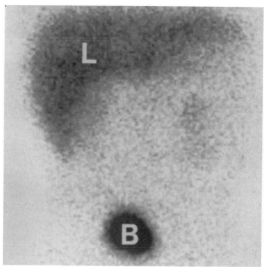

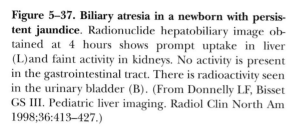

Figure 5–37. Biliary atresia in a newborn with persistent jaundice. Radionuclide hepatobiliary image obtained at 4 hours shows prompt uptake in liver (L)and faint activity in kidneys. No activity is present in the gastrointestinal tract. There is radioactivity seen in the urinary bladder (B). (From Donnelly LF, Bisset GS III. Pediatric liver imaging. Radiol Clin North Am 1998;36:413–427.)

present early in life. Presenting symptoms include jaundice (80%), an abdominal mass (50%), or abdominal pain (50%). Ultrasonography demonstrates a cystic mass in the region of the porta hepatis that is separate from an identifiable gallbladder (Fig. 5–38). The presence of a dilated common bile duct or cystic duct or visualization of the hepatic duct directly emptying into the cystic mass confirms the diagnosis. When there is a nonspecific cyst within the region of the porta hepatis, hepato-

biliary scintigraphy can be used to demonstrate radiotracer accumulation within the cyst, confirming the diagnosis (see Fig. 5–38).

LIVER MASSES

Hepatic masses constitute only 5 to 6% of all intraabdominal masses in children, and primary hepatic neoplasms constitute only 0.5 to 2% of all pediatric malignancies. Primary hepatic neoplasms are the third most common

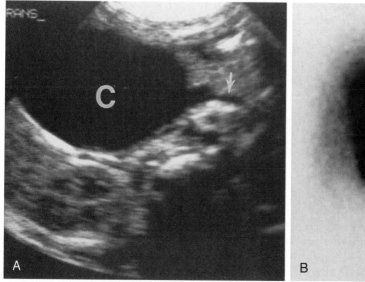

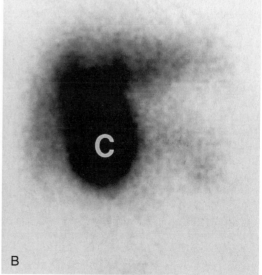

Figure 5–38. Choledochal cyst in an infant girl with jaundice and a palpable right upper quadrant mass. *A,* Transverse ultrasonogram shows large cystic structure (C) in region of the porta hepatis. Medially, the cyst appears to connect with the common bile duct *(arrow). B,* Radionuclide hepatobiliary scan shows radioactivity accumulating in cyst *(arrow),* confirming the diagnosis. (From Donnelly LF, Bisset GS III. Pediatric liver imaging. Radiol Clin North Am 1998;36:413–427.)

abdominal malignancy in childhood, after Wilms tumor and neuroblastoma, and are by far the most common primary malignancy of the GI tract.

Most children with benign or malignant liver masses present with a palpable mass on physical examination. Other presenting symptoms include pain, anorexia, jaundice, paraneoplastic syndromes, hemorrhage, or congestive heart failure. Although it is often obvious that these children have an upper abdominal mass, the organ of origin often is not clear without imaging. Whether CT or magnetic resonance imaging (MRI) is the modality of choice for definitive imaging of liver masses is a controversial issue. There are no pathognomonic imaging features for hepatic malignancies. The major role of imaging is to define the extent of the lesion accurately in relation to hepatic lobar anatomy and vascular and biliary structures for preoperative planning and to monitor tumor response to chemotherapy or radiation therapy. For most hepatic malignancies, complete tumor resection or liver transplantation is essential for cure. The types of liver resection performed include left lobectomy, left lateral segmentectomy, right lobectomy, or trisegmentectomy (right lobe and medial segment of the left lobe). Therefore, a mass must be confined to the left or right lobe or the right lobe plus the medial segment of the left lobe to be considered resectable. If a lesion does not meet anatomic requirements for resectability at initial imaging, the child is often treated initially with chemotherapy, with or without radiation, and then reimaged.

The differential diagnosis for liver masses in children includes benign and malignant neoplasms such as hepatoblastoma, hemangioendothelioma, mesenchymal hamartoma, hepatocellular carcinoma, hemangiomas, lymphoproliferative disorder, lymphoma, hepatic adenomas, metastatic disease, and uncommon sarcomas such as undifferentiated embryonal sarcoma and angiosarcoma. Nonneoplastic causes of liver masses include abscesses (fungal, bacterial, or granulomatous) and hematoma. Several factors help focus the differential diagnosis: the age of the child, presentation, alpha-fetoprotein level, and whether the lesion is solitary or multiple (Table 5–3). The differential diagnosis of liver tumors is different in younger than in older children. The most common hepatic tumors in children less than 5 years include hepatoblastoma, hemangioendothelioma, mesenchymal hamartoma, and metastatic disease from neuroblastoma or Wilms tumor. In chil-

TABLE 5–3. **Causes of Pediatric Hepatic Masses**

Age less than 5 years

Hepatoblastoma (+ AFP)
Hemangioendothelioma
Mesenchymal hamartoma
Metastatic disease (Wilms, neuroblastoma)

Age greater than 5 years

Hepatocellular carcinoma (+ AFP)
Undifferentiated embryonal sarcoma
Hepatic adenoma
Metastatic disease
Lymphoma

Immunocompromised

Lymphoproliferative disorder
Fungal infection

dren older than 5 years, the preceding lesions are uncommon, and the most common tumors include hepatocellular carcinoma (see Fig. 5–32), undifferentiated sarcoma, hepatic adenoma, and metastatic disease. Liver tumors that are associated with an elevated serum alpha-fetoprotein level include hepatoblastoma and hepatocellular carcinoma. Hemangioendothelioma can have an elevated serum alpha-fetoprotein level in a minority (less than 3%) of lesions. Other liver masses are not associated with an elevated serum alpha-fetoprotein level. The presence of multiple liver lesions favors metastatic disease (Fig. 5–39), abscesses, cat scratch disease, lymphoproliferative disorder, or hepatic adenomas associated with a predisposing syndrome (Fanconi anemia, Gaucher disease).

Hepatoblastoma

Hepatoblastoma is the most common primary liver tumor of childhood, composing 43% of total liver masses. Hepatoblastoma is usually seen in infants and young children and occurs primarily in children younger than 3 years. Predisposing conditions include Beckwith-Wiedemann syndrome, hemihypertrophy, familial polyposis coli, Gardner syndrome, Wilms tumor, and biliary atresia. The most common presentation is a painless mass. There is usually no history of underlying liver disease. Serum alpha-fetoprotein levels are elevated in more than 90% of patients. Therefore, a liver mass presenting in a child less than 3 years of age with an elevated alpha-fetoprotein level is almost always hepatoblastoma.

On imaging, the lesions are most commonly well defined and have a tendency to displace rather than invade adjacent structures such as the falciform ligament (Fig. 5–40). The lesions

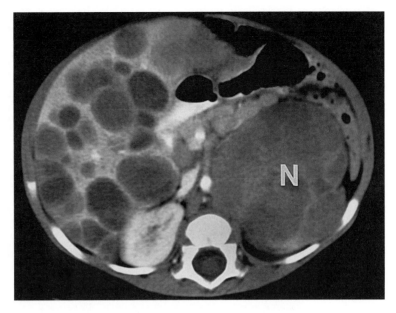

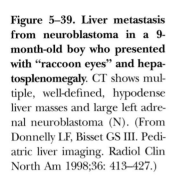

Figure 5–39. Liver metastasis from neuroblastoma in a 9-month-old boy who presented with "raccoon eyes" and hepatosplenomegaly. CT shows multiple, well-defined, hypodense liver masses and large left adrenal neuroblastoma (N). (From Donnelly LF, Bisset GS III. Pediatric liver imaging. Radiol Clin North Am 1998;36: 413–427.)

may be heterogeneous related to necrosis or hemorrhage. Overall survival rate for hepatoblastoma is 63 to 67%.

Infantile Hemangioendothelioma

Infantile hemangioendothelioma is the most common symptomatic vascular lesion of infancy. The lesions most commonly present in young infants as abdominal masses associated with high-output congestive heart failure, consumptive coagulopathy (thrombocytopenia), or hemorrhage. Eighty-five percent of the lesions present by 6 months of age. The imaging appearance is variable, and lesions can be well defined or diffuse. The appearance is most often heterogeneous. There may be prominent vessels within the lesions (Fig. 5–41). On all imaging modalities, the descending aorta superior to the level of the hepatic branches of the celiac artery may appear abnormally enlarged compared with the infrahepatic aorta related to flow phenomena.

Hemangioendotheliomas tend to involute spontaneously without therapy over a course of months to years. Sequential ultrasonography is often used to follow lesions, and the ultrasonograms most often demonstrate a progressive decrease in size and an increase in the degree of calcification.

Mesenchymal Hamartoma of the Liver

Mesenchymal hamartoma of the liver is a rare, benign, predominantly cystic liver mass that most commonly presents in infancy, almost always before 2 years of age. The lesion is considered a developmental anomaly rather than a true neoplasm. Patients usually present with a large, painless abdominal mass and a normal serum alpha fetoprotein level. At imaging, lesions appear as large, multilocular, cystic masses with thin internal septations (Fig. 5–42). Occasionally, the solid component of the lesion can be more predominant, with multiple smaller cysts, giving the lesion a "Swiss cheese" appearance.

BLUNT ABDOMINAL TRAUMA

Blunt abdominal trauma is a common indication for CT of the abdomen and pelvis in children. The most common cause of such trauma in children is motor vehicle accidents. Other causes include a direct blow from abuse or from a handlebar when falling from a bicycle. Many aspects of imaging of pediatric trauma, such as the appearance of parenchymal lacerations, are similar in children and adults and are not discussed in detail. However, several significant differences are emphasized.

Parenchymal Organ Injuries

The order of frequency of parenchymal organ injuries in children is liver (36%), spleen (34%), kidney (22%), adrenal gland (11%),

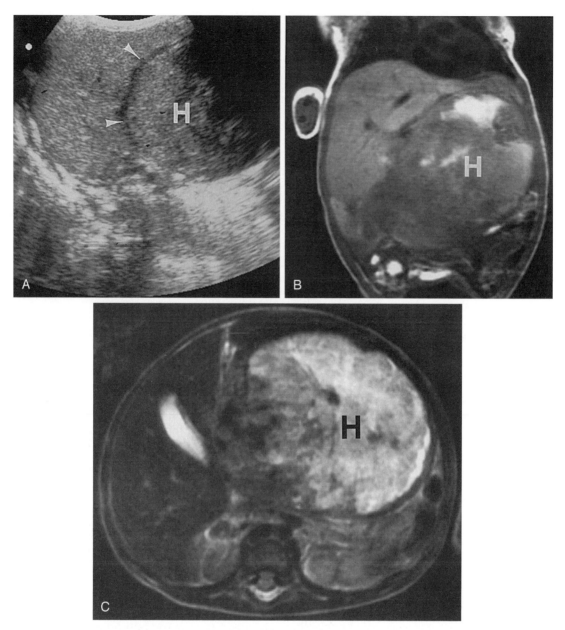

Figure 5–40. Hepatoblastoma in a 4-day-old girl who presented with an abdominal mass. *A*, Transverse ultrasonogram shows well-defined, heterogeneous mass (H), isoechoic to liver, arising from the left lobe of the liver. The falciform ligament is displaced rightward *(arrowheads)*. *B*, Coronal T1-weighted (500/11, TR/TE) magnetic resonance (MR) image shows large mass (H) arising from left lobe of liver with heterogeneous high and low signal probably related to intratumoral hemorrhage. *C*, Axial T2-weighted (3000/85 TR/TE) image shows heterogeneous high signal mass (H) displacing rather than invading falciform ligament. (From Donnelly LF, Bisset GS III. Pediatric liver imaging. Radiol Clin North Am 1998;36:413–427.)

and pancreas (6%). Injury of multiple organs occurs in up to 21% of incidences of trauma. Most solid organ injuries are treated conservatively, with surgery reserved for patients who are hemodynamically unstable. It has been shown that the size and appearance of the parenchymal organ injury are not accurate predictors of which patients will need surgery. The visualization of active extravasation of contrast from a lacerated organ (density as high as the enhancing aorta seen within the peritoneum) has been advocated as a predictor of

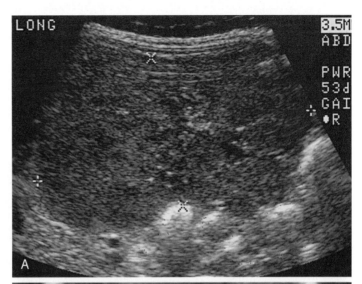

Figure 5–41. Hemangioendothelioma in a 5-week-old boy. *A*, Longitudinal ultrasonogram shows heterogeneously echogenic mass involving the left lobe of the liver. *B*, Coronal T1-weighted image shows a predominantly low-signal, well-defined mass (H) containing some heterogeneous high-signal inferiorly. *C*, Axial T2-weighted (2000/ 85 TR/TE) image shows a well-defined, high-signal mass (H) confined to left lobe of the liver. There are prominent vascular structures within the mass suggesting the diagnosis. (From Donnelly LF, Bisset GS III. Pediatric liver imaging. Radiol Clin North Am 1998;36:413–427.)

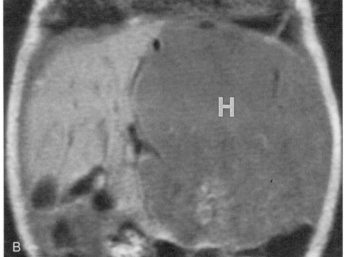

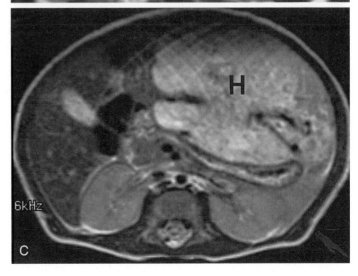

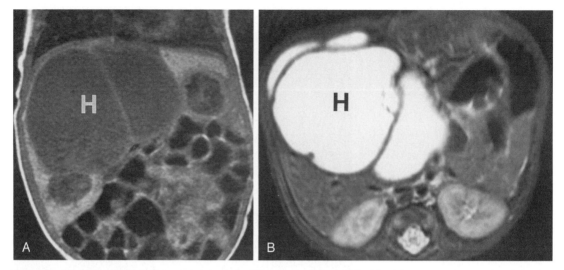

Figure 5–42. Mesenchymal hamartoma of the liver in a 3-week-old girl with an asymptomatic abdominal mass. *A,* Coronal T1-weighted (300/8, TR/TE) MR image shows a well-defined, large, predominantly cystic mass (H) with internal septations, involving the medial segment of the left lobe of the liver and anterior segment of the right lobe of the liver. *B,* Axial T2-weighted (3500/85, TR/TE) image shows a homogeneous high signal (H) of the multiple cysts. (From Donnelly LF, Bisset GS III. Pediatric liver imaging. Radiol Clin North Am 1998;36:413–427.)

the high likelihood of a need for surgery (Fig. 5–43).

There can be artifactual areas of low attenuation seen within the spleen—transient splenic heterogeneity, which is a normal flow phenomenon often seen during the arterial phase of contrast enhancement. These artifacts should not be mistaken for splenic injury. Patterns of splenic heterogeneity include archiform (alternating bands of low and high attenuation) (Fig. 5–44), focal, and diffuse heterogeneity.

Bowel Injury

Injury to the bowel is seen in approximately 8% of abdominal injuries after trauma. Bowel injury is more common in children who have had lap belt–type injuries. The most commonly encountered computed tomographic findings include focal bowel wall thickening, associated prominence of bowel wall enhancement, mesenteric soft tissue stranding, and unexplained free peritoneal fluid (fluid in the absence of solid organ injury) (Fig. 5–45). When subtle, these findings may be suggestive of, but not diagnostic of, a bowel injury. It is inappropriate to send all such patients to the operating room. More often, the findings are communicated to the surgical team and are kept in mind if the patient develops increasing

abdominal symptoms. More specific findings of bowel injury are less common and include free intraperitoneal air, extraluminal bubbles of gas in the vicinity of the injury and, much less commonly, extraluminal extravasation of enteric contrast.

Patients who receive a focal, direct blow to the upper abdomen, most commonly from a handlebar when falling from a bicycle or from abuse, are at increased risk of having a duodenal hematoma-laceration or pancreatitis (Figs. 5–46 and 5–47). On CT, duodenal hematomas appear as high- or low-attenuation masses or wall thickening in the third portion of the duodenum.

Hypoperfusion Complex

It is suggested that children can mask the clinical findings of hypovolemic shock longer than adults can through more pronounced peripheral vasospasm and tachycardia. The appearance of such children on CT has been referred to as the *hypoperfusion complex* or as *shock bowel.* Computed tomographic findings include abnormal intense enhancement of the bowel wall (Fig. 5–48), mesentery, adrenal glands, liver, kidneys, and pancreas; intense enhancement and decreased caliber of the inferior vena cava (IVC) and aorta; and diffusely di-

Figure 5–43. Active arterial extravasation from splenic rupture in a 7-year-old victim of a motor vehicle accident. *A* and *B*, Computed tomographic scans of the upper abdomen show a ruptured spleen with adjacent areas of high attenuation from extravasated intravascular contrast *(large arrows).* Attenuation of extravasated contrast is equal to that of the aorta. There is hemoperitoneum. Note computed tomographic findings of hypoperfusion complex, including intense enhancement of the right adrenal gland *(arrowhead* on *A),* liver, aorta, and inferior vena cava (IVC) as well as the small-caliber IVC *(small arrow* on *A).* By the time that CT was completed, the patient had developed hypotension. Emergent splenectomy was successful. (From Donnelly LF, Frush DP, O'Hara SM, et al. CT appearance of clinically occult abdominal hemorrhage in children. AJR Am J Roentgenol 1998;170:1073–1076.)

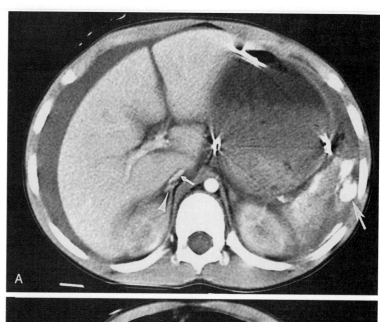

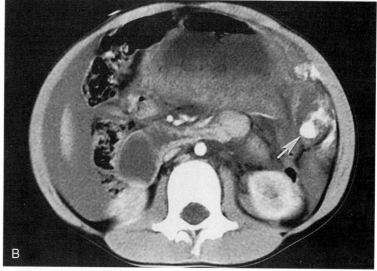

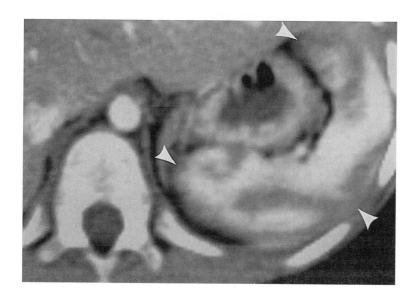

Figure 5–44. Heterogeneous splenic enhancement related to imaging during arterial phase of enhancement. CT shows bizarre pattern of low and high attenuation throughout the spleen *(arrowheads).* This should not be mistaken for splenic laceration or a mass.

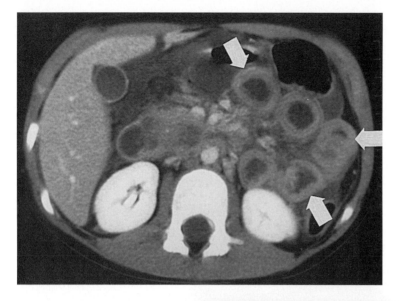

Figure 5–45. Jejunal laceration in a 12-year-old boy after a motor vehicle accident. CT shows bowel wall thickening and abnormal enhancement of loops of jejunum *(arrows)*. The mesentery located central to the abnormal bowel loops demonstrates soft tissue attenuation surrounding the mesenteric vessels. (From Zarewych ZM, Donnelly LF, Frush DP, Bisset GS III. Imaging of pediatric mesenteric abnormalities. Pediatr Radiol 1999; 29:711–719.)

Figure 5–46. Duodenal hematoma and laceration in a 6-year-old boy who had a "handle bar" injury 2 days before and presented with progressively increasing vomiting and a tense abdomen on physical examination. Computed tomographic scan shows intramural hematoma as wall thickening of the second portion of the duodenum *(arrows)*. There is also extraluminal gas and extravasation of orally administered contrast *(arrowhead)* adjacent to the duodenum, which is consistent with perforation.

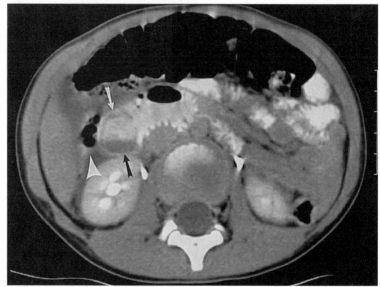

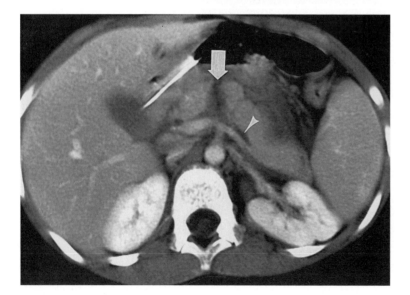

Figure 5–47. Traumatic pancreatic transection in an 11-year-old girl after a "handle bar" injury. CT shows low-attenuation cleft *(arrow)* traversing the pancreas and soft tissue stranding in the peripancreatic portion of the anterior pararenal space. There is also fluid *(arrowhead)* between the pancreas and splenic vein, which is a sensitive finding of pancreatic injury.

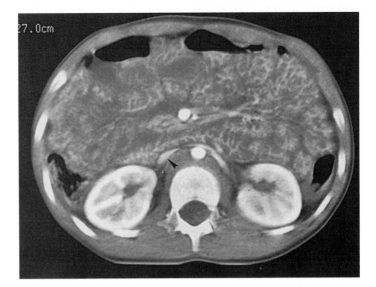

Figure 5–48. Hypoperfusion complex in an 8-year-old child after a high-speed collision. CT shows diffuse abnormal bowel enhancement, intense enhancement of the aorta and IVC, and a small-caliber IVC *(arrowhead)*.

lated fluid-filled bowel loops (see Figs. 5–43 and 5–48). This appearance on CT may be identified before clinical findings of shock and is associated with a poor prognosis. The bowel findings, bowel wall enhancement and dilation over diffuse distribution, should not be confused with the focal dilatation and bowel wall thickening-enhancement that is more typical of bowel injury. When the cause of the bowel findings is unclear, identifying other findings of the hypoperfusion complex is helpful.

THE IMMUNOCOMPROMISED CHILD

The population of immunocompromised children has greatly increased. The causes of immunosuppression can be related to therapy for malignancy, bone marrow transplantation, solid organ transplantation, primary immunodeficiency, and acquired immunodeficiency syndrome (AIDS). These patients can have problems related to immunodeficiency (infection, lack of neoplasm surveillance); thrombocytopenia (bleeding) (Fig. 5–49); other complications related to therapy, including mucositis, radiation injury, and the development of secondary neoplasm; recurrence of the primary neoplasm; and illnesses that occur in childhood unrelated to the oncologic problems. The GI tract is commonly involved with such processes. Often, these patients present with nonspecific symptoms, and imaging, usually CT, is requested. Immunocompromised children are of-

ten referred for abdominal CT imaging to "rule out abscess." However, drainable focal intraabdominal fluid collections are uncommon in immunocompromised children. More often, the abdominal source of sepsis is related to bowel wall compromise secondary to various types of enterocolitis. Common causes of bowel conditions are listed in Table 5–4. Most of these causes of enterocolitis are managed medically

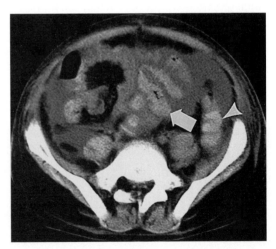

Figure 5–49. Acute gastrointestinal bleeding in a 9-year-old boy with graft-versus-host disease and thrombocytopenia. At the time of scanning, gastrointestinal bleeding was not suspected. The study was performed to rule out abscess. CT, performed without enteric contrast, shows high-attenuation fluid within the small *(arrow)* and large *(arrowhead)* bowel due to acute intraluminal gastrointestinal bleeding.

TABLE 5–4. **Computed Tomographic Findings Helpful in Differentiating Between Bowel Diseases in Immunocompromised Children**

Entity	Typical Distribution	Imaging Features
Pseudomembranous colitis	Pancolitis	Marked bowel wall thickening Nonprominent pericolonic inflammatory changes
Neutropenic colitis	Cecum, ascending colon, terminal ileum	Bowel wall thickening Pericolonic inflammatory changes
CMV colitis	Cecum, ascending colon, terminal ileum	Bowel wall thickening Pericolonic inflammatory changes
Mucositis	Small and large bowel	Fluid-filled, dilated small and large bowel Thin but enhancing bowel wall Absent: bowel wall thickening or adjacent inflammatory changes
Graft-versus-host disease	Diffuse small and large bowel	Mucosal enhancement Fluid-filled dilated bowel Wall thickening mild, isolated to small bowel Prominent mesenteric inflammatory changes
Lymphoproliferative disorder	Focal involvement, typically small bowel	Marked, focal bowel wall thickening Aneurysmal dilatation bowel lumen Parenchymal (liver) masses Lymphadenopathy-mesenteric masses
GI bleeding	Anywhere	High-attenuation fluid or heterogeneous mass (solid thrombus) within lumen Associated underlying enterocolitis

CMV = cytomegalovirus; GI = gastrointestinal.

unless there is evidence of perforation (extraluminal gas, fluid collection). When intraabdominal abscesses are present, they are often related to systemic fungal infection with organisms such as *Candida albicans* or to aspergillosis. These abscesses appear as multiple small, low-attenuation lesions within the liver and spleen (Fig. 5–50).

Pseudomembranous Colitis

Because immunocompromised patients often receive antibiotics, they are at risk for the development of pseudomembranous colitis. This condition is related to the overgrowth of, and toxin production by, *Clostridium difficile*, most often related to the use of antibiotics. On gross

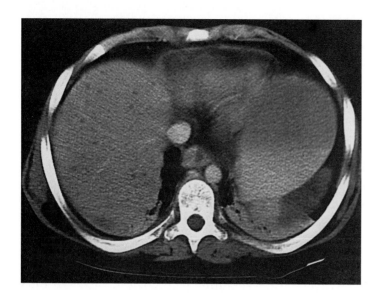

Figure 5–50. Multiple hepatic and splenic fungal abscesses in a 13-year-old boy with *Candida albicans* sepsis. CT shows multiple small (1 to 2 mm), low-attenuation lesions diffusely located throughout the liver and spleen. (From Donnelly LF, Bisset GS III. Pediatric liver imaging. Radiol Clin North Am 1998;36:413–427.)

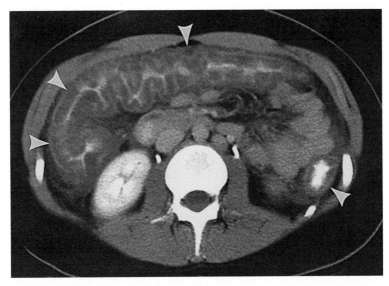

Figure 5–51. Pseudomembranous colitis in an 18-year-old girl with abdominal pain, diarrhea, leukocytosis, and a history of recent antibiotic use. CT shows pancolitis characterized by marked bowel wall thickening and low attenuation within the bowel wall and inflammatory changes in the adjacent fat of the ascending, transverse, and descending colon *(arrowheads)*. Intraluminal contrast is interposed between markedly thickened haustra (the "accordion" sign), which is highly suggestive of pseudomembranous colitis. (From Donnelly LF. CT imaging of immunocompromised children with acute abdominal symptoms. AJR Am J Roentgenol 1996;167:909–913.)

inspection of the colon, there are discrete, yellow plaques (pseudomembranes) involving the mucosal surface. The plaques are usually separated by normal-appearing mucosa. The computed tomographic findings, although nonspecific, are often highly suggestive of pseudomembranous colitis (Fig. 5–51). In the majority of cases, there is diffuse colonic involvement (pancolitis). There is marked colonic wall thickening (average, 15 mm), that is greater in degree than that seen in most other types of colitis. Often, contrast material insinuates between the pseudomembranes and swollen haustra, creating an "accordion sign," which is highly suggestive of the diagnosis (see Fig. 5–51). Because pseudomembranous colitis predominantly involves the mucosa and submucosa, the degree of inflammatory change in the pericolonic fat is often disproportionately subtle compared with the degree of colonic wall thickening (see Fig. 5–51).

Neutropenic Colitis

Neutropenic colitis (typhlitis, necrosing enteropathy) is a life-threatening right-sided colitis associated with severe neutropenia. Pathologically, there is necrosing inflammation of the cecum and ascending colon, with associated ischemia and secondary bacterial invasion. CT shows bowel wall thickening, pericolonic fluid, and inflammation of the pericolonic fat, usually isolated to the cecum and ascending colon (Fig. 5–52). The adjacent terminal ileum may also appear abnormal, but involvement of other portions of the small bowel or descending colon is unusual.

Graft-Versus-Host Disease

Acute graft-versus-host disease (GVHD) is a disease process specific to bone marrow transplant recipients, in which donor T lymphocytes cause selected epithelial damage of recipient target organs. Histopathologically, there is extensive crypt cell necrosis and, in severe cases, diffuse destruction of the mucosa throughout both the large and small bowel, with replacement by a thin layer of highly vascular granulation tissue. Computed tomographic findings include diffuse enterocolitis from the duodenum to the rectum. Compared with the previously discussed causes of enterocolitis, bowel wall thickening may be mild, isolated to the small bowel, or absent. More characteristically, there is abnormal bowel wall enhancement in a central, mucosal location corresponding pathologically with the thin

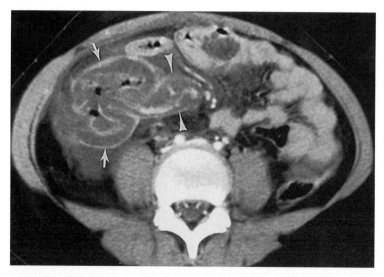

Figure 5–52. Neutropenic colitis in an 11-year-old girl with a history of acute lymphocytic leukemia and right lower quadrant pain and diarrhea. CT shows marked bowel wall thickening, adventitial enhancement, low attenuation of the central bowel wall, and a pericolonic inflammatory change involving both cecum *(arrows)* and terminal ileum *(arrowheads)*. The descending colon and remainder of small bowel appear to be normal. (From Donnelly LF. CT imaging of immunocompromised children with acute abdominal symptoms. AJR Am J Roentgenol 1996;167:909–913.)

layer of vascular granulation tissue replacing the destroyed mucosa (Fig. 5–53). Both the small and large bowel are usually filled with fluid and dilated. There is often prominent infiltration of the mesenteric fat with soft tissue attenuation (see Fig. 5–53).

Mucositis

Gut toxicity has been described in association with multiple chemotherapeutic agents. Dam-

age to the mucosa, impaired ability of the bowel to regenerate its protective cell lining (mucosa), and resultant inflammation is often referred to as *mucositis*. Patients present with nonspecific abdominal complaints including nausea, vomiting, and abdominal pain and demonstrate an ileus pattern on abdominal radiographs. The symptoms may be severe and difficult to separate clinically from the previously discussed processes. On CT, the predominant finding of mucositis is dilated, fluid-

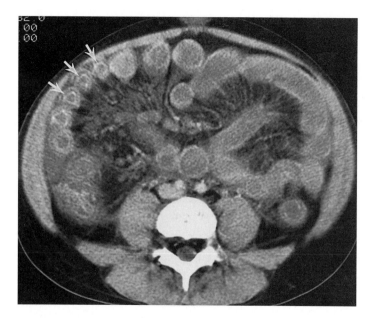

Figure 5–53. Acute graft-versus-host disease in a 9-year-old boy. CT image in midabdomen shows multiple, fluid-filled loops of both large bowel and small bowel with mild small bowel wall thickening. Central ring enhancement in region of mucosa *(arrows)* corresponds histologically to thin layer of highly vascular granulation tissue replacing destroyed mucosa. Note infiltration of mesenteric fat with soft tissue attenuation.

filled loops of small and large bowel. There may be associated mild small bowel wall enhancement. Marked bowel wall thickening, predominance of colonic involvement, and marked abdominal inflammatory changes suggest other diagnoses. Treatment for mucositis is supportive.

Lymphoproliferative Disorders

Lymphoproliferative disorders are lymphoma-like diseases related to an uncontrolled proliferation of Epstein-Barr virus–infected cells in an immunocompromised host. Although they can occur in any immunocompromised individual, they are most commonly encountered after solid organ transplantation. Similar to the variable appearance of lymphoma, abdominal involvement with lymphoproliferative disorders shows a spectrum of imaging findings, including focal parenchymal mass, diffuse lymphadenopathy, mesenteric mass, and bowel wall thickening, and associated aneurysmal dilatation of the small bowel lumen (Fig. 5–54). In contrast to typical non-Hodgkin lymphoma, which manifests more commonly as abdominal lymphadenothy, lymphoproliferative disorder

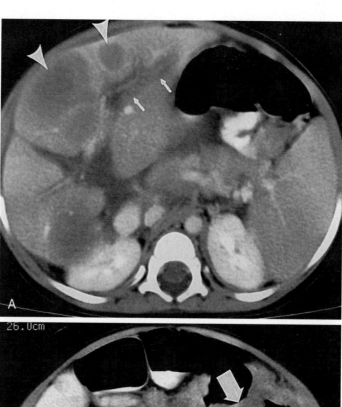

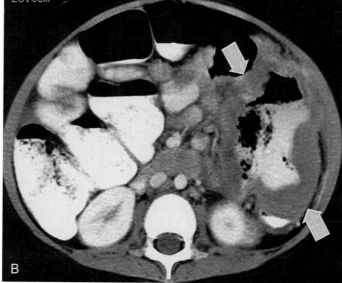

Figure 5–54. Lymphoproliferative disorder. *A,* CT shows multiple low-attenuation liver lesions *(arrowheads)* and periportal low attenuation *(arrows)* in a 1-year-old boy after segmental liver transplantation. *B,* CT shows marked bowel wall thickening and associated aneurysmal dilatation of a focal loop of small bowel *(arrows)* in an 8-year-old with Wiskott-Aldrich syndrome. (From Donnelly LF, Frush DP, Marshall KW, White KS. Lymphoproliferative disorders: CT findings in immunocompromised children. AJR Am J Roentgenol 1998; 171:725–731.)

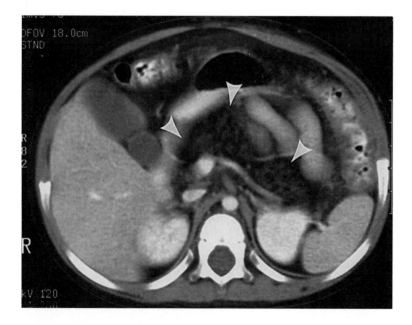

Figure 5–55. Pancreatic atrophy in a patient with cystic fibrosis. CT shows replacement of the normal soft tissue attenuation of the pancreas with fat attenuation *(arrowheads)*.

is associated more commonly with involvement of the parenchymal organs, most commonly the liver, than with lymphadenopathy. In solid organ transplant recipients, the distribution of disease tends to occur in the vicinity of the transplant organ. Therefore, liver transplant recipients are more likely to have abdominal disease than are heart transplant recipients. Therapeutic options include reduction of immunosuppressive therapy, when possible, and chemotherapy.

COMPLICATIONS RELATED TO CYSTIC FIBROSIS

Newborn infants with cystic fibrosis presenting with meconium ileus have already been discussed. Older children and adults can present with a similar syndrome—distal intestinal obstruction syndrome (DIOS), also known as *meconium ileus equivalent*. These children develop obstruction secondary to inspissated, tenacious intestinal contents lodging within the bowel lumen. On radiographs, there is abundant stool within the ascending colon and distal small bowel as well as findings of obstruction. When other therapy fails to resolve the obstruction, contrast enemas with diatrizoate meglumine (Gastrografin) are sometimes requested. It should be noted that it has been reported that patients with cystic fibrosis who develop pseudomembranous colitis can experience abdominal pain and bloating, much like the presentation of those with DIOS, and often do not have the diarrhea typically seen with pseudomembranous colitis. If colonic wall thickening is identified on imaging studies such as CT or contrast enemas, this diagnosis should be considered. Enemas are contraindicated in such patients.

Another cause of bowel pathology in cystic fibrosis is the development of colonic thickening or stricture from iatrogenic damage caused by pancreatic enzyme replacement therapy. Other gastrointestinal problems associated with cystic fibrosis include cirrhosis, portal hypertension and varices, gallstones, and pancreatic atrophy (Fig. 5–55). Patients with cystic fibrosis may have striking atrophy and fatty replacement of the pancreas on imaging studies such as CT, ultrasonography, and MRI.

Suggested Reading

Berdon WE, Baker DH, Santulli TV, et al. Microcolon in newborn infants with intestinal obstruction: its correlation with the level and time of onset of obstruction. Radiology 1968;90:878–885.

Buonomo C. Neonatal gastrointestinal emergencies. Radiol Clin North Am 1997;35:845–864.

Donnelly LF. CT imaging of immunocompromised children with acute abdominal symptoms. AJR Am J Roentgenol 1996;167:909–913.

Donnelly LF, Bisset GS III. Pediatric liver imaging. Radiol Clin North Am 1998;36:413–427.

Donnelly LF, Foss JN, Frush DP, Bisset GS III. Heterogeneous splenic enhancement patterns on spiral CT in children: minimizing misinterpretation. Radiology 1999;210:493–497.

Donnelly LF, Frush DP, Bisset GS III. The appearance

and significance of extrapleural fluid after esophageal atresia repair. AJR Am J Roentgenol 1999;172:231–233.

Donnelly LF, Frush DP, Marshall KW, White KS. Lymphoproliferative disorders: CT findings in immunocompromised children. AJR Am J Roentgenol 1998;171:725–731.

Donnelly LF, Frush DP, O'Hara SM, et al. CT appearance of clinically occult abdominal hemorrhage in children. AJR Am J Roentgenol 1998;170:1073–1076.

Frush DP, Donnelly LF. State of the art: spiral CT: technical considerations and applications in children. Radiology 1998;209:37–48.

Kirks DR. Air intussusception reduction: "the winds of change." Pediatr Radiol 1995;25:89–91.

Kliegman RM, Fanaroff AA. Necrotizing enterocolitis. N Engl J Med 1984;310:1093–1103.

Long FR, Kramer SS, Markowitz RI, et al. Intestinal obstruction in children: tutorial on radiographic diagnosis in difficult cases. Radiology 1996;198:775–780.

Sivit CJ, Taylor GA, Bulas DI, et al. Post traumatic shock in children: CT findings associated with hemodynamic instability. Radiology 1992;182:723–726.

Teele RL, Smith EH. Ultrasound in the diagnosis of idiopathic hypertrophic pyloric stenosis. N Engl J Med 1977;296:1149–1150.

Zarewych ZM, Donnelly LF, Frush DP, Bisset GS III. Imaging of pediatric mesenteric abnormalities. Pediatr Radiol 1999;29:711–719.

Chapter

6

Genitourinary Tract

URINARY TRACT INFECTIONS

Urinary tract infection (UTI) is the most common problem of the genitourinary system encountered in children. The urinary tract is the second most common site of infection in children, after the upper respiratory tract. The incidence of UTIs is higher in girls than in boys, most likely related to the short length of the female urethra. There is some controversy about when children with UTIs should be imaged. Most physicians would agree that boys should be studied after the first UTI and girls should be studied after the second UTI. There are some physicians who advocate that all children should be studied with imaging after the first UTI. The goals of imaging in children with UTIs include identifying underlying congenital anomalies predisposing the child to UTI, identifying vesicoureteral reflux, identifying and documenting any renal cortical damage, providing a baseline of renal size for subsequent evaluation of renal growth, and establishing prognosticating factors. The underlying goal is to eliminate the chance of renal damage that can lead to chronic renal disease.

The work-up of a child with a UTI typically involves both a renal ultrasound and a voiding cystourethrogram.

Renal Ultrasonography

At Children's Hospital Medical Center in Cincinnati, renal ultrasonography is performed with a patient in both the supine and prone positions. Transverse and longitudinal images are obtained of the kidney and bladder. Renal lengths are measured in both the prone and supine positions but are often more accurately assessed with the patient in the prone position.

In every case, it is important to compare the patient's renal length with tables that plot normal renal length according to age. The length of the kidneys should normally be within 1 cm of each other, left to right. If there is a greater than a 1-cm size discrepancy, an underlying abnormality should be suspected. Something may be causing one of the kidneys to be too small—for example, global scarring—or something may be making one of the kidneys too large, such as pyelonephritis or renal duplication. The kidneys of infants have several characteristics that are different from those of older children and adults. Often, infant kidneys have a prominent undulating contour. This is a normal appearance secondary to fetal lobulation. In addition, infant kidneys can demonstrate prominence of hypoechoic renal pyramids (Fig. 6–1), in contrast to the more echogenic renal cortex. These findings should not be mistaken for hydronephrosis.

Voiding Cystourethrogram

A voiding cystourethrogram (VCUG) is most commonly performed in the evaluation of UTI. Other indications include voiding dysfunction, enuresis, and the work-up of hydronephrosis. The VCUG demonstrates the presence or absence of vesicoureteral reflux and documents anatomic abnormalities of the bladder and urethra. Because catheterization is used for the procedure, there can be a great deal of anxiety for both the patient and parents. Education of the parents and patient before the examination is crucial to optimizing the patient's experience. VCUGs are performed under fluoroscopy with the patient awake. The patient is catheterized under sterile conditions on the fluoroscopy table. Typically an 8 French catheter is used. When

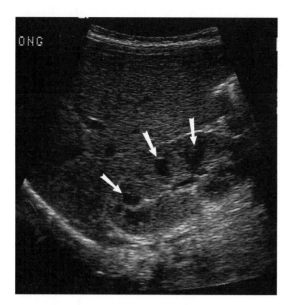

Figure 6–1. Normal ultrasonographic appearance of neonatal kidneys. Note the prominent hypoechoic renal pyramids *(arrows)*. This normal finding should not be mistaken for hydronephrosis.

performing a VCUG, I usually obtain a precontrast scout view of the abdomen to evaluate for calcifications, document the bowel pattern so that this is not later mistaken for vesicoureteral reflux, and to document the catheter position within the bladder. Contrast is then instilled into the bladder. An early filling view of the bladder should be obtained. The main purpose for this view is to exclude a ureterocele, which appears as a round, well-defined filling defect on early filling views. On later full views of the bladder, a ureterocele can be compressed and obscured. Once the patient's bladder is full, bilateral oblique views are obtained, visualizing the regions of the ureteral vesicular junctions. I obtain these views with the collimators open from top to bottom, with the bladder positioned at the inferior aspect of the screen and the expected path of the ureter included on the film. During voiding, the male urethra is optimally imaged with the patient in oblique projection. The female urethra is best seen on the anteroposterior view. It is critical to obtain an image of the urethra during voiding, particularly in males. To play it safe, I typically obtain a view of the urethra with the catheter in place and then obtain a second view after the catheter has been removed. After the patient has completed voiding, images are obtained of the pelvis and over the kidneys, documenting the presence or absence of vesicoureteral reflux and evaluating

the extent of postvoid residual contrast within the bladder. The use of fluoroscopy should be brief and intermittent during bladder filling.

Sometimes, particularly in older children, it may be difficult to get the child to void on the table. Almost all children eventually void and a great deal of patience is required during such prolonged examinations. There are several maneuvers that may help the child void. These include placing warm water on the patient's perineum or toes, placing a warm, wet washcloth on the patient's lower abdomen, tilting the table with head up, running water in a sink so that the patient can hear it, and dimming the lights.

The expected bladder capacity of small children can be calculated by adding 2 to the patient's age in years and multiplying that number by 30. This yields the bladder capacity in milliliters. Obviously, this formula works only up to a certain age.

Acute Pyelonephritis

There is some confusion concerning the terminology for infections of the urinary tract in children. The definition of UTI is *the presence of bacteria in the urine* and the term typically refers to infections of the lower urinary tract. Acute pyelonephritis is defined as *a UTI that involves the kidney*. Young children may present with nonspecific symptoms such as fever, irritability, and vague abdominal pain. In older children, the findings may be more specific, such as fever associated with flank pain. When the diagnosis is straightforward, no imaging is needed during the acute infection. Patients are then imaged later as the standard workup for UTI. When there is a clinical issue of distinguishing an upper UTI from a lower UTI, cortical scintigraphy using dimercaptosuccinic acid (DMSA) has been advocated as the most sensitive test. This study demonstrates a single or multiple areas in which there is no or decreased uptake of radiotracer. These areas tend to be triangular and peripheral (Fig. 6–2). Other imaging studies that have been advocated as able to detect acute pyelonephritis include color Doppler ultrasonography or contrast-enhanced spiral computed tomography (CT). These studies typically demonstrate lack of color flow or contrast enhancement of triangular, peripheral portions of the kidney (see Fig. 6–2). However, pyelonephritis can be focal and can mimic a mass on all these studies (Fig. 6–3). Ultrasonography and CT may also demonstrate disproportionate enlargement

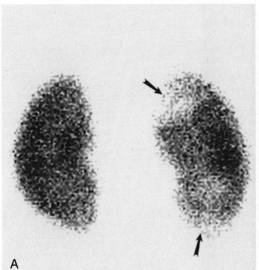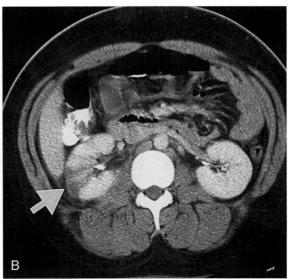

Figure 6–2. Acute pyelonephritis. *A,* Nuclear scintigraphy with dimercaptosuccinic acid (DMSA) shows areas of decreased uptake *(arrows)* in the upper and lower poles of the right kidney consistent with pyelonephritis in a child with known reflux and flank pain. *B,* Computed tomography (CT) shows a wedge-shaped peripheral area of decreased enhancement *(arrow)* within the right kidney of a 15-year-old boy initially thought to have appendicitis. (*A* Courtesy of Sara M. O'Hara, M.D.)

and swelling of the affected kidney as compared with the contralateral side. Sometimes the finding of pyelonephritis will be encountered on these imaging studies when they were obtained for other causes of suspected abdominal pain, such as appendicitis (see Fig. 6–2).

Chronic Pyelonephritis

Chronic pyelonephritis is defined as the loss of renal parenchyma resulting from previous bacterial infection. It is synonymous with renal scarring. Normally, the renal cortical thickness should be symmetric and equal within the upper, middle, and lower poles of the kidneys. The loss of renal cortical substance as seen on ultrasonography, most commonly at one of the renal poles, is suggestive of the diagnosis (Fig. 6–4). This should not be confused with an interrenicular septum (Fig. 6–5), which is a normal variant. In pyelonephrotic scarring, the indentations of the renal contour tend to overlie the renal calyces, whereas with an interrenicular septum, the indentations are between renal calyces.

Evaluation of Prenatally Diagnosed Hydronephrosis

Because of the increasing use of prenatal ultrasonography, one of the scenarios to which pe-

diatric radiologists are increasingly exposed to is the postnatal work-up of prenatally diagnosed hydronephrosis. Such patients are typically evaluated with both ultrasonography and a VCUG. The controversy revolves around the timing of the ultrasonographic evaluation. In neonates, there is a relative state of dehydration that occurs after the first 24 hours of life. Reports have shown that this relative state of dehydration can lead to ultrasonographic underestimation or nondetection of hydronephrosis. Therefore, it is recommended that the postnatal evaluation of prenatally diagnosed hydronephrosis be performed during the first 24 hours of life or after 1 week of age. The disadvantage of performing ultrasonography during the first 24 hours of life is related to interruption of mother-child bonding, whereas the major disadvantage of doing the examination at 7 days of life is the potential of parental noncompliance and losing the patient for follow-up.

CONGENITAL ANOMALIES

Congenital anomalies of the genitourinary tract are often encountered during the work-up of UTIs or other abnormalities.

Vesicoureteral Reflux

Vesicoureteral reflux (VUR) is defined as retrograde flow of urine from the bladder into

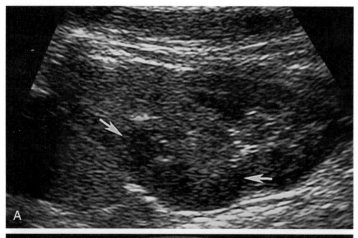

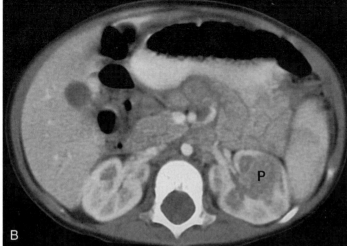

Figure 6–3. Acute pyelonephritis appearing as a focal mass in a 16-year-old girl. *A,* Longitudinal ultrasonogram shows focal mass *(arrows)* within midpole of kidney. Computed tomographic images obtained during cortical phase of enhancement *(B)* and excretory phase *(C)* show persistent focal mass *(P).* Follow-up CT after treatment with antibiotics showed resolution of mass.

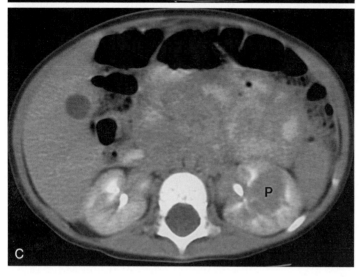

the ureter. It is thought to be a primary abnormality related to immaturity or maldevelopment of the ureterovesicular junction. Normally, the ureter enters the ureterovesicular junction in an oblique manner so that the intramural ureter traverses the bladder wall for an adequate length to create a passive antireflux valve. When the angle of the entrance

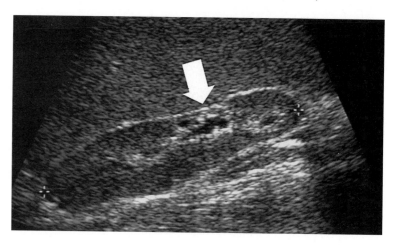

Figure 6–4. Global renal scarring shown on longitudinal ultrasonography of the left kidney. There is diffuse thinning of the renal parenchyma, most striking in the lower pole *(arrow),* where the renal surface is in close approximation to the collecting system.

to the ureter is abnormal, it is thought to result in VUR. The incidence of VUR is less than 0.5% of asymptomatic children, and it is present in up to 50% of children with UTI. There is an increased incidence of VUR in siblings of other children with VUR, in non–African Americans compared with African Americans, and in children of parents who

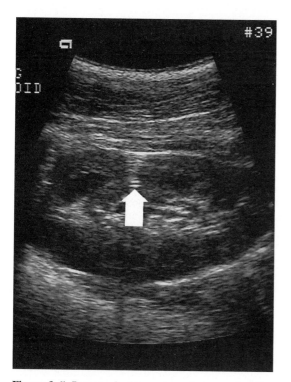

Figure 6–5. Interrenicular septum shown on longitudinal ultrasonogram. The wedge-shaped defect *(arrow)* in the renal parenchyma is a normal variant and occurs between calyces, as compared with scarring, which tends to occur over renal calyces.

had VUR. The importance of VUR is its association with renal parenchymal scarring. VUR is present in almost all children with severe renal scarring. It has also been previously demonstrated that a direct correlation exists between the grade of VUR and the prevalence of scarring. Other complications associated with VUR include acute pyelonephritis, interference with the normal growth of the kidney, and development of hypertension. The degree of VUR is graded based on several characteristics (Fig. 6–6). They include the level to which the reflux occurs (ureteral, ureteral and collecting system), the degree of dilatation, calyceal blunting, and papillary impressions. Grade 1 reflux is confined to the ureter. Grade 2 reflux fills the ureter and collecting system; however, there is no dilatation of the collecting system. Grade 3 reflux is associated with blunting of the calyces. In reference to determining whether a calyx is dilated or not, I was taught that if it looks like you could pick your teeth with it, it is not dilated (Fig. 6–7). Grade 4 reflux is progressive tortuous dilatation of the renal collecting system. Grade 5 reflux is defined by the presence of a very tortuous dilated ureter. Both Grade 4 and Grade 5 reflux can be associated with interrenal reflux.

Most VUR resolves spontaneously by 5 to 6 years unless there is an underlying anatomic abnormality. When there is no anatomic reason prohibiting spontaneous resolution of reflux, most children are treated with prophylactic antibiotics alone. Antibiotic therapy is discontinued when the reflux has resolved. Surgical reimplantation of the ureter is considered when the degree of VUR is severe, there is evidence of renal scarring, the VUR has not resolved over a reasonable time, or breakthrough infections occur frequently.

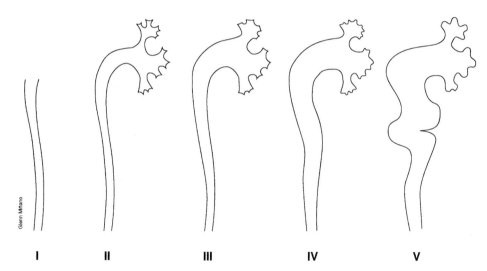

| I | II | III | IV | V |

Figure 6–6. Grading system for vesicoureteral reflux. Grade I reflux is confined to the ureter. Grade II reflux fills the ureter and collecting system without dilatation of the collecting system. Grade III reflux is associated with blunting of the calyces. Grade IV reflux is progressive tortuous dilatation of the renal collecting system. Grade V reflux is defined by the presence of a very tortuous dilated ureter.

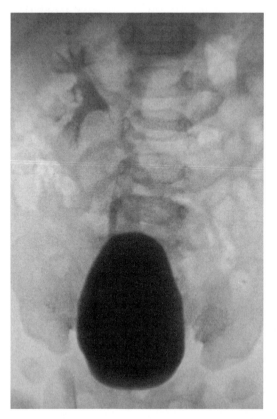

Figure 6–7. Grade II vesicoureteral reflux shown on voiding cystoureterogram. Image shows reflux of contrast filling a nondilated right ureter and renal collecting system. Note that the calyces appear sharp and are not blunted.

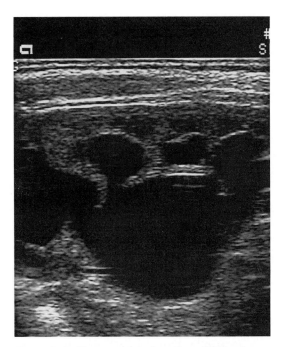

Figure 6–8. Ureteropelvic junction (UPJ) obstruction in a 10-day-old neonate with a history of prenatally diagnosed hydronephrosis. Ultrasonography shows dilatation of renal collecting system and renal pelvis. The ureter was not dilated.

Ureteropelvic Junction Obstruction

Ureteropelvic junction (UPJ) obstruction is defined as an obstruction of flow of urine from the renal pelvis into the proximal ureter. It is the most common congenital obstruction

of the urinary tract. There is an increased incidence of other congenital anomalies of the urinary tract in patients with UPJ obstruction. They include VUR, renal duplication, and ureterovesicular junction obstruction. In addition, UPJ obstruction may be present bilaterally, but the severity may be asymmetric. The cause of most UPJ obstruction is related to intrinsic narrowing at the UPJ. However, extrinsic compression secondary to anomalous vessels is also occasionally identified. On ultrasonography, there is dilatation of the renal collecting system without dilatation of the ureter (Fig. 6–8). The degree of dilatation may be severe. Renal scintigraphy with Tc-99m MAG3 with diuretic (Florosimide) challenge is often used to evaluate the severity of the UPJ obstruction. Mild to moderate UPJ obstructions are sometimes treated conservatively. Most urologists treat severe UPJ obstruction surgically.

Multicystic Dysplastic Kidney

Multicystic dysplastic kidney (MCDK) is thought to be related to severe obstruction of the renal collecting system during fetal development. The site of the obstruction determines the imaging appearance. The most common appearance of MCDK is that of a "grape-like" collection of variably sized cysts that do not appear to communicate (Fig. 6–9). There is a lack of a central dominant cyst. If the level of the fetal obstruction is within the proximal ureter, the "hydronephrotic" form of MCDK can occur when there is a central pelvis sur-

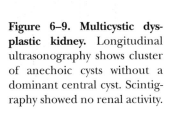

Figure 6–9. Multicystic dysplastic kidney. Longitudinal ultrasonography shows cluster of anechoic cysts without a dominant central cyst. Scintigraphy showed no renal activity.

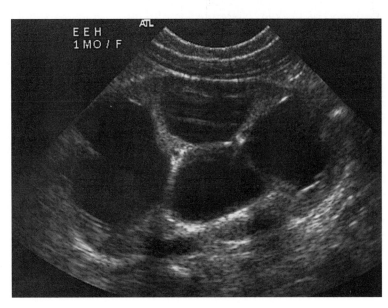

rounded by dilated cysts. In such cases, renal scintigraphy can be useful in differentiating severe UPJ obstruction from MCDK. In MCDK, no tracer accumulation is seen within the renal pelvis on 4-hour images. In patients with MCDK, it is important to exclude other associated congenital anomalies of the contralateral kidney. UPJ obstruction is frequently identified.

Most MCDKs slowly decrease in size over time. Often, the remaining residual dysplastic renal tissue is no longer visualized by imaging techniques. Although nephrectomy was previously the usual treatment for MCDK, most patients are currently treated nonoperatively and followed with ultrasonography. There is some controversy as to whether there is an increased risk of malignancy developing within an MCDK, and this is the reason for follow-up imaging. MCDK can predispose patients to hypertension, and if hypertension develops, nephrectomy is usually performed.

Ureteropelvic Duplications

The term *ureteropelvic duplication* refers to a broad range of anatomic variations ranging in severity from incomplete to complete. The incomplete forms of duplication are more common than the complete form. With incomplete duplication, there can be a bifid renal pelvis, two ureters superiorly that join in midureter, or duplicated ureters that join just before inserting into the bladder wall. With complete duplication, there are two completely separate ureters that have separate orifices into the bladder. Ureteropelvic duplication is thought to be secondary to premature division or duplication of the ureteral bud. Such duplications are five times more common unilaterally than bilaterally. On ultrasonography, incomplete renal duplication may appear as an area of echogenicity, similar to the renal cortex separating the echogenic central renal fat into superior and inferior components (Fig. 6–10). Noncomplicated, incomplete renal duplications have little significance. Children with incomplete duplication are not at increased risk for urinary tract disease compared with children without duplications.

In patients with complete pelviureteral duplication, there is a higher incidence of UTI, obstruction, VUR, and parenchymal scarring. In these patients, the ureteral orifice of the upper pole moiety inserts more medially and

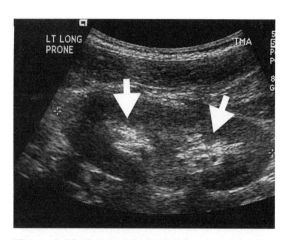

Figure 6–10. Intrarenal duplication. Longitudinal ultrasonography shows an area of echogenicity similar to the renal cortex separating the central pelvicaliceal fat into separate superior and inferior components *(arrows)*.

more inferiorly than the orifice of the upper pole ureter. This is known as the *Weigert-Meyer rule*. The lower pole system is more prone to VUR and UPJ obstruction. The upper pole system is more prone to obstruction secondary to ureterocele (Fig. 6–11).

Ureterocele

A *ureterocele* is defined as dilatation of the distal ureter. The dilated portion of the ureter lies between the mucosa and the muscular layers of the bladder. The ureteral orifice is usually stenotic or obstructed. Ureteroceles are defined as simple when they are positioned at the expected orifice of the ureter at the lateral aspect of the trigone. They are defined as ectopic when they are associated with an ectopic insertion of the ureter. Ectopic ureteroceles are almost always associated with a duplicated collecting system (see Fig. 6–11). The ureter from the upper pole moiety is associated with the ureterocele. There can be marked associated dilatation of that ureter in the upper pole moiety collecting system. Ectopic ureteroceles can be large. On VCUG, ureteroceles appear as round, well-defined filling defects, best visualized on early filling views (see Fig. 6–11). Ureteroceles may not be visualized when the bladder is distended with contrast. Sometimes the ureteroceles can invert and appear as a diverticulum. On ultrasonography, a dilated ureter typically is seen to terminate in a round anechoic intravesicular

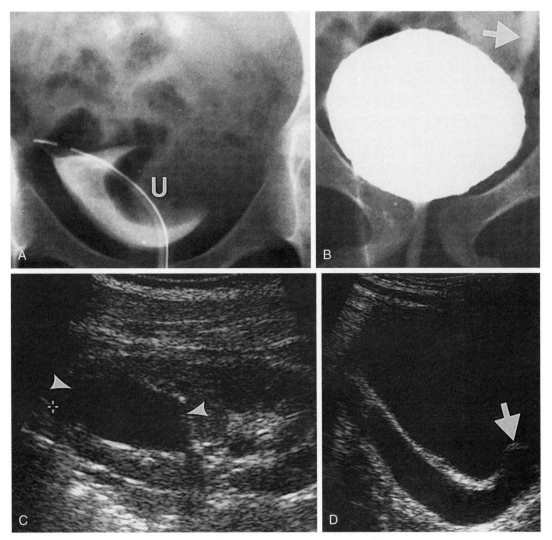

Figure 6–11. Duplicated left renal collecting system with ureterocele causing obstruction of upper pole seen in a 4-year-old girl with urinary tract infection. *A,* Early filling view from voiding cystourethrogram (VCUG) shows ureterocele as mass (U) in leftward aspect of bladder. *B,* Image obtained with bladder distended no longer shows ureterocele. Note vesicoureteral reflux into nondilated lower pole ureter *(arrow).* *C,* Longitudinal ultrasonogram of left kidney shows dilated upper pole *(arrowheads)* secondary to obstructing ureterocele. *D,* Longitudinal ultrasonogram of pelvis shows dilated left upper pole ureter ending within ureterocele *(arrow).*

cystic structure (see Fig. 6–11). Usually there is associated dilatation of the upper pole moiety.

Renal Ectopia and Fusion

Renal ectopia and fusion result from either failure of separation of the primitive nephrogenic cell masses into two separate left and right blastemas or abnormal migration from their fetal position within the pelvis to their expected position in the renal fossa. *Renal ec-*

topia is defined as abnormal position of the kidney. *Renal fusion* is defined as a connection between the two kidneys. With ectopia, the ectopic kidney most commonly lies within the pelvis. Most ectopic kidneys are also malrotated. With cross-fused renal ectopia, both kidneys lie on the same side of the abdomen and are fused (Fig. 6–12). The ureter from the ectopic kidney crosses the midline and enters the bladder in the expected location of the contralateral ureterovesicular junction. The most common type of renal fusion is horse-

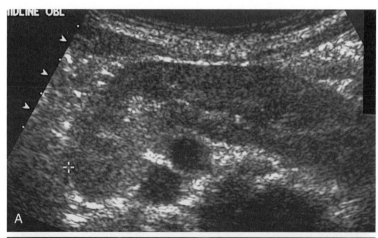

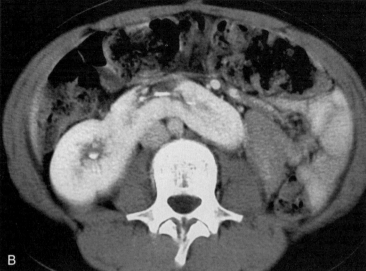

Figure 6–12. Cross-fused renal ectopia. This is demonstrated as fusion of the left and right kidneys to the right of the midline on ultrasonography *(A)* and CT *(B)* in a 12-year-old girl.

shoe kidney, which occurs in approximately 1 in 600 births. With horseshoe kidney, there is fusion of the lower pole of the two kidneys across the midline. The connecting isthmus may consist of functional renal tissue or fibrous tissue and cross at the midline anterior to the aorta and inferior vena cava (IVC). Most horseshoe kidneys are located more inferiorly than normal. The number of ureters arising from a horseshoe kidney is variable, and they exit the kidney ventrally rather than ventromedially. Horseshoe kidneys and other types of renal fusions are at increased risk of infection, injury from mild traumatic events (Fig. 6–13), renal vascular hypertension, and stone formation, and there is a slight increase in the incidence of Wilms tumor and adenocarcinoma. Ultrasonographically, horseshoe kidney may be difficult to diagnose on the standard longitudinal and axial planes. It may be difficult to

obtain accurate measurements of the kidneys in the longitudinal plane because of the poorly defined inferior pole. If the ultrasonographic probe is moved posterior laterally and the patient is scanned in the coronal plane, the two kidneys and connecting isthmus can be visualized on a single image (Fig. 6–14). Such images are most easily obtained in infants. Horseshoe kidneys are readily visualized on CT.

Primary Megaureter

Primary megaureter can be thought of as the ureteral equivalent of Hirschsprung disease. With primary megaureter, there is an aperistaltic segment of the distal ureter, which results in a relative obstruction. The normal, more proximal ureter dilates as a consequence of the relative obstruction. It is more common on the left and in boys. Children affected with

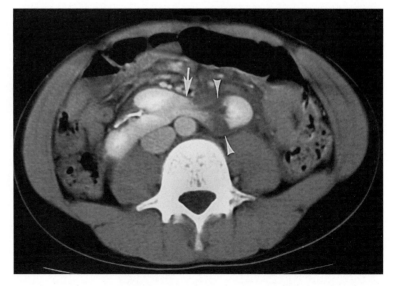

Figure 6–13. Horseshoe kidney with laceration from minor injury in a 12-year-old boy. CT shows parenchymal isthmus *(arrow)* connecting right and left kidneys. There is a laceration *(arrowheads)* of the kidney, just to the left of the isthmus.

primary megaureter may present with infection or may be diagnosed prenatally. Ultrasonography demonstrates hydronephrosis and enlargement of the ureter above the aperistaltic segment (Fig. 6–15).

Posterior Urethral Valves

Posterior urethral valves are the most common cause of urethral obstruction in male infants. Affected children can be diagnosed prenatally or can present with renal failure or UTI. The high back pressure and associated reflux can damage the kidneys and result in renal failure.

Posterior urethral valves present most commonly in infancy but can present in older children.

The typical ultrasonographic features include a thick wall bladder, with associated bilateral dilatation of the renal collecting system and ureters (Fig. 6–16). Occasionally, a dilated posterior urethra can be identified inferior to the bladder (see Fig. 6–16). On VCUG, the posterior urethra appears very dilated. The actual valve itself may be difficult to visualize but can appear as a membrane-like obstruction. Again, the bladder is trabeculated. VUR is present in only approximately 50% of patients with posturethral valves.

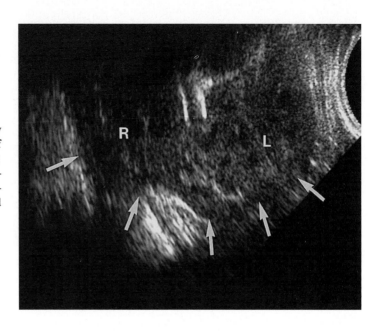

Figure 6–14. Horseshoe kidney shown on coronal ultrasonogram of an infant. The right (R) and (L) kidneys are connected by a parenchymal isthmus *(arrows)*. Inferior margin of horseshoe kidney is denoted with arrows.

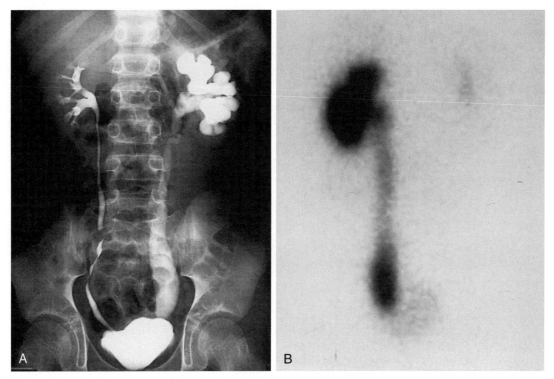

Figure 6–15. Primary megaureter in a 10-year-old boy. He presented with flank pain and had dilatation of the left renal collecting system and ureter seen on a helical computed tomographic scan performed to rule out stones. *A,* Intravenous pyelogram (IVP) shows dilatation of the left renal collecting system and ureter to the level of the ureterovesicular junction. *B,* Image from Tc-99m MAG3 nuclear medicine study obtained 30 minutes after the administration of furosemide (Lasix) shows persistent activity in left collecting system and ureter consistent with obstruction at the ureterovesicular junction.

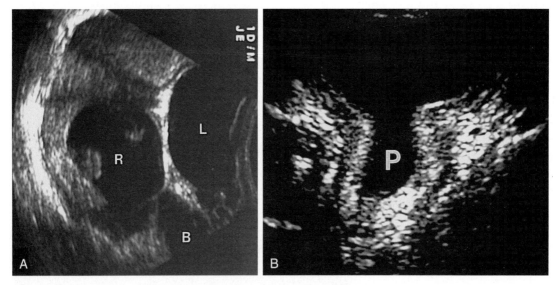

Figure 6–16. Posterior urethral valves in a newborn with renal failure. *A,* Coronal ultrasonogram shows marked dilatation of the right (R) and (L) renal collecting systems. The bladder (B) was also persistently dilated. *B,* Transverse image through inferior bladder shows dilated posterior urethra (P).

Anything that relieves the increased pressure within the urinary system of patients with posturethral valves protects against renal failure and is associated with a better prognosis. Such entities include unilateral VUR (with protection of the kidney contralateral to the reflux) (Fig. 6–17), large bladder or calyceal diverticuli, or development of intrautero ascites. It is the potential presence of posturethral valves that make obtaining an image of the urethra during voiding a vital part of every VCUG performed on boys.

Urachal Abnormalities

The urachus is an embryologic structure that communicates between the apex of the bladder and the umbilicus. Normally, it closes by birth. If any portion of this embryologic structure remains patent, a urachal abnormality results. The type of the anomaly is determined by which portion of the urachus remains patent (Fig. 6–18). If the urachus remains patent in its entirety from the umbilicus to the bladder, it is a patent urachus. Such neonates have urine draining from the umbilicus. Patent urachus can be demonstrated by VCUG, fistula tract injection, or ultrasonography. If the urachus remains patent only at the bladder end of the urachus, a urachal diverticulum results. On ultrasonography or VCUG, a diverticulum of variable size is seen arising from the anterosuperior aspect of the dome on the bladder. Ultrasonography may also demonstrate a fibrous tract extending from the diverticulum to the umbilicus (Fig. 6–19). If the umbilicus remains patent only at the umbilical end, a urachal sinus results. If the urachus remains patent only at its midportion and is closed at both the umbilical and bladder ends, a urachal cyst results. Urachal cysts may present as palpable masses; more commonly, they present with inflammatory changes after becoming infected. Ultrasonography or CT shows a cystic mass anterosuperior to the bladder dome in the midline (see Fig. 6–19). Urachal carcinoma is rare in adults and extraordinarily rare in children.

Prune-Belly Syndrome

Prune-belly syndrome, or *Eagle-Barrett syndrome,* is the name given to the triad of hypoplasia of

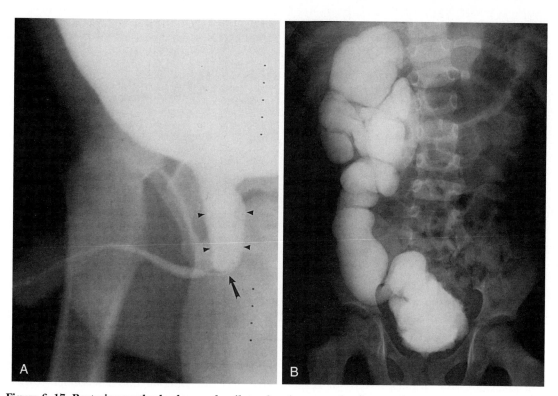

Figure 6–17. Posterior urethral valves and unilateral vesicoureteral reflux serving as a protective mechanism for the contralateral kidney in a 3-year-old boy. *A,* VCUG reveals dilated posterior urethra *(arrowheads)* and posterior urethral valve *(larger arrow)*. *B,* There is unilateral right grade V vesicoureteral reflux.

Illustration continued on following page

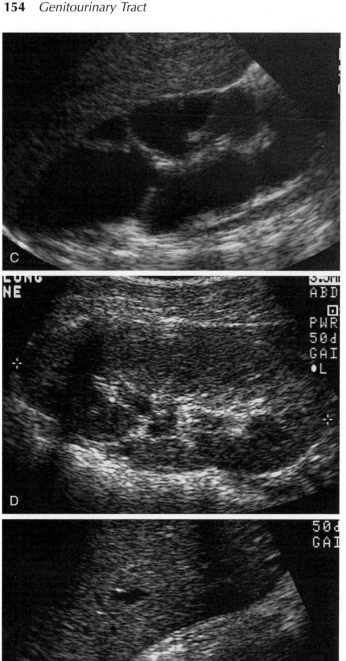

Figure 6–17 *Continued. C,* Initial longitudinal ultrasonogram of right kidney shows marked dilatation of renal collecting system and marked cortical thinning. *D,* Initial longitudinal ultrasonogram of protected left kidney shows normal kidney. *E,* Follow-up ultrasonogram of right kidney shows small kidney with loss of corticomedullary differentiation consistent with scarring. The left kidney (not shown) appeared normal with interval growth. (From Donnelly LF, Gylys-Morin VM, Wacksman J. Unilateral vesicoureteral reflux: association with protected renal function in patients with posterior urethral valves. AJR Am J Roentgenol 1997; 168:823–826.)

the abdominal muscles, cryptorchidism, and abnormalities of the urinary tract system. Potential urinary tract abnormalities include severe bilateral hydronephrosis, a trabeculated and hypertrophied bladder, urachal diverticulum, and hydroureter. Radiographic manifestations include bulging flanks secondary to the abdominal wall, hypoplasia, and the ultrasonographic features of the previously described renal manifestations. There are multiple asso-

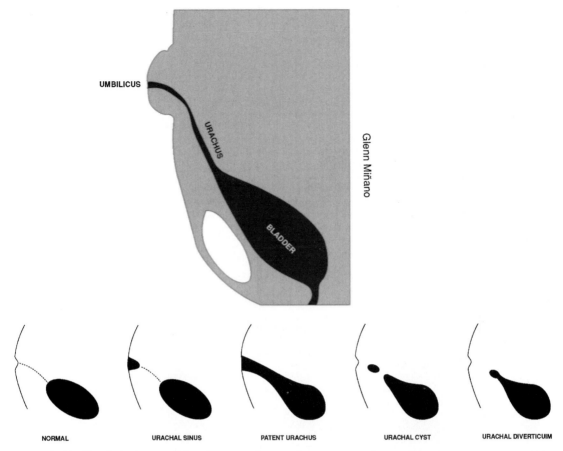

Figure 6–18. Urachal abnormalities. The top image demonstrates the urachus as a patent connection between the umbilicus and the bladder during fetal life. The bottom row of images demonstrates the potential urachal anomalies that occur when a portion or all of the urachus remains patent after birth. The type of urachal abnormality present depends on which portion of the urachus remains patent.

ciated congenital anomalies. Rarely, the syndrome can be incomplete (pseudo prune-belly syndrome) occurring in girls, who obviously cannot have cryptorchidism, or occurring unilaterally.

Hydrometrocolpos

Hydrometrocolpos is the term given to dilatation of the vagina and uterus with blood products secondary to a congenital obstruction. The condition typically presents during infancy, secondary to influences of maternal hormones, or during puberty with a palpable, fixed midline mass. The mass can become large enough to cause ureteral obstruction and resulting hydronephrosis. Plain radiography or ultrasonography can demonstrate the midline abdominal mass. On ultrasonography, the mass appears tubular in the midline and

has heterogeneous echogenicity secondary to the underlying hemorrhage (Fig. 6–20). Often, the uterus can be identified as a small, C-shaped cavity arising from the anterosuperior aspect of the distended vagina. Ultrasonography also can reveal the degree of obstructive hydronephrosis. In problematic cases, magnetic resonance imaging (MRI) can be helpful in confirming the cause and anatomic features of the lesion (see Fig. 6–20).

Renal Cystic Disease

In children, renal cysts can be secondary to polycystic kidney disease, associated with multiple syndromes, secondary to cystic neoplasms, or related to other cystic processes such as MCDK (Table 6–1). The categorization and nomenclature for renal cystic disease in children can sometimes be confusing. In addition,

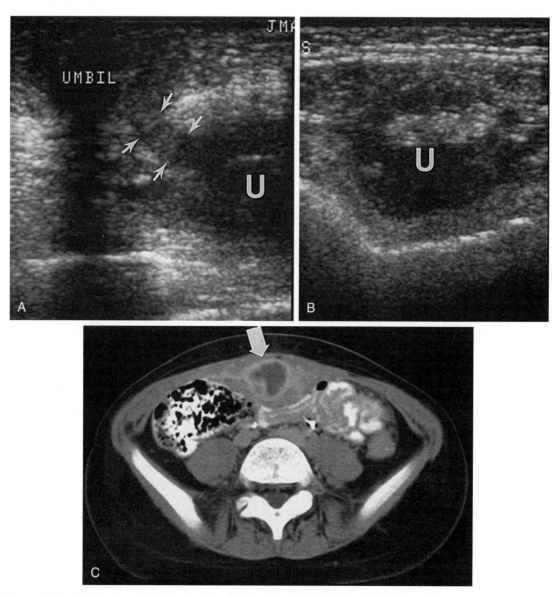

Figure 6–19. Infected urachal remnant in a 3-year-old girl with palpable fullness, fevers, and urinary tract infection. *A,* Ultrasonogram in the midline, longitudinal plane shows a hypoechoic tract *(arrows)* extending inferiorly and posteriorly from the umbilicus (UMBIL) to a cystic-appearing mass (U). *B,* Ultrasonogram in the transverse plane shows a heterogeneous complex cystic-appearing mass (U). *C,* CT shows a low-attenuation mass *(arrow)* with peripheral enhancement in the midline, anterior and superior to the bladder.

it is important to note that although they are much less common than in adults, solitary simple renal cysts are not uncommonly identified in children. When such unilocular, solitary cysts are encountered during the work-up or in the presence of a UTI or hematuria, such simple cysts are usually of no clinical significance and do not necessarily suggest underlying developing polycystic kidney disease. As in adults, the ultrasonographic criteria for a simple renal cyst include an anechoic, well-

defined, round lesion with an imperceptible wall and increased through transmission. No central echoes or vascular flow is present within the lesion or within its walls.

Autosomal Recessive Polycystic Kidney Disease

Autosomal recessive polycystic kidney disease, also known as *infantile polycystic kidney disease,*

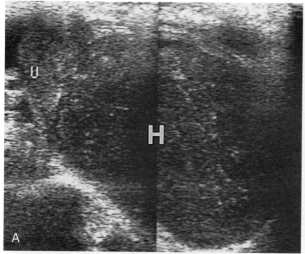

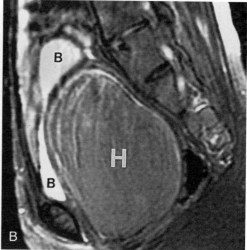

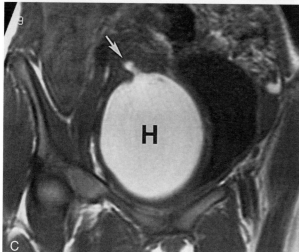

Figure 6–20. Hydrometrocolpos in a 15-year-old girl who presented with a new pelvic mass on one of a series of sequential renal ultrasonograms performed to follow renal scarring. *A,* Ultrasonogram performed in midline sagittal plane shows large, heterogeneous mass (H) displacing uterus (U) superiorly. *B,* Sagittal T2-weighted MR image (TR 4500, TE 85) shows mass (H) to have a low signal, consistent with hemorrhage. The bladder (B) is compressed by the mass and displaced anteriorly. *C,* Coronal T1-weighted MR image (TR 500, TE 9) shows mass (H) to have a high signal, again consistent with hemorrhage. The uterine cavity *(arrow)* is seen to be slightly dilated and continuous with the blood-filled and distended vagina.

encompasses a range of recessive diseases that are associated with varying amounts of cystic disease within the kidneys and hepatic fibrosis. When the renal findings (severe renal tubular ectasia) predominate, the disease most com-

TABLE 6–1. **Renal Cyst Disease in Children**

Solitary simple cyst
Autosomal recessive polycystic renal disease
Autosomal dominant polycystic renal disease
Multicystic dysplastic kidney
Syndromes
   Tuberous sclerosis
   von Hippel–Lindau disease
   Meckel-Gruber syndrome
Cystic neoplasms
   Wilms tumor
   Multilocular cystic nephroma
Calyceal diverticulum

monly presents during infancy (infantile polycystic kidney disease). When the liver disease (severe fibrosis) predominates and there is minimal renal disease, the disease usually presents later in childhood and is referred to as *juvenile polycystic kidney disease.* In the infantile form, the kidneys are markedly enlarged and replaced with numerous small, 1- to 2-mm cysts throughout the cortex and medulla. On ultrasonography, the kidneys are grossly enlarged and demonstrate diffuse increased echogenicity (Fig. 6–21). Discrete cystic structures usually are not identified because of the small nature of the cysts. In the juvenile form, patients usually present with hepatosplenomegaly and portal hypertension. The kidneys may demonstrate enlargement, with cysts of varying size, but may also appear normal. The liver is usually of increased echogenicity related to the diffuse hepatic fibrosis.

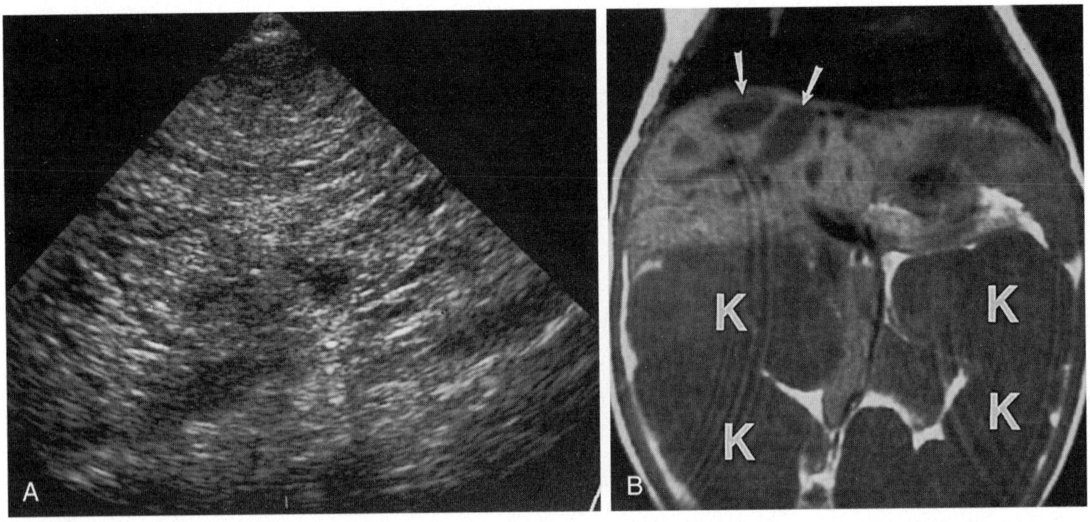

Figure 6–21. Recessive polycystic kidney disease in an infant girl. *A,* Ultrasonogram showed diffuse enlargement of the bilateral kidneys (longitudinal image of left kidney shown here) with markedly increased and heterogeneous echogenicity. No normal renal architecture is identified. *B,* Coronal T1-weighted (TR600, TE 20) MR image shows massive enlargement of the bilateral kidneys (K) and cystic dilatation of the biliary structures *(arrows).*

Autosomal Dominant Polycystic Kidney Disease

Autosomal dominant polycystic kidney disease, also known as *adult polycystic kidney disease,* is a dominantly inherited disease with variable penetrance. Usually, the diagnosis is first encountered in early adulthood with hypertension, hematuria, or renal failure. However, the cysts can be encountered during childhood. Some patients even present during the neonatal period. During childhood, several cysts of varying size may be identified in both the cortex and the medulla. The intervening renal parenchyma appears normal. The cysts gradually grow in size and number, and the normal renal parenchyma can be compressed and destroyed. Cysts may also be found in other organs, most commonly within the liver or pancreas. There is an association between the disease and the presence of intracranial berry aneurysms (10% of cases).

RENAL TUMORS

Wilms Tumor

Wilms tumor is the most common renal malignancy in children. It accounts for approximately 8% of all childhood malignant tumors. Also referred to as *nephroblastoma,* Wilms tu-

mor is a malignant embryonal neoplasm. Its peak incidence is at approximately 3 years with approximately 80% of cases detected between 1 and 5 years of age. Most commonly, Wilms tumor presents as an asymptomatic abdominal mass but may present with abdominal pain, particularly when there is intratumoral hemorrhage (Fig. 6–22). Although most cases of Wilms tumor occur in otherwise normal children, there is an association between the development of Wilms tumor and overgrowth disorders (congenital hemihypertrophy, Beckwith-Wiedemann syndrome), sporadic aniridia, and other malformations. Wilms tumor is bilateral in approximately 5% of cases. Invasion of the renal vein and extension into the renal vein or IVC occurs commonly in Wilms tumor. Pulmonary metastatic disease can occur in up to 20% of cases.

On ultrasonography, Wilms tumor typically appears as a large, well-defined mass arising from the kidney. The mass is typically of increased echogenicity and may show heterogeneity related to areas of intratumoral hemorrhage, necrosis, or calcification. Doppler ultrasonography is excellent in detecting extension of the tumor into the renal vein or IVC. It is especially important to document extension of the tumor thrombus into the right atrium because the cardiothoracic surgery service is usually also involved in such cases.

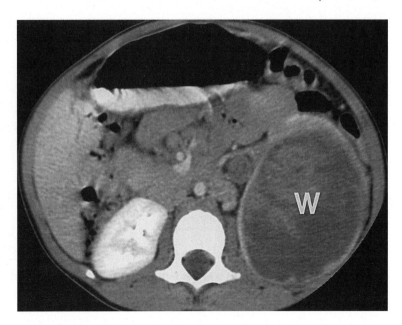

Figure 6–22. Wilms tumor presenting with acute pain in a 3-year-old girl secondary to intratumoral hemorrhage. CT shows intrarenal mass (W) within left kidney. Note ring of renal parenchyma surrounding mass, documenting that the mass arises from the kidney. There are mixed, high-attenuation areas within the lesion consistent with acute hemorrhage.

Confirmation of the lesion is usually performed with CT or MRI. When evaluating a suspected Wilms tumor with either modality, it is important to document the following features: lymph node involvement, liver and lung metastases, involvement of the contralateral kidney by a synchronous Wilms tumor, the anatomic distribution of the intrarenal tumor, involvement of the renal vein or IVC, and relationship of the path of the ureters to the mass. Identification of the ureter as anterior or posterior to the mass is important so that the ureters are not inadvertently injured when the mass is removed.

One of the most important issues when evaluating a mass in the region of the suprarenal fossa is determining whether the mass arises from the kidney and is most likely a Wilms tumor or whether it arises from the suprarenal region and represents a neuroblastoma. Differential features between these two lesions are described in Table 6–2. With Wilms tumor, the mass is usually identified on CT and MRI as a well-defined, usually large, round mass. The mass tends to grow "in a ball," displacing blood vessels rather than engulfing them as is seen with neuroblastoma. When the mass crosses the midline, the lesion usually passes anterior to the aorta as compared with neuroblastoma, which can surround the aorta posteriorly and raise it anteriorly, away from the spine. Most often, Wilms tumor is solid-appearing, but larger lesions often have areas of heterogeneity or cystic components from previous hemorrhage or necrosis (Fig. 6–23; see also Fig. 6–22).

Nephroblastomatosis

Nephroblastomatosis is a rare entity related to the persistence of nephrogenic rests within the

TABLE 6–2. **Differentiating Features Between Neuroblastoma and Wilms Tumor**

Feature	Neuroblastoma	Wilms Tumor
Age	Most common in children <2 yr	Peak incidence at 3 yr
Calcification	Calcifications common (85% on CT) and stippled	Calcifications uncommon (15% on CT) and often curvilinear or amorphous
Growth pattern	Surrounds and engulfs vessels	Grows like ball, displacing vessels
Relation to kidney	Inferiorly displaces and rotates kidney	Arises from kidney, claw sign
Lung metastasis	Uncommon	More common (20%)
Vascular invasion	Does not occur	Invasion of renal vein, inferior vena cava

CT = computed tomography.

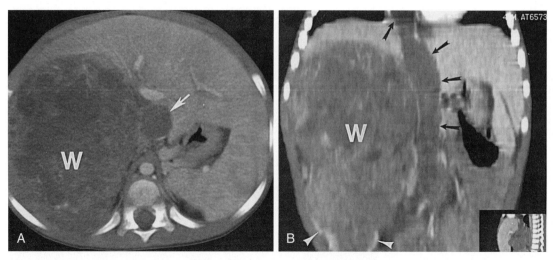

Figure 6–23. Wilms tumor in a 4-year-old boy who had a pulmonary nodule (metastatic lesion) detected on chest radiography obtained for fevers. *A,* CT shows large, heterogeneous mass (W) arising from right kidney. The lesion grows in a round, "ball-like" fashion. Note tumor thrombus *(arrow)* as low attenuation within inferior vena cava (IVC). *B,* Coronal reformatted computed tomographic image shows mass arising from right kidney with renal parenchymal "claw sign" *(arrowheads)* documenting organ of origin. Note tumor thrombus *(arrows)* extending superior within IVC to the level of the right atrium.

renal parenchyma. These nephrogenic rests are precursors of Wilms tumor. Most patients with nephroblastomatosis are monitored with ultrasonography or MRI for the development of Wilms tumor. On MRI, nephrogenic rests appear as plaque-like peripheral renal lesions and may be confluent (Fig. 6–24). Wilms tumor is suggested when a spherical-appearing lesion demonstrates an interval increase in size compared with previous studies, or when it demonstrates progressively increasing inhomogeneous enhancement as compared with the more nonenhancing nephrogenic rests.

Multilocular Cystic Nephroma

Multilocular cystic nephroma is a rare type of cystic mass containing multiple septa. The

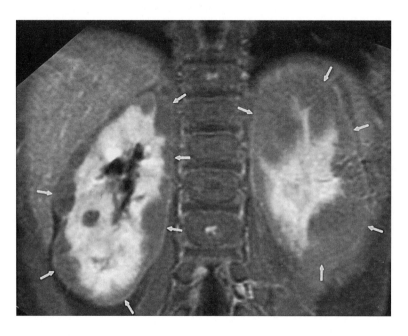

Figure 6–24. Nephroblastomatosis in an 11-month-old boy. Gadolinium-enhanced, fat-saturated T1-weighted images (TR 550, TE 8) show a diffuse ring-like mass *(arrows)* involving the cortex of both kidneys. The abnormal tissue demonstrates less enhancement than the more centrally located normal renal parenchyma.

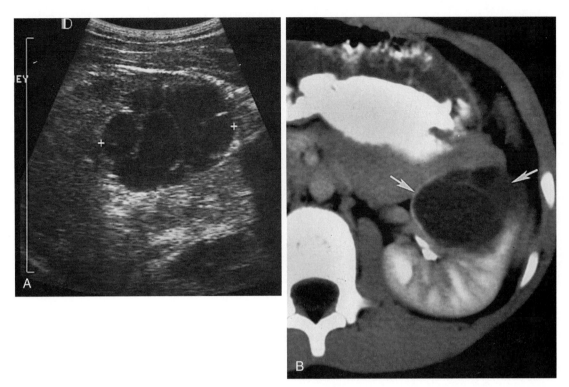

Figure 6–25. Multilocular cystic nephroma in an 8-year-old boy. *A,* Ultrasonogram shows a multiloculated cystic mass within the left kidney. *B,* CT shows well-defined water attenuation structure with internal septa *(arrows).* (Courtesy of Sara M. O'Hara, M.D.)

lesions have an unusual distribution in that they affect mainly young boys and adult women. Typically, the lesions present as a painless abdominal mass. By definition, the lesions do not contain malignant cells but can be difficult to differentiate from a well-differentiated Wilms tumor on imaging. On ultrasonography, CT, and MRI, the lesions appear as a well-circumscribed multiseptated mass (Fig. 6–25). Because the lesions cannot be differentiated from malignancy at imaging, surgical resection is performed.

Mesoblastic Nephroma

Mesoblastic nephroma, or fetal renal hamartoma, is the most common renal mass encountered in neonates. Typically, it is encountered during the first few months of life, with a mean age at diagnosis of approximately 3 months. Neonates most commonly present with a nontender palpable abdominal mass. The lesion consists of benign spindle-type cells. Ultrasonography demonstrates a mixed echogenic mass that is intrarenal in location and indistinguishable from Wilms tumor. CT demonstrates

a solid intrarenal mass with variable enhancement (Fig. 6–26).

Other Renal Tumors

Other less common causes of malignant renal lesions include renal cell carcinoma, renal lymphoma, clear cell carcinoma, and rhabdoid tumor. Although it is a much less common cause of renal malignancy than in adults, renal cell carcinoma is the most common cause of renal malignancy in older children. Ultrasound and CT typically show a nonspecific solid renal mass. Calcification is more common with renal cell carcinoma (25%) than with Wilms tumor. Patients with tuberous sclerosis are predisposed to developing angiomyelofibromas. These lesions often demonstrate fatty components on imaging (Fig. 6–27) and may spontaneously hemorrhage. Patients with tuberous sclerosis also are predisposed to developing cysts.

ADRENAL GLANDS

There are a number of pathologic processes that can involve the adrenal glands in chil-

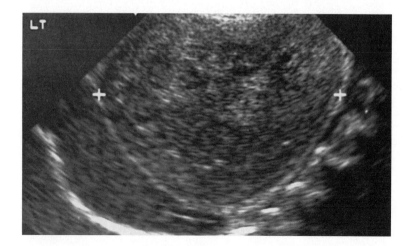

Figure 6–26. Mesoblastic nephroma in a neonate. Ultrasonogram shows well-defined, solid mass replacing the majority of the upper pole of the left kidney.

TABLE 6–3. **Evans Anatomic Staging for Neuroblastoma**

Stage	Definition	Prognosis (% survival)
I	Tumor confined to organ of origin	90
II	Tumor extension beyond organ of origin but not crossing midline	75
III	Tumor extension crossing midline	30
IV	Disseminated disease (skeleton or distant soft tissue, lymph nodes, and organs)	10
IV-S	Age <1 yr	Near 100
	Primary tumor with metastatic disease to skin, liver, and/or bone marrow	Often, no therapy

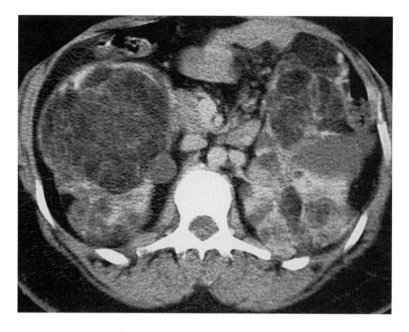

Figure 6–27. Angiomyelofibromas in a patient with tuberous sclerosis. CT shows multiple bilateral renal masses, several of which demonstrate low attenuation equal to that of subcutaneous fat.

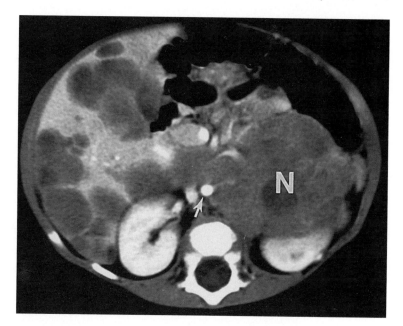

Figure 6–28. Stage IV-S neuroblastoma in a 9-month-old boy. CT shows left suprarenal mass (N) displacing the kidney posteriorly and engulfing the aorta *(arrow)*. There are multiple low-attenuation metastatic lesions within the liver.

dren. The most commonly encountered include neuroblastoma and neonatal adrenal hemorrhage.

Neuroblastoma

Neuroblastoma is a malignant tumor of primitive neural crest cells that most commonly arises in the adrenal gland but can occur anywhere along the sympathetic chain. It is differentiated from its more benign counterparts, ganglioneuroma and ganglioneuroblastoma, by the degree of cellular maturation. Neuroblastoma is an aggressive tumor with a tendency to invade adjacent tissues. The tumor metastasizes most commonly to liver and bone. It is the most common extracranial solid malignancy in children and the third most common malignancy of childhood, with only leukemia and primary brain tumors being more common. Approximately 90 to 95% of patients with neuroblastoma have elevated levels of catecholamines (vanillylmandelic acid, VMA) in their urine, which is a useful diagnostic tool.

Neuroblastoma is an unusual tumor in that prognosis and patterns of distribution of disease are age-dependent. Children who are less than 1 year tend to have a better prognosis; their disease tends to spread to liver and skin. Those older than 1 year of age tend to have a poor prognosis, and their disease tends to spread to bone. The staging (Evans) system for neuroblastoma is unique (Table 6–3). There is

a special stage IV-S that is given to children less than 1 year of age with metastatic disease confined to skin, liver, and bone marrow (Fig. 6–28). Cortical bone involvement demonstrated by radiography or nuclear bone scintigraphy is not considered stage IV-S. It is intriguing that patients with stage IV disease have a very poor prognosis (see Table 6–3) and often require therapy such as bone marrow transplantation, whereas patients with stage IV-S disease have an excellent prognosis, and at many institutions are watched with imaging and receive no therapy. Other factors associated with a better prognosis are listed in Table 6–4.

Although neuroblastoma may be encountered initially on imaging as a calcified mass seen on abdominal radiographs or a mass seen on ultrasonography, confirmation of the diagnosis and definition of the exact extent of disease is obtained with either CT or MRI. Some investigators have advocated MRI over CT because of its superior ability to identify tumor extension into the neuroforamina. Neu-

TABLE 6–4. **Features Associated with a Better Prognosis in Patients with Neuroblastoma**

Age at diagnosis <1 yr
Histologic grade
Decreased *n-myc* amplification
Stage IV-S
Thoracic primary

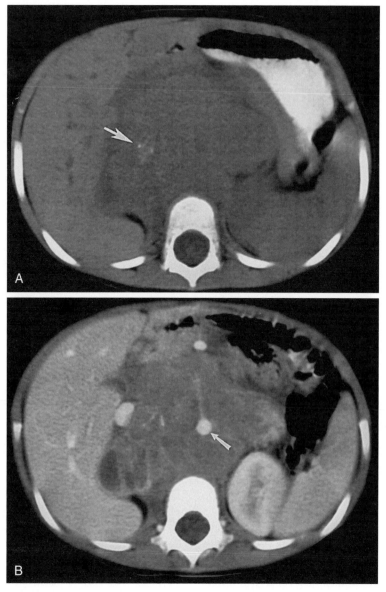

Figure 6–29. Neuroblastoma in a 2-year-old girl. *A,* Non-contrast-enhanced computed tomographic scan shows retroperitoneal mass with calcifications *(arrows). B,* Contrast-enhanced computed tomographic scan shows heterogeneously enhancing retroperitoneal mass that surrounds and anteriorly displaces the abdominal aorta *(arrow)* and its branches.

roforaminal involvement is important to identify because, at many institutions, neurosurgery services will also become involved in surgical resection. In my experience, both CT and MRI are excellent at identifying neuroforaminal and spinal canal involvement.

On CT, neuroblastoma is detected with a sensitivity near 100%. The tumors tend to appear lobulated and grow in an invasive pattern, surrounding and engulfing, rather than

displacing, vessels such as the celiac axis, superior mesenteric artery, and aorta (Fig. 6–29). The mass is often inhomogeneous secondary to hemorrhage, necrosis, and calcifications. Calcifications are seen by CT in up to 85% of cases (see Fig. 6–29). On MRI, neuroblastoma, like most other malignancies, appears high on T2-weighted images and can be heterogeneous in signal (Fig. 6–30). Calcifications are less commonly seen with MRI. During the staging

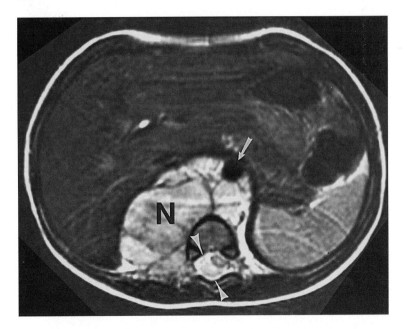

Figure 6–30. Neuroblastoma in a 1-year-old girl. T2-weighted MR image (TR 3000, TE 119) shows lobulated right suprarenal mass (N) that displaces and engulfs the aorta *(arrow)*. There is intraspinal extension *(arrowheads)* with displacement of the spinal cord to the left.

of neuroblastoma, most patients also undergo evaluation with metaiodobenzylguanidine (MIBG) and bone scintigraphy.

Other adrenal tumors that occur in childhood, but much less frequently than neuroblastoma, include pheochromocytoma and adrenal carcinoma.

Neonatal Adrenal Hemorrhage

Adrenal hemorrhage can occur in neonates secondary to birth trauma or stress. Like neuroblastoma, adrenal hemorrhage may present as an asymptomatic flank mass and can be seen on imaging as an adrenal mass. Adrenal hemorrhage is actually a more common cause of adrenal mass than is neuroblastoma in newborn infants. Since surgical intervention is unnecessary in adrenal hemorrhage, differentiation from neuroblastoma is important. Ultrasonography can usually differentiate the two. Neuroblastoma typically appears as an echogenic mass with diffuse vascularity (color Doppler), whereas adrenal hemorrhage typically appears as an anechoic, avascular mass (Fig. 6–31). Serial ultrasonograms over time (see Fig. 6–31) is an acceptable way to differentiate problematic cases, since the prognosis of stage I neuroblastoma in neonates is excellent. With time, adrenal hemorrhages will decrease in size. MRI can also be useful in differentiating adrenal hemorrhage (low T2-weighted signal, blood product signal) from neuroblastoma

(high T2-weighted signal) (Fig. 6–32) in very problematic cases.

PELVIC RHABDOMYOSARCOMA

Rhabdomyosarcoma is a highly malignant tumor that can occur in numerous locations throughout the body. It is the most common malignant sarcoma of childhood and typically presents during the first 3 years of life. Its most common locations include the pelvis and genitourinary tract (39%) and the head and neck (39%). The most common locations within the genitourinary tract are the bladder, prostate (Fig. 6–33), spermatic cord, paratesticular tissues (Fig. 6–34), uterus, vagina, and perineum. It affects girls and boys equally. When the lesion involves the bladder, it typically appears as a multilobulated mass, which has been likened to a bundle of grapes. The pelvic masses may result in hydronephrosis (Fig. 6–35).

SCROTUM

The two major problems that can be encountered in the pediatric scrotum are testicular neoplasm and an acutely painful scrotum. Ninety percent of testicular neoplasms are germ cell in origin. Less than 10% of testicular tumors are metastatic, from leukemia or lymphoma. Most primary testicular tumors pre-

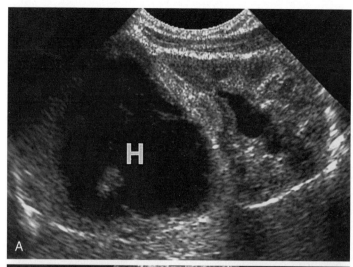

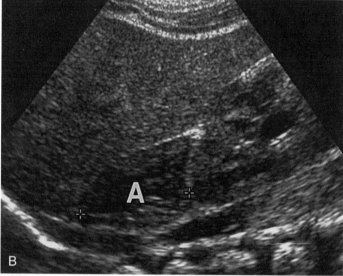

Figure 6–31. Adrenal hemorrhage in a 4-day-old neonate. *A,* Initial ultrasonogram shows a predominantly cystic-appearing, hypoechoic mass (H) in a suprarenal location. The kidney is displaced inferiorly. *B,* Follow-up ultrasonogram from approximately 1 month later shows a marked interval decrease in the size of the adrenal gland (A), more adeniform shape, and resolution of the cystic appearance.

sent with a nontender, firm scrotal mass. Ultrasonography confirms an intratesticular mass. However, there are no ultrasonographic findings that offer a specific histologic diagnosis. If a scrotal mass is extratesticular in location, the most likely diagnosis is embryonal rhabdomyosarcoma (see Fig. 6–34), arising from the spermatic cord or epididymis.

Acute Scrotum

Because of the possibility of testicular torsion, imaging of the acutely painful scrotum is an emergency. The major differential considerations in a child with acute scrotal pain include testicular torsion, epididymoorchitis, and torsion of the testicular appendage. Testicular

hematoma is another less commonly encountered entity. It is reported that up to 40% of boys who present with an acute scrotum have testicular torsion. However, in the experience at the Children's Hospital Medical Center in Cincinnati, epididymoorchitis is overwhelmingly the most common diagnosis.

Testicular torsion occurs when the testis and cord twist within the serosal space, leading to ischemia. Prompt diagnosis and therapy are important because preservation of the testis is possible only in patients whose torsion is relieved within 6 to 10 hours. Color Doppler ultrasonography has replaced testicular scintigraphy as the modality of choice in evaluating the acute scrotum. Color Doppler demonstrates absence of flow or asymmetrically decreased flow within the affected testis (see Fig.

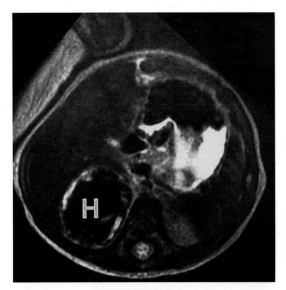

Figure 6–32. Adrenal hemorrhage in a 4-day-old neonate. T2-weighted MR image (TR1800, TE 80) shows right adrenal mass (H) that demonstrates a heterogeneous low signal. This is consistent with adrenal hemorrhage and in contrast to the high T2-weighted signal typically seen with neuroblastoma.

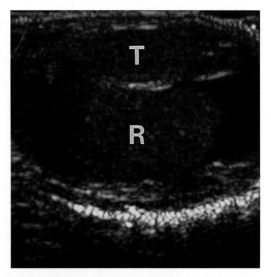

Figure 6–34. Extratesticular rhabdomyosarcoma. Ultrasonogram shows testis (T) with adjacent extratesticular mass (R) and surrounding hydrocele.

6–35). Demonstration of flow within a normal testis may be difficult in children less than 2 years. Gray scale ultrasonography may demonstrate asymmetric enlargement and a slight decreased echogenicity of the affected testis. With progressive ischemia or infarction, hem-

orrhage and necrosis may cause increasing asymmetric heterogeneity.

Epididymoorchitis is usually of unknown cause. In contrast to testicular torsion, the affected testis and epididymis in epididymoorchitis demonstrate asymmetric and sometimes strikingly increased flow on Doppler ultrasonography (Fig. 6–36). Gray scale ultrasonography demonstrates enlargement and decreased

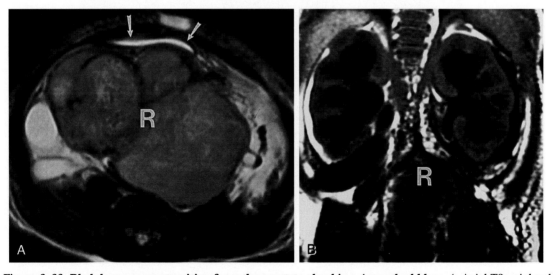

Figure 6–33. Rhabdomyosarcoma arising from the prostate gland in a 4-month-old boy. *A,* Axial T2-weighted MR image (TR5000, TE 87) shows large mass (R) extending superiorly from pelvis and compressing and displacing the bladder anteriorly *(arrows). B,* Coronal T1-weighted MR image (TR 350, TE 14) shows bilateral hydronephrosis. The superior aspect of the mass (R) is seen splaying the aortic bifurcation.

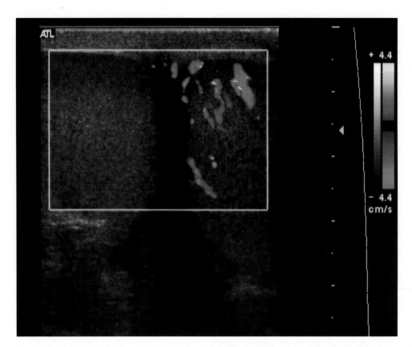

Figure 6–35. Testicular torsion in a 15-year-old boy who was awakened from sleep by severe right testicular pain. Transverse color Doppler–enhanced image shows absence of detectable flow within the right testis and detectable flow within the asymptomatic left testis.

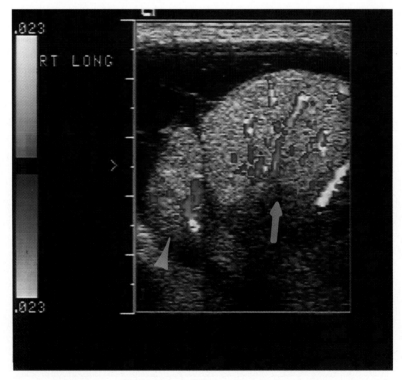

Figure 6–36. Epidydymoorchitis in a 16-year-old boy with acute onset of right scrotal pain. Color Doppler ultrasonogram shows enlargement of the right epididymis *(arrowhead)* and right testis *(arrow)*. There is an adjacent complex hydrocele. There is increased vascular flow to both the epididymis and the testis.

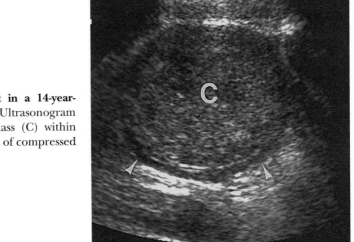

Figure 6–37. Large hemorrhagic cyst in a 14-year-old girl with left lower quadrant pain. Ultrasonogram shows a heterogeneous, echogenic mass (C) within the left adnexa with a surrounding rim of compressed ovarian tissue *(arrowheads).*

echogenicity of the testis and epididymis. Reactive hydroceles are common.

Another cause of acute scrotum is torsion of the testicular appendage, a vestigial remnant of the mesonephric ducts. A mass of increased echogenicity may be seen next to the testicle. The testis appears normal with normal flow. However, enlargement and increased flow to the epididymis, indistinguishable from epididymoorchitis, may be the only findings.

Trauma may result in testicular hematoma. On ultrasonography, hematomas appear as avascular masses of abnormal echogenicity. Associated hematoceles are common.

Acute Pelvic Pain in Older Girls and Adolescents

Acute pain in older girls and adolescents is a commonly encountered problem with multiple possible causes. Pain can be related to menstruation or ovarian pathology, for example, ovarian cysts, hemorrhagic cysts, ectopic pregnancy, ovarian torsion, endometriosis, pelvic inflammatory disease, or other masses such as teratoma and other neoplasms. In girls with right lower quadrant pain, appendicitis is also a possibility. The high incidence and variety of pathologic processes that may involve the ovary make many use ultrasonography as the primary imaging modality for right lower quadrant pain in girls. Hemorrhagic cyst is a common cause of pelvic pain. On ultrasonography, the lesion appears as an echogenic mass (Fig. 6–37) that often has enhanced through transmission. Sometimes the masses can be

quite large. In difficult cases, MRI can be helpful (Fig. 6–38). Ovarian torsion, which is less common, appears as an enlarged, echogenic ovary, secondary to edema. There are often prominent, peripheral follicular cysts, which are highly suggestive of the diagnosis (Fig. 6–39). However, a hemorrhagic cyst compress

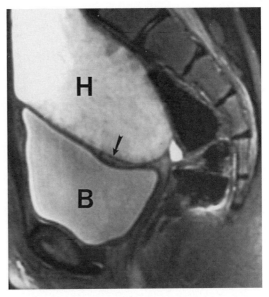

Figure 6–38. Large hemorrhagic cyst in a 9-year-old girl who was suspected to have hydrometrocolpos on physical and ultrasonographic examinations. Sagittal T2-weighted MR image (TR 3000, TE 80) shows a large, heterogeneous high-signal mass (H) posterior to the bladder (B). The uterus *(arrow)* is seen as a separate structure between the bladder and the mass.

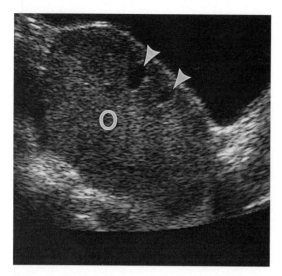

Figure 6–39. Ovarian torsion in an 11-year-old girl with acute left lower quadrant pain. Ultrasonogram shows enlargement of the left ovary (O) with increased echogenicity and peripheral cysts *(arrowheads)*. Doppler evaluation (not shown) showed no vascular flow.

ing the ovarian parenchyma peripherally can have a similar appearance.

Suggested Reading

Daneman A, Alton DJ. Radiographic manifestations of renal anomalies. Radiol Clin North Am 1991;29:351–363.

Donnelly LF, Gylys-Morin VM, Wacksman J. Unilateral vesicoureteral reflux: association with protected renal function in patients with posterior urethral valves. AJR Am J Roentgenol 1997;168:823–826.

Han BK, Babcock DS. Sonographic measurements and appearance of normal kidneys in children. AJR Am J Roentgenol 1985;145:611–618.

Hartman DS. Renal cystic disease in multisystem conditions. Urol Radiol 1992;14;13–17.

Kirks DR, Kaufman RA, Babcock DS. Renal neoplasms in infants and children. Semin Roentgenol 1987;22:292–302.

Lebowitz RL, Olbing H, Parkkulainen KV, et al. International system of radiographic grading of vesicoureteral reflux. International Reflux Study in Children. Pediatr Radiol 1985;15:105–109.

Ng YY, Kingston JE. The role of radiology in the staging of neuroblastoma. Clin Radiol 1993;47:226–235.

Sty JR, Wells RG, Schroeder BA, Starshak RJ. Diagnostic imaging in pediatric renal inflammatory disease. JAMA 1986;256:895–899.

Musculoskeletal System

NORMAL VARIANTS AND COMMON BENIGN ENTITIES

Probably more than in any other organ system, the normal appearance of the skeletal system on imaging is strikingly different in children than in adults. This is related to the changing appearance of growing and maturing bone. The more striking changes occur in the vicinity of physes and apophyses. Many of the more common mistakes made in pediatric skeletal radiology are related to the misinterpretation of normal structures as abnormal. There are textbooks dedicated to the normal appearance and variation of the radiographic appearance of bones in children. The details of the normal changes in the radiographic appearance throughout the maturing skeleton cannot be covered here. The following sections describe several normal variants and commonly encountered benign entities.

Apophyseal Irregularity

In the growing child, apophyses in different parts of the body can have variable and often somewhat irregular appearances. Separate ossicles of an apophysis can mimic fragments, irregularity can mimic periosteal reaction, and mixed sclerosis and lucency can be confused with findings of an inflammatory or neoplastic process. Common apophyses that may have this appearance include the tibial tuberosity, ischial tuberosity, ischial pubic synchondrosis, and posterior calcaneal apophyses (Fig. 7–1). Irregularity and fragmentation are often normally seen in the tibial tuberosity. The calca-

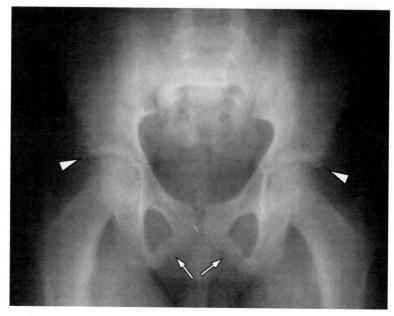

Figure 7–1. Normal variants within the pelvis of a 14-year-old boy. Note irregular ossicles along lateral aspect of acetabuli *(arrowheads)* and prominent ischial pubic synchondroses *(arrows)*.

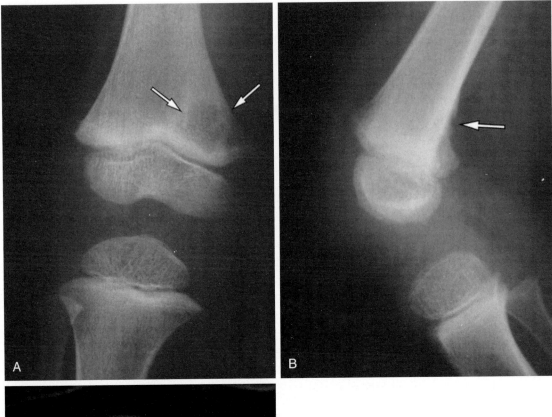

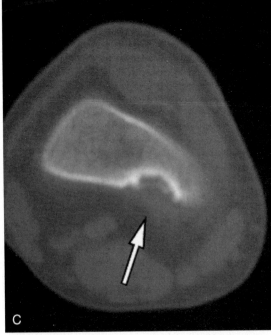

Figure 7–2. Distal femoral metaphyseal irregularity in a 5-year-old boy. *A,* Frontal radiograph shows well-defined lucency *(arrows)* with sclerotic rim in medial femoral metaphysis. *B,* Lateral radiograph shows irregularity *(arrow)* along posterior cortex of distal femoral metaphysis. *C,* Computed tomographic scan shows characteristic "scoop-like" defect *(arrow)* with associated irregularity of the cortex.

neal apophysis can normally demonstrate a strikingly sclerotic appearance. The ischial pubic synchondrosis can appear prominent and asymmetric (see Fig. 7–1).

Distal Femoral Metaphyseal Irregularity (Cortical Irregularity Syndrome)

Distal femoral metaphyseal irregularity, also called *cortical desmoid,* refers to the presence of irregular cortical margination and associated lucency involving the posteromedial aspect of the distal femoral metaphysis. Although debated, its presence is thought to be related to chronic avulsion at the insertion of the adductor magnus muscle. Although this lesion can be associated with pain, its significance lies in its alarming, and often incidental, radiographic appearance. It occurs in up to 11% of boys aged 10 to 15 years. On radiography, there is cortical irregularity along the posteromedial cortex of the distal femoral metaphysis, best seen on the lateral view (Fig. 7–2). On frontal radiographs, there may be an associated lucency (see Fig. 7–2). Familiarity with the typical location and appearance of the lesion and the age of the patient is important so that these lesions are not confused with aggressive malignancies. Because the lesions are often bilateral, confirmation of the benign nature of these lesions can be made by demonstrating a similar lesion on radiographs of the opposite knee. In problematic cases, computed tomography (CT) can be used to demonstrate characteristic findings: a characteristic "scoop"-like defect with an irregular but intact cortex, no associated soft tissue mass, and sometimes a subtle contralateral lesion (see Fig. 7–2).

Benign Cortical Defects

Benign cortical defects and nonossifying fibroma are commonly encountered lesions of no clinical significance. They are seen in up to 40% of children at some time in development and are most common at 5 to 6 years of age. The term *nonossifying fibroma* is typically reserved for larger lesions, which most commonly occur within the bones around the knee, particularly the distal femur. They appear as lucent, eccentric, well-defined lesions with thin cortical rims. They are typically

round or oval. Over time they become more sclerotic and eventually resolve. When the characteristic pattern is identified, no further imaging or follow-up is necessary.

TRAUMA

Fractures in children differ from those in adults for multiple reasons. Children's bones are more porous and have a greater propensity to deform prior to breaking in comparison with those of adults. Therefore, incomplete fractures are more common in children than in adults. The incomplete fracture may be purely a "bowing-type" fracture (Fig. 7–3), may be associated with a buckling of the cortex on the concave margin of the bowing (torus fracture), or may demonstrate an incomplete fracture along the cortex of the convex margin

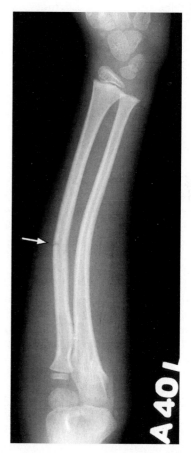

Figure 7–3. Incomplete fractures of the radius and ulna. The radius demonstrates a greenstick-type fracture *(arrow)* with an incomplete fracture along the convex margin of the cortex. The ulna demonstrates a bowing fracture.

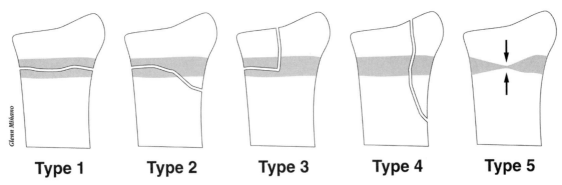

Type 1 **Type 2** **Type 3** **Type 4** **Type 5**

Glenn Miñano

Figure 7–4. Salter-Harris classification. This diagram shows the Salter-Harris classification for fractures involving the physis.

of the bowing (greenstick fracture) (see Fig. 7–3).

Another difference between adults and children is the rate of and potential for healing. Younger children heal quickly. Periosteal reaction can be expected to be radiographically present 7 to 10 days after an injury in children. They also tend to heal completely. Nonunited fractures are uncommon in children. Fracture remodeling is also rapid and impressively complete with fractures of pediatric long bones. Normal alignment is typically restored.

Involvement of the Physis

One of the other major potential differences between fractures in adults and children and one of the ways in which fractures in children can be more problematic than those in adults is fracture involvement of the physis. The physis is involved in up to 18% of fractures that involve the long bones of children. Involvement of the growth plate may result in arrest of growth in that limb and a higher rate of necessary internal fixation. The standard classification for physeal fractures is that by Salter and Harris. It divides fractures into types 1 to 5 based on whether there is involvement of the physis, epiphysis, or metaphysis as determined by radiography (Fig. 7–4). The higher numbers have a greater incidence of complications. Type 1 refers to fracture that involves only the physis. Type 1 fractures tend to occur in children younger than 5 years. On radiography, the epiphysis may appear to be displaced in comparison to the metaphysis (Fig. 7–5). However, type 1 fractures often will reduce before the radiograph is obtained, and the only imaging finding will be soft tissue swelling adjacent to the physis. Type 2 fractures involve

the metaphysis and the physis but do not involve the epiphysis (Fig. 7–6). They are the most common type of physeal injury (up to 75% of physeal injuries). On radiography, there is typically a triangular fragment of bony metaphysis attached to the physis and epiphysis. Type 3 fractures involve the physis and epiphysis but not the metaphysis. Type 3 injuries have a greater predisposition for growth

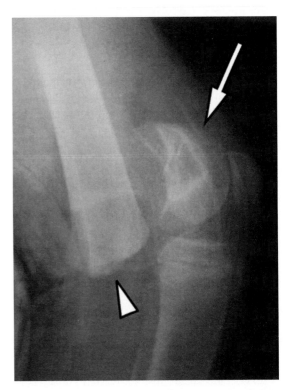

Figure 7–5. Salter type 1 fracture of the distal tibia in a child struck by a car. Radiograph shows displacement of the epiphysis *(arrow)* from the metaphysis *(arrowhead)*.

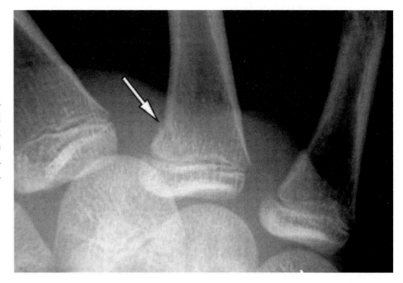

Figure 7–6. Salter type 2 fracture of the fourth proximal phalanx. Radiograph shows oblique fracture line *(arrows)* extending through metaphysis, abutting physis, and not involving epiphysis.

arrest. Type 4 injuries involve the epiphysis, physis, and metaphysis and, like type 3 injuries, have a high rate of growth arrest. Type 5 fractures consist of a crush injury to part or all of a physis. Posttraumatic growth arrest may be detected radiographically by demonstration of a bony bridge across the physis.

Commonly Encountered Fractures by Anatomic Location

There are unique features of pediatric fractures in almost all locations. The following sections review several of the more commonly encountered areas.

Wrist

The wrist is the most common area of fracture in children. Most fractures of the distal forearm are buckle or transverse fractures of the distal metaphysis of the radius with or without fracture of the metaphysis of the distal ulna. However, the distal radius is also the most common area of physeal fracture (28% of physeal injuries). Displacement or obliteration of the pronator fat pad is indicative of a fracture or deep soft tissue injury. The normal pronator fat pad is visualized on a lateral view of the forearm as a thin line of fat with a mildly convex border. With most distal forearm fractures, the pronator fat pad is of increased convexity or becomes obliterated with soft tissue attenuation.

Elbow

There are several unique features that make elbow injuries different in children than in adults. In contrast to adults, in whom fracture of the radial neck is the most common injury, supracondylar fractures are the most common fractures in children. They usually occur secondary to hyperextension from falling on an outstretched arm. Up to 25% of such fractures are incomplete and may be subtle on radiography. On radiographs, there is typically posterior displacement of the distal fragment such that a line drawn down the anterior cortex of the humerus (anterior humeral line) no longer bisects the middle third of the capitellum (Fig. 7–7). The fracture line is usually best seen through the anterior cortex of the distal humerus on the lateral view (see Fig. 7–7). A joint effusion is typically evident. Elbow effusions are identified when there is displacement of the posterior fat pad, resulting in its visualization on a lateral view (see Fig. 7–7). Normally, the posterior fat pad rests within the olecranon fossa and is not visible on a true lateral view of the elbow. The anterior fat pad, which is often visible normally, may become prominent and have a prominent apex anterior convexity.

There is much debate over the significance of a traumatic elbow effusion in the absence of a visualized fracture. It is often taught that such a joint effusion is synonymous with an occult fracture. However, studies have shown that fractures are probably present in the minority rather than the majority of such cases.

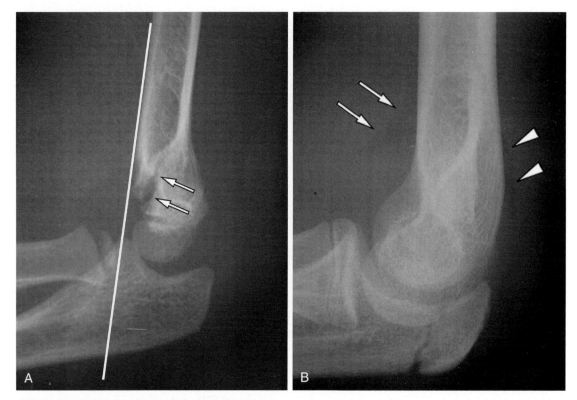

Figure 7–7. Manifestations of elbow trauma. *A,* Supracondylar fracture. Lateral radiograph shows fracture line through anterior cortex *(arrow).* There is posterior displacement of the capitellum in relation to the anterior humeral line. *B,* Elbow effusion. Lateral radiograph of the elbow shows elevation of both the anterior *(arrows)* and posterior *(arrowheads)* fat pads.

It is a moot point anyway, because traumatic injury to the elbow is treated with splinting whether a subtle fracture is identified or not. Therefore, obtaining additional oblique views or follow-up studies to document the presence or absence of a fracture exposes the patient to additional radiation and does not alter subsequent care.

Other elbow injuries include fractures of the lateral condyle (Fig. 7–8) and avulsion of the medial epicondyle ("little league elbow"). With avulsion of the medial epicondyle (10% of elbow injuries), the medial epicondyle may become displaced (Fig. 7–9). To avoid mistaking the displaced apophysis for one of the other ossicles of the elbow, it is important to know the predictable order of ossification of the elbow ossification centers. The order can be remembered by "CRITOEcal" (capitellum, radial head, internal epicondyle, trochlea, olecranon, external epicondyle).

Toddler's Fracture

When a child first begins to walk, there may be a nondisplaced oblique or spiral fracture of the midshaft of the tibia (Fig. 7–10). Such an injury is common and is referred to as a *toddler's fracture.* Most children present refusing to continue to walk or bear weight on that extremity. Oblique views often demonstrate the fracture better than do frontal or lateral views. Toddlers can suffer from similar types of fractures involving the calcaneus and cuboid.

Avulsive Fractures in Adolescents

An avulsion injury is a structural failure of bone at a tendon or aponeurotic insertion related to a tensile force applied from a musculoskeletal unit. Adolescents are prone to avulsive injuries because of a combination of their propensity for great strength, ability to sustain extreme levels of activity, and immature growing apophyses. The growing apophysis is often more prone to injury than are the adjacent tendons. The insertions of muscles capable of generating great forces are most predisposed to avulsion injuries.

Radiologists may encounter findings of

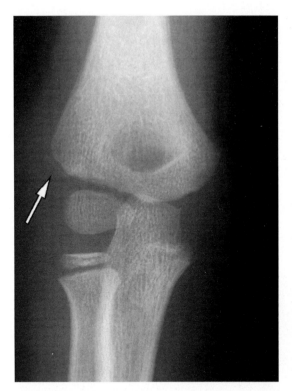

Figure 7–8. Fracture of the lateral condyle in a 6-year-old boy. Radiograph shows avulsed sliver of bone *(arrow)* arising from lateral condyle.

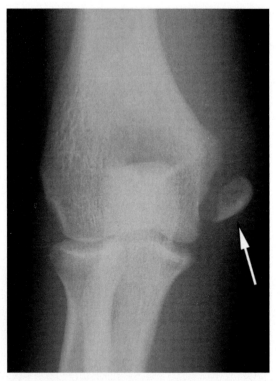

Figure 7–9. Avulsion of the medial epicondyle in a 14-year-old baseball pitcher. Frontal radiograph shows displacement of medial epicondyle *(arrow)* and overlying soft tissue swelling.

Figure 7–10. Toddler's fracture in a 1-year-old girl. Radiograph shows subtle oblique, nondisplaced fracture *(arrows)* through tibial shaft.

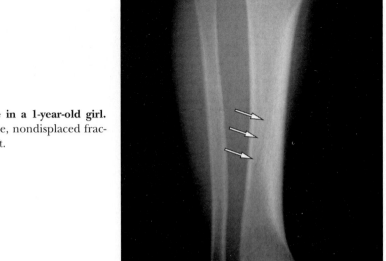

chronic avulsion when patients are imaged for pain or when the avulsions are seen incidentally when imaging is performed for other reasons. The irregularity and periostitis that can be associated with chronic avulsions should not be misinterpreted as suspicious for malignancy. In addition, if unwarranted biopsies of these areas are performed, the histologic changes associated with the healing callus of the avulsion injury may be misinterpreted as malignancy. The most common sites of avulsion occur within the pelvis, where muscles capable of great force attach. Sites at which apophyseal avulsions most commonly occur, along with the associated muscular attachments, include the iliac crest (transversalis, in-

ternal oblique abdominal muscle, external oblique abdominal muscle), anterior superior iliac spine (sartorius), anterior inferior iliac spine (rectus femoris), ischial apophyses (hamstring muscles: biceps femoris, gracilis, semimembranosus, semitendinosus) (Fig. 7–11), and lesser trochanter (iliopsoas) (Fig. 7–12). The radiographic findings of avulsion injuries include displacement of the ossified apophysis from a normal position and variable, often exuberant amounts of associated periosteal new bone formation.

The extensor mechanism of the knee consists of the quadriceps femoris muscles, quadriceps tendon, the patella, the patellar tendon, and the patellar tendon insertion on the tibial

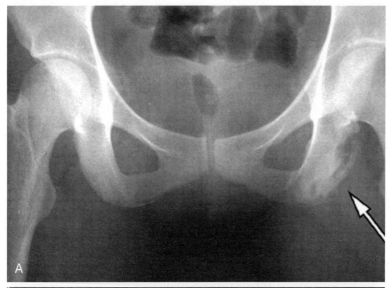

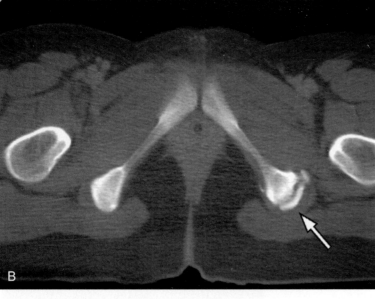

Figure 7–11. Avulsion injury of the ischial apophysis in a 15-year-old girl. *A,* Radiographs show irregularity and mixed sclerosis and lucency involving the left ischium *(arrow)*. *B,* Computed tomographic scan further shows the fragmentation and irregularity of the region *(arrow)*. There is no soft tissue mass or findings to suggest other causes, such as malignancy, as a cause of the pain.

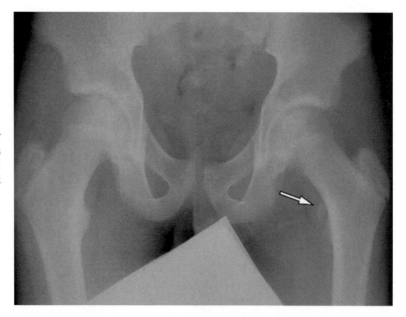

Figure 7–12. Avulsion injury of the lesser trochanter in a 14-year-old boy. Radiograph shows displacement of the left lesser trochanter *(arrow)*.

tuberosity; this mechanism can also be involved by avulsion injuries. Chronic avulsion of the patellar tendon at its proximal attachment to the patella is call *Sinding-Larsen-Johansson syndrome.* It occurs most commonly in children between the ages of 10 and 14 years. Symptoms include localized pain and swelling over the inferior aspect of the patella associated with restricted knee motion. Radiography demonstrates irregular bony fragments at the inferior margin of the patella associated with adjacent soft tissue swelling and thickening and indistinctness of the patellar tendon (Fig. 7–13). Chronic avulsive injury of the patellar tendon and its inferior attachment is referred to as *Osgood-Schlatter disease* (tibial tuberosity avulsion). It is a common disorder that most often affects active adolescent boys. Symptoms include pain and swelling over the tibial tuberosity. Radiography demonstrates bony fragmentation of the tibial tuberosity, associated adjacent soft tissue swelling, and thickening and indistinctness of the patellar tendon (see Fig. 7–13).

Child Abuse

Child abuse, also referred to by the more politically correct and less graphic term *nonaccidental trauma,* is unfortunately common. It is estimated that more than 1 million children are seriously injured and 5000 killed secondary to abuse each year in the United States alone. Most of the children are younger than 1 year,

and almost all are younger than 6 years. When clinical or imaging findings are suspicious for potential abuse, a radiographic skeletal survey is typically obtained. The purpose of the skeletal survey is to document the presence of findings of abuse for legal reasons so that the child can be removed from exposure to the abuser. Other tests that are sometimes used include a repeat skeletal survey in approximately 2 weeks to look for healing injuries not seen on the initial skeletal survey, skeletal scintigraphy, abdominal CT, and magnetic resonance imaging (MRI) of the brain. The identification and reporting of findings of child abuse by the radiologist is an important task. False-positive findings can cause a nonabused child to be removed from the family, whereas false-negative findings can result in returning a child to a potentially life-threatening environment.

The radiographic findings of abuse vary in their specificity. One of the highly specific findings is the presence of posterior rib fractures occurring near the costovertebral joints (Fig. 7–14). They are thought to occur from an adult squeezing the infant's thorax. Such rib fractures may be subtle prior to the development of callus formation. The evaluation of rib fractures should be a routine part of the evaluation of the chest radiograph of any infant. Another finding highly specific of abuse is the metaphyseal corner fracture (see Fig. 7–14). This fracture extends through the primary spongiosa of the metaphysis, the weakest portion, and is most likely secondary to a forceful pulling of an extremity. The broken

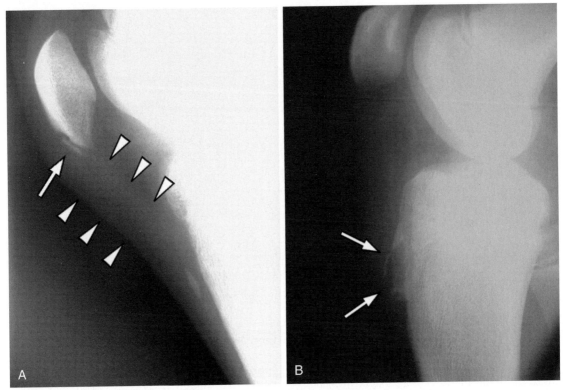

Figure 7–13. Avulsion injuries to the extensor mechanism of the knee. *A,* Findings of chronic avulsion of the patellar tendon at its proximal attachment to the patella (Sinding-Larsen-Johansson syndrome) shown as thickening of the patellar tendon *(arrowheads)* and irregularity at the attachment to the patella *(arrow).* *B,* Findings of chronic avulsion of the patellar tendon at its distal attachment to the tibial tuberosity (Osgood-Schlatter lesion) shown as irregularity and fragmentation of the tibial tuberosity *(arrows)* with overlying soft tissue swelling.

metaphyseal rim will appear as a corner fracture (triangular piece of bone) when seen tangentially or as a crescentic rim of bone (the "bucket handle fracture") when seen obliquely. Other specific fractures include those of the scapula, spinous process, and sternum. In fact, any fracture seen in an infant should be viewed with suspicion because up to 30% of fractures seen in infants are secondary to abuse. Spiral long bone fractures in nonambulatory children are highly suspicious. Multiple fractures of different ages (some with callus and some acute) as well as multiple fractures of different body parts are highly suspicious for abuse (see Fig. 7–14). Extraskeletal findings seen in abuse include acute or chronic subdural hematomas, cerebral edema (asphyxia), intraparenchymal brain hematoma, lung contusions, duodenal hematoma, solid abdominal organ laceration, and pancreatitis.

The clinical and imaging findings of abuse do not usually require a differential diagnosis.

However, other entities that may cause multiple fractures or radiographic findings that could be confused with injury, such as periosteal reaction, should always be considered. The primary entities that may present with multiple fractures in an infant are osteogenesis imperfecta and Menkes syndrome. Both of these entities are also associated with excessive wormian bones and osteopenia.

Periosteal Reaction in the Newborn

When periosteal reaction is encountered in the newborn, there are a number of entities that must be considered (Table 7–1), for example, physiologic new bone formation, TORCH (see below), prostaglandin therapy, Caffey disease, metastatic disease from neuroblastoma, and abuse. Physiologic periosteal new bone formation can commonly be seen in infants during the first few months of life. It typically involves long bones of rapid

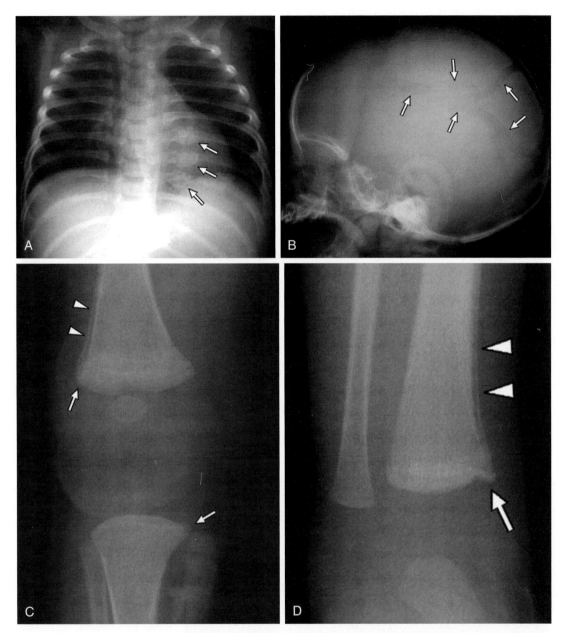

Figure 7–14. Multiple findings of abuse on skeletal survey of a 3-month-old infant. *A,* Chest radiograph shows callus formation along fractures of multiple posterior medial ribs *(arrows).* *B,* Skull radiograph shows "eggshell"-type fractures *(arrows)* throughout skull. *C,* Radiograph of the knees shows corner fracture of the metaphyses *(arrows)* of the distal femur and proximal tibia. There is an associated periosteal reaction *(arrowheads)* of the fracture of the femur. *D,* Radiograph of the tibia demonstrates additional corner fracture *(arrow)* and periosteal reaction *(arrowheads).*

growth, such as the femur, tibia, and humerus. Differential features that support physiologic growth as the cause of periosteal reaction as opposed to a pathologic cause include a symmetric distribution, benign appearance of the periosteal reaction, and appropriate age of the child. When periosteal reaction involves the femur, tibia, or humerus, the other two of the three bones are also usually involved. On radiographs, there are one or more dense lines of periosteal reaction paralleling the cortex of the diaphysis of the long bones. Neonates with congenital heart disease are often treated with prostaglandins in order to main-

TABLE 7–1. **Differential Diagnosis for Periosteal Reaction in the Newborn**

Physiologic growth
TORCH infections
  Syphilis, rubella
Prostaglandin therapy
Caffey disease (infantile cortical hyperostosis)
Neuroblastoma metastasis
Abuse

TORCH = toxoplasmosis, other infections, rubella, cytomegalovirus infection, and herpes simplex (association).

tain patency of the ductus venosus. Children on such therapy often demonstrate prominent periosteal reaction.

TORCH Infections

The differential diagnosis for transplacentally acquired infections can be remembered by TORCH: toxoplasmosis, other (syphilis), rubella, cytomegalovirus infection, and herpes simplex. *Congenital rubella syndrome* is the most common of the transplacental viral infections. Features include eye abnormalities, deafness, hepatosplenomegaly, aortic and pulmonic stenosis, and intrauterine growth retardation. Bone changes are present in up to 50% of

cases. These changes include irregular fraying of the metaphyses of long bones and generalized lucency of the metaphyses. The findings have been likened to a "celery stalk" appearance (Fig. 7–15). These radiographic findings are most apparent during the first few weeks of life.

Syphilis

Congenital syphilis occurs secondary to transplacental infection, usually during the second or third trimester. Clinical findings include hepatosplenomegaly, rash, rhinorrhea, anemia, and ascites. Bony changes are present in up to 95% of patients but often do not occur until 6 to 8 weeks after the time of infection. The radiographic findings may be present before blood serologic test results are positive. Findings include nonspecific metaphyseal lucent bands and periosteal reaction involving multiple long bones (Fig. 7–16). The Wimberger corner sign is the most specific finding of syphilis and consists of destruction of the medial portion of the proximal metaphysis of the tibia, resulting in an area of irregular lucency (see Fig. 7–16).

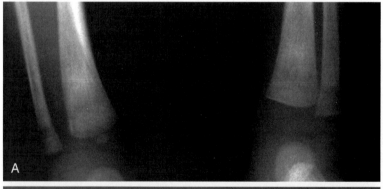

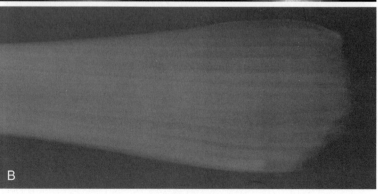

Figure 7–15. Congenital rubella in a 6-week-old infant. *A,* Radiograph shows irregular fraying of the metaphyses and alternating longitudinal dark and light bands of density, or "celery stalking." *B,* Radiograph of a celery stalk for comparison.

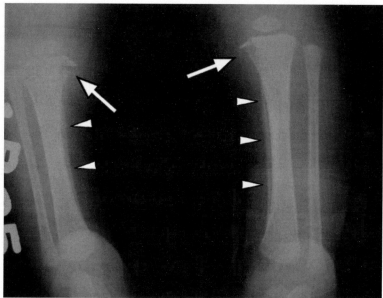

Figure 7–16. Congenital syphilis in a 6-week-old girl. Radiograph shows periosteal reaction along the shafts of the bilateral tibias *(arrowheads)*. There is also characteristic lucency of medial proximal femoral condyles *(arrows)*, which is called the *Wimberger corner sign*.

Caffey Disease (Infantile Cortical Hyperostosis)

Caffey disease is an idiopathic syndrome that consists of periosteal reaction seen on radiographs, irritability, fever, and soft tissue swelling over the areas of periosteal reaction. It occurs during the first few months of life. The most common bones involved include the mandible, clavicles, ribs, humerus, ulna, femur, scapula, and radius. Imaging shows periosteal new bone formation, sclerosis, and adjacent soft tissue swelling (Fig. 7–17). The disease is self-limited and is currently seen much less frequently than in the past.

LUCENT PERMEATIVE LESIONS IN CHILDREN

A bone lesion is considered permeative when it has ill-defined borders, a wide zone of transition, and consists centrally of multiple, small, irregular holes. As in adults, a permeative bone lesion in a child is consistent with an aggressive inflammatory or neoplastic lesion. The finding is nonspecific. The more common causes of a permeative lesion in a child include osteomyelitis, Langerhans cell histiocytosis (LCH), neuroblastoma metastasis, Ewing sarcoma, and lymphoma or leukemia. The differential diagnosis can be limited to most likely diagnoses even further by considering the patient's age (Table 7–2). If the patient is younger than 5 years, the most likely diagnoses include osteomyelitis, LCH, and metastatic neuroblastoma. Ewing sarcoma and lymphoma are exceedingly rare in children younger than 5 years. In older children, Ewing sarcoma and lymphoma or leukemia become candidates, and metastatic neuroblastoma becomes much less likely.

Osteomyelitis

Acute osteomyelitis is a relatively common cause of clinically significant bone pathology in children. It is primarily a disease of infants and young children, with one third of cases occurring before 2 years and one half of cases occurring before 5 years. Because of the young age of most of the children, the presentation is often nonspecific, and diagnosis delayed. The erythrocyte sedimentation rate is elevated

TABLE 7–2. **Differential Diagnosis for a Permeative Bone Lesion in a Child Based on Age**

Less than 5 Yr
Osteomyelitis
Langerhans cell histiocytosis
Neuroblastoma metastasis
Greater than 5 Yr
Ewing sarcoma
Lymphoma and leukemia
Osteomyelitis
Langerhans cell histiocytosis

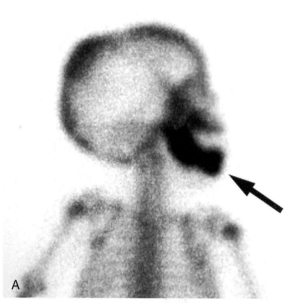

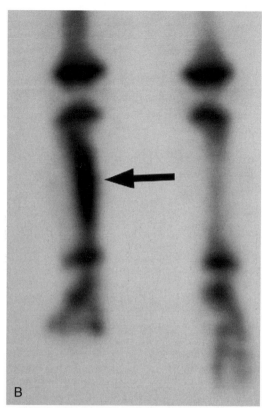

Figure 7–17. Caffey disease in an infant. Skeletal scintigraphy shows marked increased uptake *(arrows)* in the mandible *(A)* and tibia *(B)*.

in the overwhelming number of cases. Most cases of osteomyelitis are hematogenous in origin, with many patients having a recent history of preceding respiratory tract infection or otitis media. *Staphylococcus aureus* is the most common cause.

Osteomyelitis has a tendency to occur in the metaphyses or metaphyseal equivalents of children. This is thought to be related to the rich but slow-moving blood supply to these regions. Approximately 75% of cases will involve the metaphyses of long bones, with the most common sites being the femur, tibia, and humerus. The other 25% of cases occur within metaphyseal equivalents of flat bones, most typically involving the bony pelvis.

The earliest radiographic finding of osteomyelitis is deep soft tissue swelling, evident by displacement or obliteration of fat planes, adjacent to a metaphysis (Fig. 7–18). Bony changes may not be present until 10 days after the onset of symptoms. Initial bony changes consist of poorly defined lucency involving a metaphyseal area. There is often progressive bony destruction (see Fig. 7–18). Periosteal new bone formation occurs at approximately 10 days. Osteomyelitis can appear as sclerotic, rather than lucent, when it is a chronic process

(see Fig. 7–18). Other imaging modalities that are used in the evaluation of suspected osteomyelitis include skeletal scintigraphy, MRI, and occasionally CT. On skeletal scintigraphy, osteomyelitis appears as a focal area of increased activity on the angiographic, soft tissue, and skeletal phase images. Skeletal scintigraphy becomes positive early after the onset of osteomyelitis and is often positive before the development of radiographic changes. Another advantage of scintigraphy is the ability to evaluate for multiple sites of involvement. MRI also demonstrates abnormal findings early after the onset of osteomyelitis. Osteomyelitis appears as an area of increased T2-weighted signal within a metaphysis. There are usually large areas of surrounding edema, shown as an increased T2-weighted signal, within the adjacent bone marrow and soft tissues. Gadolinium administration may show areas of nonenhancement suspicious for necrosis or abscess formation.

Langerhans Cell Histiocytosis

LCH, also know as *eosinophilic granuloma* and *histiocytosis X*, is an idiopathic disorder that

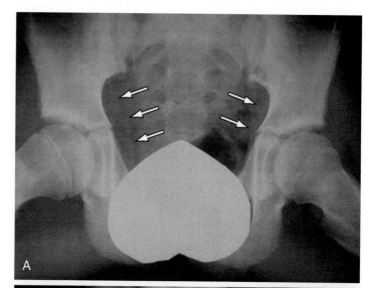

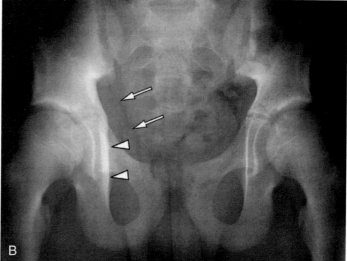

Figure 7–18. Osteomyelitis in a 14-year-old boy. *A,* Initial pelvic radiograph shows asymmetric thickening *(arrows)* displacing the right obturator fat pad in comparison to the left. The finding was not noted. *B,* Repeat pelvic radiograph obtained 5 months later demonstrates persistent asymmetric thickening *(arrows)* displacing the right obturator fat pad. There are now sclerosis and thickening of the right ilioischial line *(arrows)*. *C,* Computed tomographic scan shows defect *(arrow)* in right posterior acetabulum with surrounding sclerosis. The surrounding soft tissues are thickened *(arrowheads)*, displacing the adjacent fat pads and illustrating why displaced fat pads are seen on radiographs.

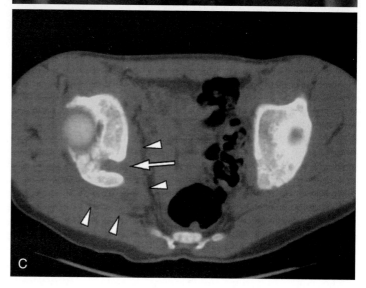

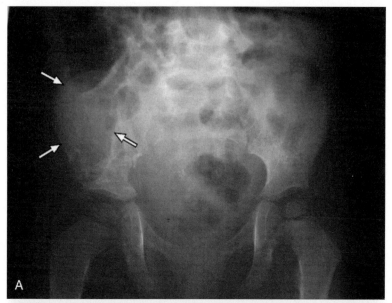

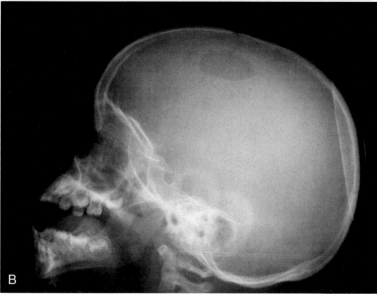

Figure 7–19. Langerhans cell histiocytosis in a 2-year-old girl. *A,* Radiograph shows lytic destructive lesion of right ilium *(arrows). B,* Radiograph shows well-defined lytic lesion of skull.

may manifest as focal, localized, or systemic disease. It remains unclear whether the disease process is inflammatory or neoplastic. It is characterized by abnormal proliferation of Langerhans cells. The disease is twice as common in boys than in girls and occurs most commonly in whites. Although the degree of disease from focal to systemic is a spectrum, there are several specific categories of disease. *Letterer-Siwe disease* is an acute disseminated form of LCH that occurs in children younger than 1 year. There is an acute onset of hepatosplenomegaly, rash, lymphadenopathy, marrow failure, and pulmonary involvement. Skeletal involvement may not be present. The prognosis is poor, with most children dying within 1 to 2 years. *Hand-Schüller-Christian disease* is the chronic form of systemic LCH. Most of these patients have skeletal involvement. Other manifestations include hepatosplenomegaly, diabetes insipidus, exophthalmos, dermatitis, and growth retardation. These patients typically present at 3 to 6 years of age, and morbidity is high. *Eosinophilic granuloma* is the term used when the process is isolated to bone or lung. Such cases make up to 70% of cases of LCH, and the prognosis is excellent. Most patients have a single site of bony involvement.

The radiographic appearance of skeletal manifestations in LCH is extremely variable. Lesions may be lucent or sclerotic, permeative or geographic, and have a sclerotic or poorly defined border. The most common sites of LCH, in decreasing order of frequency, include the skull (Fig. 7–19), ribs, femur, pelvis (see Fig. 7–19), spine, and mandible. Skull lesions may have a "beveled edge," related to uneven destruction of the inner and outer tables of the skull. Rib lesions may be multiple and often have an expanded appearance. When the spine is involved, a classic finding is vertebral plana (vertebral destruction with severe collapse).

Most children who present with a lesion suspicious for LCH will be evaluated with a skeletal survey to identify other bony lesions, a chest radiograph to exclude pulmonary involvement, and often MRI or CT (Fig. 7–20) to characterize and evaluate the anatomic extent of disease.

Ewing Sarcoma

Ewing sarcoma is the second most common primary malignancy of bone after osteosarcoma. It is an aggressive, small, round, blue cell tumor similar to a primitive neuroectodermal tumor. Ewing sarcoma most commonly occurs in the second decade of life and occurrence at less than 5 years of age is exceedingly rare. The most common sites of involvement in decreasing order of frequency include the femur, pelvis, tibia, humerus, and ribs. Two thirds of cases involve the pelvis or femur.

The radiographic appearance of Ewing sarcoma is variable. Most lesions involve the metaphysis, but diaphyseal involvement is more common than with other bone malignancies. Most lesions have an aggressive appearance: a lucent lesion with poorly defined borders and a permeative appearance to the cortex (Figs. 7–21 and 7–22). Aggressive-appearing periosteal new bone formation (spiculated, onion skin, Codman triangle) is often present. However, Ewing sarcoma can appear predominantly sclerotic in up to 15% of cases. MRI demonstrates a destructive bony mass, often with an associated soft tissue component (see Figs. 7–21 and 7–22). The 5-year survival rate for Ewing sarcoma is 70% for localized disease and 30% when metastatic disease is present.

Metastatic Disease

In children, most cases of metastatic disease are from small round blue cell tumors. The most common primary neoplasms to metastasize to bone are neuroblastoma and leukemia or lymphoma. In any child younger than 5 years with a neoplastic bony lesion, metastatic neuroblastoma (Fig. 7–23) should be considered and is much more likely than a primary bone neoplasm. Leukemia and lymphoma may deposit in the regions of the metaphyses and cause bony destruction. The appearance is often that of lucent metaphyseal bands (Fig. 7–

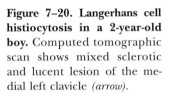

Figure 7–20. Langerhans cell histiocytosis in a 2-year-old boy. Computed tomographic scan shows mixed sclerotic and lucent lesion of the medial left clavicle *(arrow)*.

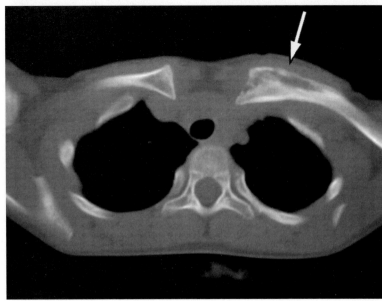

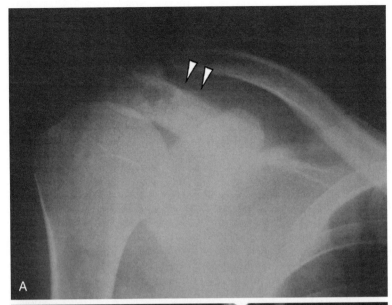

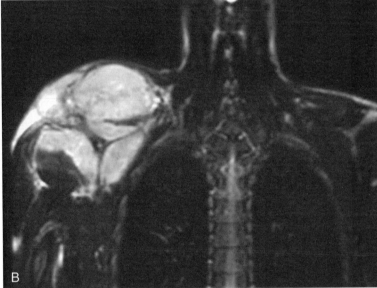

Figure 7–21. Ewing sarcoma in a 17-year-old boy who was treated by a chiropractor for shoulder pain for almost 2 years. *A,* Radiograph shows permeative lucency within right acromion with associated periosteal reaction *(arrowheads).* *B,* Coronal T2-weighted image shows large soft tissue mass arising from and surrounding the right scapula.

24). These bands are nonspecific but are often referred to as leukemic lines. Primary bone lymphoma is rare in children.

FOCAL SCLEROTIC LESIONS IN CHILDREN

There are multiple causes of focal sclerotic bone lesions in children. The more common causes are listed in Table 7–3.

Osteoid Osteoma

Osteoid osteoma is a relatively common lesion of bone. Most cases occur in the second de-

cade of life and usually present with pain. Classically, the pain is worse at night and is relieved with aspirin. The lesions are more common in boys. The cause is unknown, and it is currently unclear whether the lesion is a benign neoplasm or an inflammatory lesion. Most commonly, osteoid osteomas occur

TABLE 7–3. **Common Causes of Focal Sclerotic Lesions in Children**

Osteoid osteoma
Chronic osteomyelitis
Stress fracture
Osteosarcoma

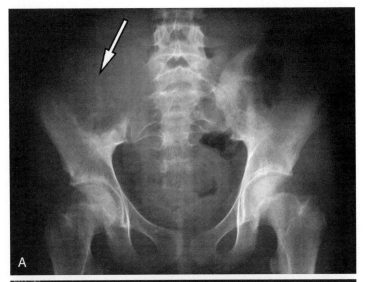

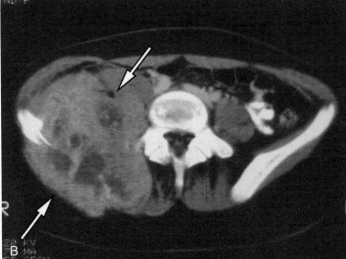

Figure 7–22. Ewing sarcoma in a 13-year-old girl who was treated by a chiropractor for hip pain for almost 1 year. *A,* Radiograph shows lucency destroying right iliac wing *(arrow).* CT *(B)* and T2-weighted axial MRI *(C)* show large soft tissue mass *(arrows)* arising out of and destroying right iliac wing.

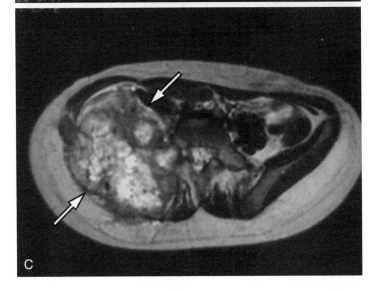

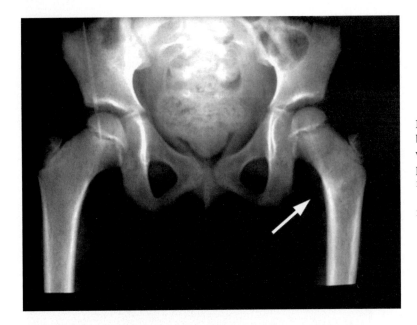

Figure 7–23. Metastatic neuro-blastoma in a 5-year-old girl who presented with left hip pain. Radiograph shows asymmetric permeative lucency *(arrow)* within the left proximal femur.

within the cortex of the metadiaphyses or diaphyses of the long bones of the lower extremities.

On radiography, osteoid osteomas appear as a lucent cortical nidus surrounded by an area of reactive sclerosis (Fig. 7–25). The nidus is typically less than 1.5 cm in diameter. Classically, a punctate radiodensity is identified within the central lucency (a dense dot within a lucent area, surrounded by sclerotic density). CT is often used to further characterize the lesion (the punctate central radiodensity and

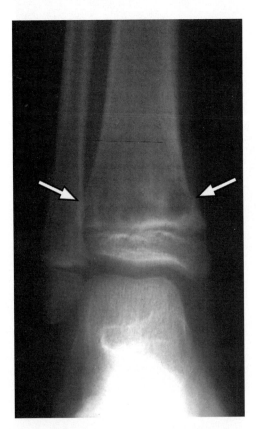

Figure 7–24. Leukemia in a 7-year-old girl. Radiograph shows irregular lucent metaphyseal band (leukemic line) *(arrows)* involving distal tibia.

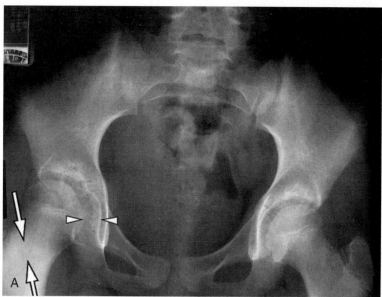

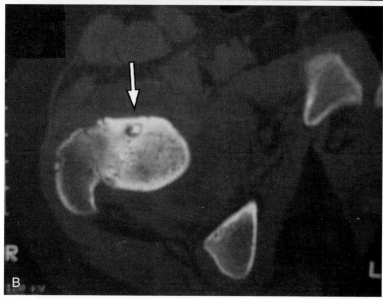

Figure 7–25. Osteoid osteoma in an 11-year-old girl. *A,* Radiograph shows increased sclerosis of intertrochanteric region of right femur. Within this area of sclerosis is a round central lucency *(arrows)* containing a central punctate density. There is an associated joint effusion identified by asymmetric widening of the right joint space *(arrowheads)*. *B,* Computed tomographic scan shows dense nidus *(arrow)* within central lucency and surrounding sclerosis.

lucency are often better demonstrated on CT than on radiography) (see Fig. 7–25) and to define the anatomic position of the nidus. At some institutions, CT is used for guidance in percutaneous drill removal of the osteoid osteoma. Skeletal scintigraphy demonstrates a "double-density sign" of intense increased uptake by the nidus surrounded by less intense but abnormally increased uptake by the surrounding sclerotic bone.

Stress Fracture

A stress fracture is defined as an injury from repetitive trauma. It usually occurs when a new

or intense activity has recently been initiated. The most common sites of stress fractures in children, in decreasing order of frequency, include the tibia, fibula, metatarsals, and calcaneus. Stress fractures appear on radiographs as a transverse or oblique band of sclerosis or a lucent line surrounded by sclerosis or periosteal new bone formation (Fig. 7–26). Periosteal new bone formation may be the only finding. In the tibia, the most common location is the proximal posterior cortex, but the anterior cortex can also be involved. In the calcaneus, there is typically a vertical sclerotic band paralleling the posterior cortex. Calcaneal stress fractures most commonly occur

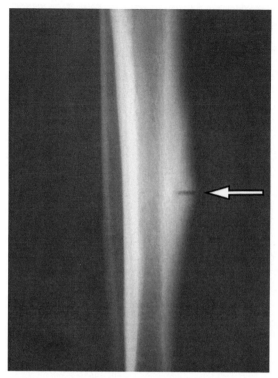

Figure 7–26. Stress fracture of the tibia in a 16-year-old boy. Radiograph shows marked cortical thickening and sclerosis surrounding a horizontal lucency *(arrow)* through the anterior cortex of the tibia.

after a child has a cast removed and returns to activity after a period of prolonged disuse (Fig. 7–27). Skeletal scintigraphy demonstrates stress fracture as an area of focal increased

uptake days to weeks before the development of radiographic findings. CT may be helpful in demonstrating a linear nature of the lesion when a sclerotic lesion is being evaluated for stress fracture, osteoid osteoma, or osteomyelitis.

Osteosarcoma

Osteosarcoma, or osteogenic sarcoma, is the most common primary bone malignancy of childhood. It occurs most commonly in patients between 10 and 15 years. Although most cases of osteosarcoma arise in otherwise healthy children, there are certain predisposing conditions, such as hereditary retinoblastoma or previous radiation therapy. It is more common in boys than in girls. Osteosarcoma is a malignant lesion that uniquely gives rise to neoplastic osteoid and bone. The majority of osteosarcoma cases arise from the medullary cavity, but the lesion may arise from the surface of bone. The latter scenario gives rise to the periosteal and parosteal forms. The most common sites for development are the metaphyses of long bones. More than 60% of cases of osteosarcoma arise in the region of the knee (distal femur or proximal tibia).

The radiographic appearance of osteosarcoma is dependent on the amount of bony destruction and new bone formation. The lesions are typically large at the time of presentation. The destruction component of the tumor is demonstrated by lucent destruction of a metaphysis with aggressive features (aggressive periosteal reaction, poorly defined borders).

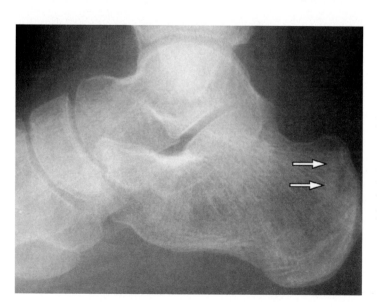

Figure 7–27. Stress fracture of the calcaneus in a 10-year-old boy. He had pain following return to activity after lower extremity was casted for different fracture. Radiograph shows vertical sclerotic band *(arrows)* in posterior calcaneus.

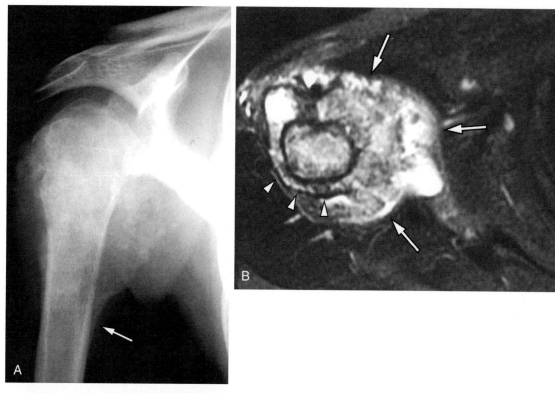

Figure 7–28. Osteosarcoma of the proximal humerus in a 16-year-old boy. *A,* Radiograph shows permeative lucency in the proximal shaft of the humerus, new bone formation, and periosteal reaction. There is a Codman triangle *(arrow).* *B,* Axial, T2-weighted MR image shows high signal mass *(arrows)* surrounding the proximal humeral shaft. The elevated periosteum appears as a black line *(arrowheads).* There is also an abnormal high signal within the marrow.

Tumor bone is seen in more than 90% of cases of osteosarcoma and helps differentiate this tumor from other types of bone malignancies (Fig. 7–28). It appears as a cloud-like density. A feature that helps differentiate tumor bone from sclerotic reactive bone is that tumor bone often extends beyond the expected confines of the bony shaft. In most cases of osteosarcoma, there is a large soft tissue mass present at the time of diagnosis. In poorly differentiated, aggressive lesions, tumor bone may not be present, and the lesion appears as a nonspecific, aggressive lucent lesion.

MRI is used to evaluate the extent of bone and soft tissue involvement for presurgical planning. The extent of marrow abnormality, soft tissue mass, and cortical destruction is well demonstrated as an abnormal, increased T2-weighted signal on MRI. This modality is not accurate in differentiating peritumoral marrow edema from tumor-involved marrow. Therefore, any abnormal signal within the marrow is generally considered to be involved by tumor in regard to surgical planning. MRI

is accurate in depicting the relationship between the soft tissue mass and adjacent nerves and vascular structures. It is important to image the entire length of the long bone involved by the tumor because osteosarcoma can occasionally have discontinuous involvement of a bone (skip lesions), and identification of such skip lesions affects surgical planning. Surgery in conjunction with chemotherapy is standard therapy, with limb salvage procedures currently being performed in up to 80% of patients. Five-year survival has increased to 77% since the late 1990s. Often, a course of chemotherapy is administered and the patient reimaged before surgery. MRI has been shown to be useful in predicting chemotherapeutic response by demonstrating a decrease in the size of the soft tissue mass and amount of peritumoral edema. The most common type of metastatic disease is pulmonary (lung nodules), which is evaluated with CT. Skeletal metastatic disease is reported to be present in up to 15% of patients and is evaluated with skeletal scintigraphy.

TABLE 7–4. **Multifocal Bone Lesions in Children**

Multifocal osteomyelitis
Langerhans cell histiocytosis
Metastatic disease
Multiple hereditary exostoses (osteochondromatosis)
Enchondromatosis (Ollier disease, Maffucci syndrome)
Polyostotic fibrous dysplasia (McCune-Albright syndrome)
Neurofibromatosis

MULTIFOCAL BONE LESIONS IN CHILDREN

The presence of multifocal involvement narrows the differential diagnosis for bone lesions in children (Table 7–4). Osteomyelitis, Langerhans cell histiocytosis, and metastatic disease have already been discussed. In addition, there are several hereditary syndromes that cause multifocal bone lesions in children.

In *multiple hereditary exostoses (osteochondromatosis)*, there is a propensity for the development of multiple bilateral osteochondromas. These lesions appear as bony growths that arise from the metaphysis and are continuous with the adjacent bony cortex. They have a tendency to "point" away from joints. The most common location is the bones around the knee. With osteochondromatosis, the lesions can lead to a number of problems, including limb shortening, leg length discrepancy, bowing and deformity, compression of adjacent nerves and vessels, and malignant degeneration into chondrosarcoma (5% of patients with osteochondromatosis). The more proximal lesions have a greater propensity for malignant degeneration.

With *enchondromatosis (Ollier disease)*, there is a propensity for the development of multiple enchondromas. Although the lesions have a propensity to be on one side of the body, they are usually seen bilaterally. Although solitary enchondromas tend to occur in the hands and feet, lesions of enchondromatosis tend to be located in the metaphyses of long bones. With growth, the lesions may take on an oblong or flame-shaped linear configuration, perpendicular to the physis (Fig. 7–29). Malignant de-

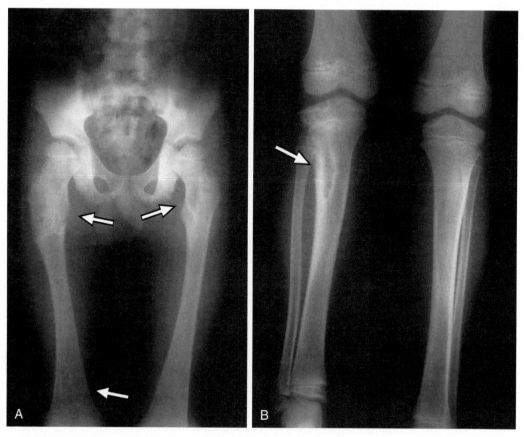

Figure 7–29. Enchondromatosis shown as multiple lucent lesions *(arrows)*. They are predominantly on the right side, involving the femur *(A)* and tibia *(B)*. The lesions have a flame-shape appearance perpendicular to the physis.

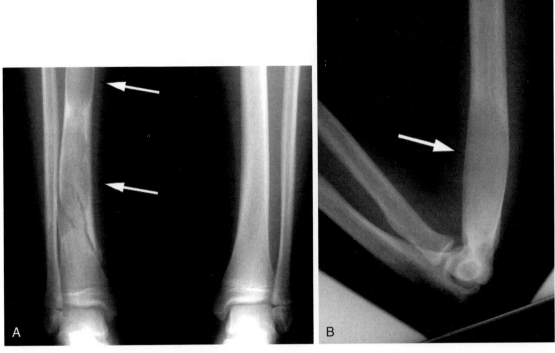

Figure 7–30. Polyostotic fibrous dysplasia in a 7-year-old girl with precocious puberty (McCune-Albright syndrome). Radiographs of the tibia *(A)* and humerus *(B)* show multiple unilateral lesions *(arrows)* consistent with fibrous dysplasia. There is a pathologic fracture through the tibia. Note the ground-glass appearance, most notably in the lesion within the humerus. The lesions are slightly expansile.

generation is higher than seen with osteochondromatosis, occurring in approximately 30% of lesions. When soft tissue venous malformations are seen in conjunction with multiple enchondromas, the syndrome is called *Maffucci syndrome*. Phleboliths may be seen in soft tissue masses on radiographs. Patients with Maffucci syndrome have a higher incidence of malignant degeneration than do those with Ollier syndrome and also are at increased risk for malignant neoplasms of the abdomen and central nervous system.

McCune-Albright syndrome is the presence of polyostotic fibrous dysplasia, skin pigmentation abnormalities, and endocrine abnormalities. The most common endocrine abnormality is precocious puberty in girls. Polyostotic fibrous dysplasia most commonly involves the facial bones, pelvis, spine, and proximal humeri. There is a tendency for the lesions to be unilateral. Many patients present with pathologic fracture by 10 years (Fig. 7–30). There is no predisposition to malignancy. Fibrous dysplasia has a variable appearance radiographically. It can be purely lytic or sclerotic and expansile or nonexpansile. The classic descrip-

tion is that of "ground glass opacity" (see Fig. 7–30). This is a smudged and somewhat dense appearance to the central portion of the lesion. Periosteal reaction should be present only if there is a pathologic fracture.

CONSTITUTIONAL DISORDERS OF BONE

The term *constitutional disorder of bone* refers to a developmental abnormality of bone resulting in diffuse bony abnormality. The skeletal dysplasias, mucopolysaccharidoses, and osteogenesis imperfecta fall into this category.

Skeletal Dysplasias

Somehow, many persons think pediatric radiology is synonymous with having a textbook knowledge of skeletal dysplasias. This unfortunate misunderstanding could not be further from the truth. Most pediatric radiologists deal with skeletal dysplasia fairly infrequently and typically know only enough about it that they can recognize that a dysplasia is present and that they need help. Most pediatric institutions have one person who is enthralled with and knowledgeable about skeletal dysplasias and that person is consulted whenever a dysplasia arises. If such a person is not available, there are excellent textbooks for consultation. I recommend the one by Taybi and Lachman. It is practical to have an approach to the dysplasias and know something about the more common ones. The radiographic identification of a particular dysplasia can be helpful for prognostication and genetic counseling for the parents (e.g., is the identified dysplasia a dominant or recessive trait?).

Radiographic evaluation of dysplasia requires images of the skull, spine, thorax, pelvis, and extremities. An important feature for categorization is identification of whether the extremities are shortened and, if so, which portion of the extremities is short. Extremity shortening can be classified as rhizomelic, mesomelic, or acromelic (Fig. 7–31). *Rhizomelic* refers to proximal (humerus, femur) shorten-

ing and is seen with achondroplasia and thanatophoric dwarfism. *Mesomelic* refers to middle (radius-ulna, tibia-fibula) narrowing. Most of the mesomelic dysplasias are rare. *Acromelic* refers to distal shortening and is seen with asphyxiating thoracic dystrophy (Jeune syndrome) and chondroectodermal dysplasia (Ellis–van Creveld syndrome). Other features that are helpful in categorizing dysplasias include determining whether there is skull enlargement, short ribs (Fig. 7–32), a short spine, abnormal vertebral bodies (see Fig. 7–32), and an abnormal pelvic configuration (Fig. 7–33). The pelvis may demonstrate abnormalities in the configuration of the iliac wings or in the appearance of the acetabulum. The iliac wings may be abnormally tall or short or have a "squared" appearance. The acetabular angle may be decreased (acetabular roof appears horizontal). *Trident acetabulum* refers to when the acetabulum demonstrates three inferior pointing spikes, resembling an upside-down "trident." This is a "buzz word" for Jeune syndrome but also can be seen with Ellis–van

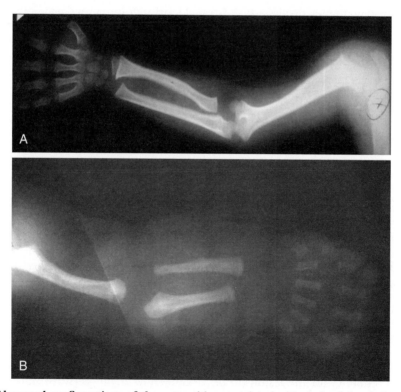

Figure 7–31. Abnormal configurations of the extremities associated with skeletal dysplasias. *A,* Rhizomelic (proximal) limb shortening demonstrated in achondroplasia, with the most severe limb shortening involving the humerus. Note the associated metaphyseal flaring. *B,* Acromelic (distal) limb shortening in chondroectodermal dysplasia, with most severe shortening involving the bones of the hands and radius and ulna. Note the polydactyly, which is also associated with chondroectodermal dysplasia.

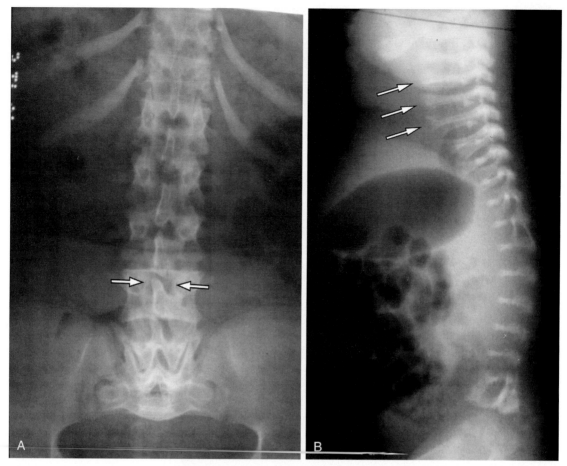

Figure 7–32. Abnormal configurations of the spine seen with skeletal dysplasias. *A*, Achondroplasia. Frontal radiograph shows that the interpediculate distance *(arrows)* becomes narrower more inferiorly. *B*, Thanatophoric dysplasia. The vertebral bodies demonstrate platyspondyly. Also, note the short ribs *(arrows)*, resulting in a narrow anterior to posterior diameter of the chest and protuberant abdomen.

Creveld syndrome and thanatophoric dysplasia. Some of the more common dysplasias and their radiographic manifestations are described in Table 7–5.

Achondroplasia

Achondroplasia is discussed in more detail because it is the most common short-limbed dwarfism. It is an autosomal dominant disease, with the heterozygous form demonstrating the clinical manifestations and the homozygous form being lethal. Patients with achondroplasia demonstrate rhizomelic limb shortening (see Fig. 7–31). There is craniofacial disproportion, an enlarged skull, small skull base, and small foramen magnum and jugular foramina. The latter may result in brainstem

compression. In the spine, the vertebral bodies are short and decreased in anterior to posterior diameter. The disk spaces are too tall. There is a decrease in the interpediculate distance on frontal radiographs, with this distance being narrower in the more inferior lumbar spine than in the more superior lumbar spine (the opposite of normal) (see Fig. 7–32). The pedicles are also short in the anterior to posterior diameter. Because of these findings, achondroplasts are prone to spinal stenosis. The shortened long bones show metaphyseal flaring (see Fig. 7–31). In infancy, there is often space between the middle fingers, resulting in a trident appearance to the hand. The iliac bones are short and the acetabular roof is horizontal (decreased acetabular angle), making the iliac bones resemble old-fashioned "tombstones" (see Fig. 7–33).

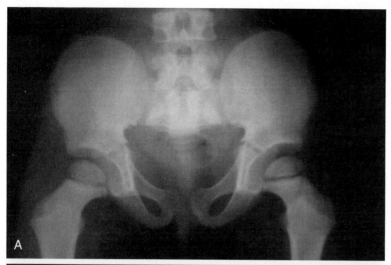

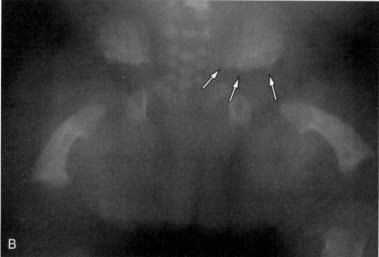

Figure 7–33. Abnormal configurations of the pelvis seen with skeletal dysplasias. *A*, Achondroplasia. Radiograph shows shallow or flat acetabular angles. The iliac angles are steep. The iliac bones are short and have a rounded top. The combination of these findings makes the iliac bone have a "tombstone" appearance. *B*, Trident acetabulum. Radiograph shows three downward spikes *(arrows)* forming an upside-down "trident." Trident acetabulum is a "buzz word" associated with Jeune syndrome, but the acetabulum often has a similar appearance in thanatophoric dysplasia and chondroectodermal dysplasia. In this patient with thanatophoric dysplasia, also note telephone receiver–shaped femurs.

Mucopolysaccharidoses

Mucopolysaccharidoses are a group of hereditary disorders related to defects in lysosomal enzymes and include disorders such as the Hunter, Hurler, and Morquio syndromes. The skeletal findings of this group of diseases are similar and have been referred to as *dysostosis multiplex*. The vertebral bodies are oval and often have an anterior beak in the anterior cortex (Fig. 7–34), which is located in the midportion of the vertebral bodies in Morquio syndrome and the inferior portion in Hurler syndrome. Beaking is most prominent in the lumbar vertebral bodies. There can be focal kyphosis (gibbus deformity) (see Fig. 7–34). The clavicles and ribs are often thickened. The ribs are narrower posteromedially, giving them a "canoe paddle" appearance. The appear-

ance of the pelvis is essentially the opposite of that in achondroplasia. The iliac wings are tall and flared and the acetabuli are shallow (increased acetabular angles) (see Fig. 7–34). The femoral heads are dysplastic, and the femoral necks are gracile and demonstrate coxa valga. The hands have a characteristic appearance, with proximal tapering of the metatarsal bones (see Fig. 7–34).

Osteogenesis Imperfecta

Osteogenesis imperfecta (OI) is a heterogeneous group of genetic disorders that result in the formation of abnormal type 1 collagen. In all types of OI, there is osteopenia and a propensity to fracture. Often, there are multiple fractures of various ages. In such cases,

TABLE 7–5. **Radiographic Manifestations of Several Skeletal Dysplasias**

Dysplasia	Type of Extremity Shortening	Pelvis	Short Ribs	Spine	Enlarged Skull	Other
Achondroplasia	Proximal	Squared iliac wings Small sacroiliac notch Decreased acetabular angle (look like tombstones)	Yes	Short vertebral bodies Narrow interpediculate distance	Yes	Metaphyseal flaring hand
Thanatophoric dysplasia	Proximal	Squared iliac wings Decreased acetabular angle Trident acetabulum	Yes	Platyspondyly	Yes	Early death Metaphyseal flaring "Telephone receiver" femurs
Chondrodysplasia punctata	Proximal	Normal	No	Stippled epiphysis	No	Stippled epiphyses
Diastrophic dysplasia	Proximal	Normal	No	Normal	No	Metaphyseal enlargement Hitchhiker thumb Enlarged ears
Mesomelic dysplasia	Middle	Normal	No	Normal	No	Mandibular hypoplasia
Asphyxiating thoracic dystrophy (Jeune syndrome)	Distal	Decreased acetabular angle Trident acetabulum	Yes	Normal	No	Very short ribs Respiratory distress Metaphyseal irregularity and beaking
Chondroectodermal dysplasia (Ellis–van Creveld syndrome)	Distal	Decreased acetabular angle Trident acetabulum	Yes	Normal	No	Polydactyly, abnormal nails Congenital ear disease Amish community
Cleidocranial dysplasia	All	Squared iliac wings Decreased acetabular angle Widened pubic symphysis	No	Abnormal ossification	Yes	Absent or small clavicles Widened pubic symphysis Wormian bones
Camptomelic dysplasia	All	Tall, narrow iliac wings Increased acetabular angle	No	Ossification defects	Yes	Bowing of long bones (campto = bent limb) Airway obstruction

other findings such as osteopenia should be clues to a diagnosis of OI rather than child abuse. There is a spectrum of clinical presentation and radiographic appearances that historically has been divided into the often fatal recessive congenital form and a dominant tarda form. With classic congenital cases, there are thick tubular bones (Fig. 7–35) that result from healing of multiple fractures, resulting in a short-limbed dwarfism. With the tarda form, there are thin bones with undertubulation (gracile). In association with OI, there is often multiple wormian bones within the skull, blue sclerae, and thin skin.

Osteopetrosis

Osteopetrosis is a rare bone disorder in which the osteoclasts are defective in resorbing and remodeling bone. As a result, bone is laid down and not resorbed. This results in dense bony sclerosis. There is often a bone-within-bone appearance on radiographs (Fig. 7–36).

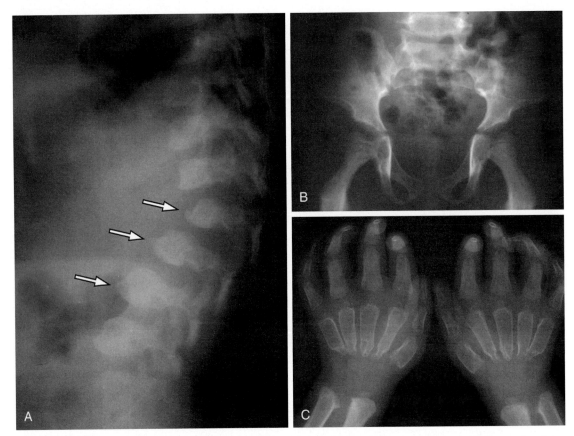

Figure 7–34. Radiographic findings in mucopolysaccharidoses (dysostosis multiplex). *A,* Radiograph of the spine demonstrates the vertebral bodies to be oval and have an anteroinferior beak *(arrows).* There is an associated focal lumbar kyphosis (gibbus deformity). *B,* Radiograph of the pelvis shows increased acetabular and iliac angles, giving the pelvis a flared appearance. The femoral necks are gracile and show coxa valgus. *C,* Radiograph of the hands show squared metacarpal bones with tapered proximal ends.

The skull base is thickened, and encroachment on the cranial nerves is a common complication. Although the total body calcium stores are increased, serum calcium levels are often paradoxically low, and radiographic findings of superimposed rickets are not uncommon (see Fig. 7–36). Lack of normal marrow space results in pancytopenia, which often leads to complications and death.

HIP DISORDERS

There are a number of unique abnormalities that can involve the pediatric hip.

Developmental Dysplasia of the Hip

Developmental dysplasia of the hip (DDH), also previously referred to as *congenital hip dis-*

location, refers to a condition related to both abnormal development and configuration of the acetabulum and increased ligamentous laxity around the hip. The cause is debated. DDH is much more common in females (up to 9:1), whites, and children born of breech deliveries. Of children with DDH, one third are affected bilaterally. Clinical evaluation for DDH is part of routine neonatal screening. Neonates may demonstrate asymmetric gluteal folds, limited abduction, positive "click" felt on Ortolani (relocation) or Barlow (dislocation) maneuvers. If not detected and treated in infancy, DDH can lead to chronic abnormalities of the hip.

At most pediatric centers, ultrasonography is used to evaluate the hips in children who have clinical findings suggestive of DDH. Ultrasonography is used both to evaluate the morphologic features of the acetabulum and to evaluate for abnormal mobility of the hip.

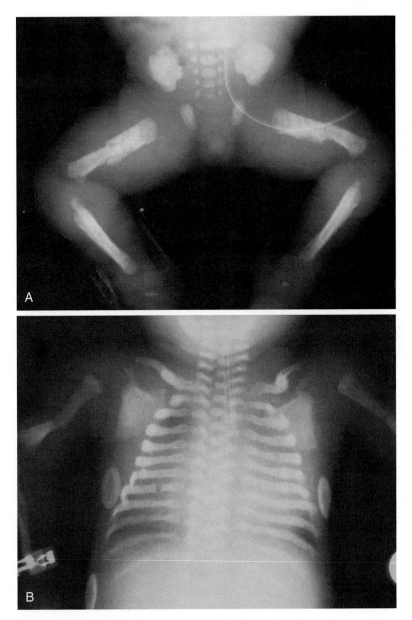

Figure 7–35. Osteogenesis imperfecta, congenital form. Radiographs of the pelvis and femurs *(A)* and chest *(B)* show multiple fractures, with healing resulting in thick tubular bones.

Because there is physiologic ligamentous laxity during the first days of life, it is better to wait 2 weeks before performing hip ultrasonography. The static morphologic evaluation is performed with the ultrasonographic probe coronal to the hip. Stress (Barlow) maneuvers are performed while evaluating the hip in the axial plane. On the static coronal view, the anatomy simulates that seen on a frontal radiograph of the pelvis (Fig. 7–37). On such a view, the iliac bone appears as an echogenic line. This line should bisect a nondislocated femoral head, which will be positioned posterolaterally (Fig. 7–38). The angle created between lines drawn along the straight part of the iliac bone and the acetabular roof form what Graf calls the alpha angle (see Fig. 7–37). An abnormal angle correlates with an increased acetabular angle seen on radiographs (see further on). Normally, the alpha angle is greater than 60 degrees (55 degrees in newborns). A shallow alpha angle may be followed on repeat static ultrasonograms during therapy to evaluate for morphologic improvement.

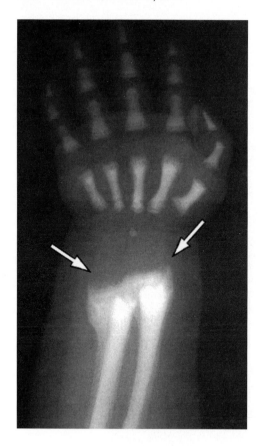

Figure 7–36. Osteopetrosis with associated rickets. Radiograph shows intense diffuse bony sclerosis with a bone-within-bone appearance. There is metaphyseal cupping and fraying *(arrows)* consistent with coexisting rickets.

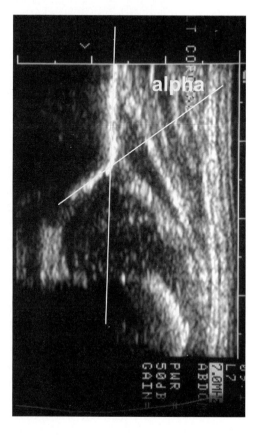

Figure 7–37. Coronal ultrasonogram of a normal hip. The iliac bone forms a straight echogenic line that bisects the femoral head (F). The alpha angle is shown by the lines drawn parallel to the roof of the acetabulum and the iliac bone. With a shallow acetabulum, this angle is decreased.

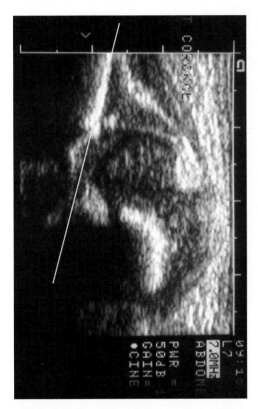

Figure 7–38. Coronal ultrasonogram of developmental dysplasia of the hip with dislocation. A line drawn along the iliac bone passes medially to the femoral head, which is dislocated superiorly and laterally.

DDH can also be evaluated with radiography. Radiographs are particularly useful after the femoral heads begin to ossify, rendering ultrasonography of limited value. Also, it is important to know the radiographic findings of DDH so that such abnormalities may be identified when evaluating other neonatal imaging studies that include the hips, such as abdominal radiographs. Because the femoral epiphysis and portions of the acetabulum are cartilaginous and not directly visualized on radiographs of the pelvis in the newborn period, landmarks are used to determine whether the hip is dislocated. With increasing age and ossification of the femoral head, direct visualization of a dislocated femoral head can be seen. Drawn lines used to evaluate for DDH include the Hilgenreiner (Y-Y) line, Perkins line, Shenton arch, and acetabular angle (Fig. 7–39). The Hilgenreiner line is a line drawn through the bilateral triradiate cartilages, touching the inferomedial aspect of each acetabulum. A second line is then drawn connecting the infero-

medial and superolateral aspects of the acetabulum, outlining the acetabular roof. The angle made between these two lines is the acetabular angle. Normally, the acetabular angle is just less than 30 degrees at birth and decreases to 22 degrees at 1 year. With DDH, acetabular angles will be abnormally increased. Other causes of increased acetabular angles include neuromuscular disorders. Abnormally decreased acetabular angles can be seen during the first year of life in Down syndrome and in multiple dysplasias, including achondroplasia (see Fig. 7–33). The vertical line of Perkins is drawn so that it is perpendicular to the Hilgenreiner line and traverses the superolateral corner of the acetabulum. When the femoral head is ossified and visible, it should lie medial to Perkins line. When the head is not ossified, the Perkins line should bisect the middle third of the metaphysis. If the metaphysis is lateral to this position, the hip is subluxated or dislocated (Fig. 7–40). The Shenton arch is a continuous smooth arch connecting the medial cortex of the proximal metaphysis of the femur and the inferior edge of the superior pubic ramus. With DDH and dislocation, the arch is discontinuous (see Fig. 7–40).

Proximal Focal Femoral Deficiency

Proximal focal femoral deficiency (PFFD) is a congenital disorder consisting of a range of hypoplasia or absence of the proximal portions of the femur (Fig. 7–41). In its most severe form, the acetabulum, femoral head, and proximal femur may be absent. There is often a varus deformity associated with the deficiency. It is important not to confuse the milder forms of PFFD with DDH. In the latter, the femur is of normal length. PFFD can be associated with ipsilateral fibular hemimelia and deformity of the foot.

Septic Arthritis

There are many potential causes of painful hips in children (Table 7–6). Many of these diagnoses present at specific ages, and the differential diagnosis can often be limited on the basis of age (see Table 7–6).

Septic arthritis is often the most pertinent diagnosis to exclude in a patient with a painful joint because delay in diagnosis can lead to destruction of the joint. In children, septic arthritis is thought to occur most commonly

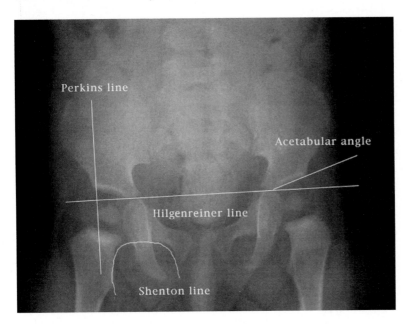

Figure 7–39. Radiograph of the normal pelvis. Anatomic landmarks are seen, including Hilgenreiner, Perkins, and Shenton lines.

TABLE 7–6. **Potential Causes of Hip Pain in Children**

Diagnosis	Typical Age at Presentation
Septic arthritis	Any age, most common in infants and teenagers
Toxic synovitis	<10 yr
Osteomyelitis	<5 yr
Langerhans cell histiocytosis	Any age, but pelvic bone involvement typically seen in those <5 yr
Slipped capital femoral epiphysis	12–15 yr
Legg-Calvé-Perthes disease	5–8 yr
Juvenile rheumatoid arthritis	1–3 yr
Ewing sarcoma	Second decade
Osteoid osteoma	Second decade

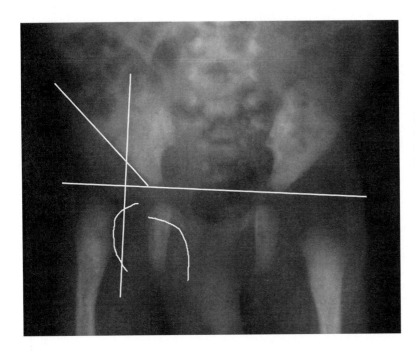

Figure 7–40. Developmental dysplasia of the hip on the right. The femoral heads are not yet ossified. The right metaphysis is displaced laterally compared with the Perkins line, and the Shenton arch is not continuous. The acetabular angle is greater than 30 degrees.

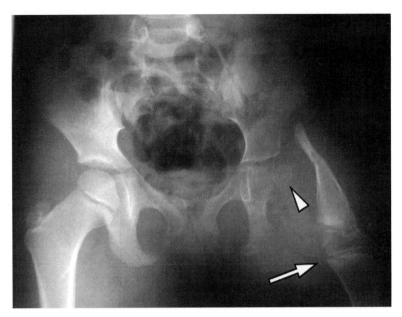

Figure 7–41. Proximal focal femoral deficiency. This is shown on the radiograph as a hypoplastic femur with the knee *(arrow)* just inferior to the hip joint. Note the presence of the femoral head *(arrowhead).*

from extension of infection from the adjacent metaphysis. In younger children, it usually occurs secondary to bacterial sepsis; most commonly, the organism is *Staphylococcus aureus* (>50% of cases) or infection with group A streptococci. Most cases of septic arthritis are monocular and involve large joints. The hip is the most common joint involved, followed by the knee.

In regard to septic arthritis of the hip, radiographs of the pelvis and hips are usually obtained to exclude other diagnoses. Many of these children present with pain, limp, or failure to bear weight. The radiographic findings of septic arthritis include asymmetric widening of the hip joint spaces by more than 2 mm on a nonrotated film (Fig. 7–42). The joint spaces are evaluated by measuring the distance between the teardrop of the acetabulum and the medial cortex of the metaphysis of the femur. Unfortunately, these findings, although important when positive, are not sensitive for a

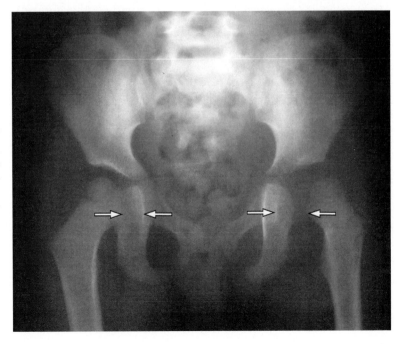

Figure 7–42. Septic arthritis of the left hip in a 3-year-old child with fever and limp. Radiograph shows marked asymmetry of the hip joint spaces *(arrows),* with the left being greater than the right.

joint effusion. Fluid tends to accumulate in the anterior recess of the hip joint before displacing the femur laterally. Other radiographic findings of septic arthritis include displacement or obliteration of the fat pads surrounding the hip, including the obturator internus, gluteus muscle, and iliopsoas fat pads (see Fig. 7–18). These findings are also insensitive. A normal pelvic radiograph in no way excludes a diagnosis of septic arthritis.

At many institutions, the presence of a hip joint effusion is evaluated with ultrasonography. The probe is placed longitudinally anterior to the hip joint. Asymmetric widening of a hypoechoic space between the shaft of the proximal femur and the joint capsule is diagnostic of a joint effusion (Fig. 7–43). The absence of fluid does exclude a diagnosis of septic arthritis. When fluid is present, ultrasonographic guidance can be used to tap the effusion. There are causes of joint effusion other than septic arthritis. They include toxic synovitis, noninfectious arthritis, and Legg-Calvé-Perthes (LCP) disease.

Toxic Synovitis

Toxic synovitis is diagnosed when there is no pain or limping on presentation, there is evidence of a joint effusion, no organisms are identified on joint aspiration, and symptoms subside with rest. It occurs in children younger than 10 years. It is a diagnosis of exclusion and is always included in the differential diagnosis of septic arthritis. It is thought to be secondary to viral infection.

Legg-Calvé-Perthes Disease

LCP is idiopathic avascular necrosis of the proximal femoral epiphysis. It occurs more commonly in boys than in girls (4:1), is most commonly seen in whites, and typically occurs between 5 and 8 years. Affected children present with pain in the groin, hip, or ipsilateral knee. The disease can be bilateral in up to 13% of cases. It is often associated with skeletal immaturity (decreased bone age). Radiographs are usually positive, even early in the disease.

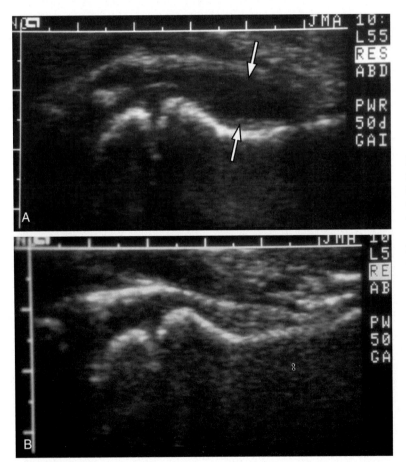

Figure 7–43. Right hip joint effusion demonstrated by ultrasonography in a 3-year-old boy with septic arthritis. Sagittal ultrasonograms of the right *(A)* and left *(B)* hips obtained from an anterior approach demonstrates hypoechoic fluid *(arrows* in *A)* anterior within the right hip. On the left, the normal appearance is demonstrated.

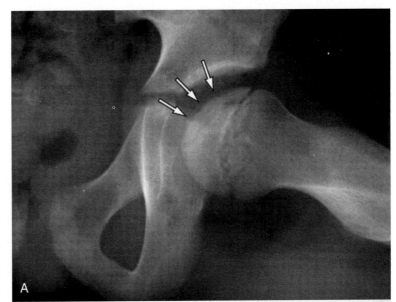

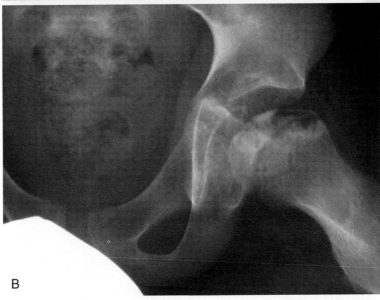

Figure 7–44. Legg-Calvé-Perthes disease in a 9-year-old boy. *A,* Radiograph of the left hip with frog leg positioning shows crescentic subchondral lucency *(arrows)* consistent with necrosis. The femoral epiphysis is irregular and sclerotic. *B,* Radiograph obtained 5 months later shows marked progression with fragmentation, mixed lucency and sclerosis, widening, and deformity of the femoral head.

Early findings include an asymmetrically small ossified femoral epiphysis, widening of the joint space as a result of either joint effusion or synovial hypertrophy, and a subchondral linear lucency. The subchondral linear lucency (crescent sign) is best seen on frog-leg views and represents a fracture through the necrotic bone (Fig. 7–44). When the diagnosis is suspected and radiographs are noncontributory to the diagnosis, LCP can be diagnosed by MRI (high-signal marrow edema, asymmetric decreased enhancement with gadolinium) or bone scintigraphy (asymmetric lack of uptake). Later evidence of LCP includes changes in the femoral epiphysis such as fragmentation, areas of increased sclerosis and lucency, and loss of height (collapse) (see Fig. 7–44). There are lucencies seen in the adjacent metaphysis in up to one third of patients. Chronic changes can include a broad, overgrown femoral head (coxa magna), short femoral neck, and physeal arrest. Problems arise when the overgrown femoral head is not covered by the acetabulum, and this scenario may require surgical reconstruction of the acetabulum.

Slipped Capital Femoral Epiphysis

Slipped capital femoral epiphysis (SCFE) is an idiopathic Salter type 1 fracture through the proximal physis of the femur, which then results in displacement (slippage of the femoral epiphysis). It is more common in boys than in girls (2.5:1), in African Americans, and in obese children. There are certain groups, such as those with renal osteodystrophy, who are predisposed. The hips can be involved bilaterally in up to one third of patients. However, involvement of both hips does not usually present at the same time.

The slippage of the femoral head in SCFE is posterior and to a lessor extent medial. Because of this, findings are more prominent on the frog leg lateral view than on the frontal anteroposterior (AP) radiograph. On the frog leg lateral view, the epiphysis is seen to be posteriorly displaced in comparison to the metaphysis. The image has been likened to an ice cream cone, with the dip of ice cream falling off the cone in SCFE. A line drawn tangential to the lateral cortex of the metaphysis on the frog leg lateral view should bisect a portion of the ossified epiphysis (Fig. 7–45). If the physis is medial to this line, it has slipped. Findings

of SCFE can be subtle on the frontal view. Findings include asymmetric widening of the physis and indistinctness of the metaphyseal border of the physis (see Fig. 7–45). SCFE is typically treated with pin fixation to prevent further slippage. The epiphysis is not moved back to its normal position, however. Potential complications of SCFE include avascular necrosis of the femoral head and chondrolysis.

METABOLIC DISORDERS

Rickets

Rickets is the bony manifestation of a heterogeneous group of problems resulting from a relative or absolute insufficiency of vitamin D or its derivatives. It may result from dietary deficiency, malabsorption, renal disease, or lack of end-organ response. The lack of vitamin D results in insufficient conversion of growing cartilage into mineralized osteoid and build-up of nonossifed osteoid. The radio-

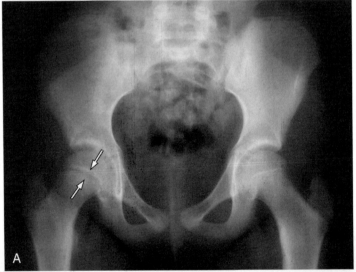

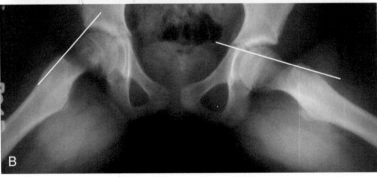

Figure 7–45. Slipped capital femoral epiphysis in an 11-year-old child with right hip pain. *A,* Frontal, neutrally positioned radiograph shows widening and indistinctness of the physis *(arrow)* of the right proximal femur. *B,* Radiograph with frog leg lateral positioning shows posterior displacement of the epiphysis in relation to the physis. A line drawn along the lateral cortex of the metaphysis does not bisect the right epiphysis, whereas a similar line does on the normal left side.

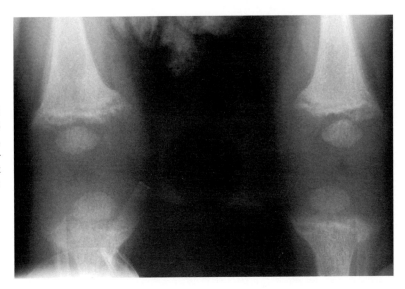

Figure 7–46. Rickets in a 1 year-old boy. Radiograph shows metaphyseal cupping, fraying, and irregularity. There is associated periosteal reaction, not uncommonly seen in severe rickets.

graphic manifestations are most prominent in bones of rapid growth, and skeletal surveys to evaluate for rickets can be confined to frontal views of the knees and wrists. Radiographic findings include metaphyseal fraying, cupping, and irregularity along the physeal margin (Fig. 7–46). There is osteomalacia with unsharp, smudged-appearing trabecular markings. Patients may be predisposed to insufficiency fractures (Looser zones) and slipped capital femoral epiphyses.

Lead Poisoning

Lead poisoning most commonly occurs in children younger than 2 years secondary to consumption of lead-containing substances such as old paint chips. It may result in broad sclerotic metaphyseal bands (lead lines). They are often best seen in areas of rapid growth such as the knee. Unfortunately, similar dense metaphyseal bands can be seen as a normal variant. One discriminating factor is that lead lines tend to affect all the metaphyses surrounding the knee, whereas the normal variant type of dense bands tends to spare the proximal fibula.

MISCELLANEOUS DISORDERS

Juvenile Rheumatoid Arthritis

Juvenile rheumatoid arthritis (JRA) is an idiopathic systemic disease that primarily affects the musculoskeletal system. It differs from adult rheumatoid arthritis in many ways. With JRA, most cases are seronegative, and the diag-

nosis is made clinically. In contrast to adult disease in which small joint involvement predominates, large joint involvement is more common in children. The most common joints involved, in descending order of frequency, include the knee, ankle, wrist, hand, elbow, and hip. In most cases, the disease is pauciarticular, with between two and four joints involved. Before the development of radiographic findings, MRI with gadolinium enhancement may show abnormal enhancing, thickened synovium in involved joints (Fig. 7–47). This may be used to aid diagnosis and in monitoring therapy. Initial radiographs may be normal or show only soft tissue swelling or joint effusion. In the knee, there may be epiphyseal overgrowth, widening of the intracondylar notch, and accelerated bony maturation. There can be an associated periosteal reaction. In the cervical spine, there is often ankylosis of the apophyseal joints. When the hands and wrists are involved, the disease is typically most severe in the carpal bones (Fig. 7–48). Findings include carpal bones that appear square and small as well as narrowing of the intracarpal joint spaces. Later changes include erosions and ankylosis. Many children also have splenomegaly or pleural effusions. *Still disease* is an acute form of JRA in which children present with fever, rash, hepatosplenomegaly, and lymphadenopathy. Skeletal involvement is rare in these children.

Hemophilia

In hemophilia, recurrent bleeding into a joint can result in a debilitating arthropathy. The

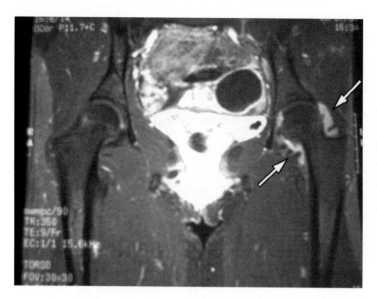

Figure 7–47. Juvenile rheumatoid arthritis in a 15-year-old girl with left hip pain. Coronal, gadolinium-enhanced, fat-saturated, T1-weighted MR image shows asymmetric enhancing synovium *(arrows)* in the left hip.

most common joints involved include, in decreasing order of frequency, the knee, elbow, and ankle. The recurrent hemorrhage deposits hemosiderin within the synovium, and there is associated hypertrophy of the synovium and destruction of the underlying articular cartilage. Radiographic findings of chronic hemophilic arthropathy include epiphyseal overgrowth; in the knee, there is often squaring of the margin of the patella and widening of the intracondylar notch (Fig. 7–49). These findings can have an appearance similar to that of JRA. On MRI, there is destruction of articular cartilage and hypertrophy of the synovium. The hypertrophied synovium may be dark on T2-weighted images secondary to the hemosiderin deposition, giving rise to an appearance similar to that of pigmented villonodular synovitis. Recurrent hematoma formation can also lead to the formation of pseudotumors, which usually occur in the soft tissues but can cause pressure necrosis and lucency of adjacent bone.

Sickle Cell Anemia and Thalassemia

With severe causes of anemia, such as sickle cell anemia or thalassemia, skeletal changes may be seen on radiography related to marrow expansion. Findings include thinning of the cortex, coarsening of the trabeculae, and bony remodeling (Fig. 7–50). The ribs appear widened. In the skull, the diploic space can become widened and have a hair-on-end appearance, particularly with thalassemia. In sickle cell anemia, there are often areas of bone infarction, which may appear as either sclerotic or lucent areas. The vertebral bodies in sickle cell anemia often demonstrate indented and flat portions of the superior and inferior

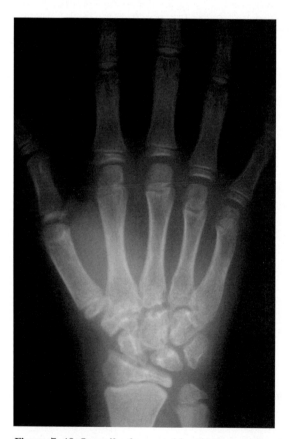

Figure 7–48. Juvenile rheumatoid arthritis involving the hand. There is joint space narrowing and erosions of the intercarpal joints.

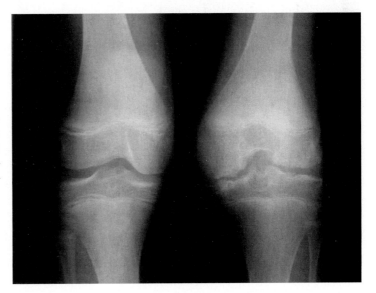

Figure 7–49. Hemophilia in a 13-year-old boy. Radiograph of the knees shows abnormal left knee with epiphyseal overgrowth, joint irregularity, and widening of the intracondylar notch.

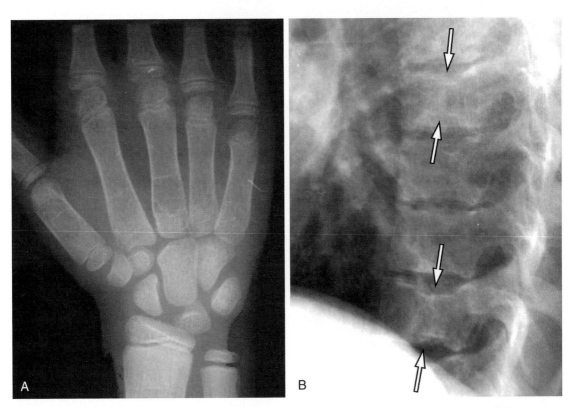

Figure 7–50. Bone changes of childhood anemias. *A,* Radiograph demonstrates expansion of the marrow cavities with associated expansion and thinning of the cortex, particularly in the metacarpal bones, in a child with thalassemia. *B,* Lateral radiograph shows "Lincoln Log" appearance of the spine in a child with sickle cell anemia. The superior and inferior end plates of multiple vertebral bodies show a concavity *(arrows)*.

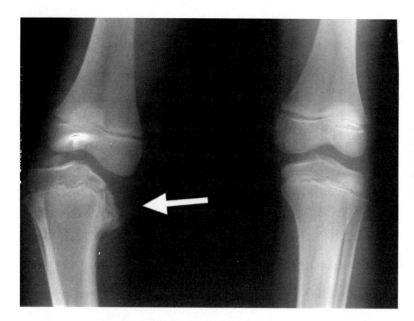

Figure 7–51. Blount disease. Radiograph demonstrates bowing of the tibia in association with irregularity and fragmentation of the tibial metaphysis *(arrow).*

end plates, giving the vertebral bodies a "Lincoln Log" appearance (see Fig. 7–50).

With severe anemia, other imaging findings may include cardiomegaly, gallstones, splenomegaly (or conversely, in sickle cell anemia, there may be autoinfarction of the spleen with a small calcified spleen), extramedullary hematopoiesis, and predisposition to osteomyelitis.

Radial Dysplasia

Radial dysplasia, often referred to as *radial array syndrome*, refers to a variable degree of hypoplasia or aplasia of the radius. Often, the first metatarsal or thumb may be hypoplastic or absent as well. Radial array syndrome may be seen in conjunction with a number of syndromes including VATERL (vertebral defects, imperforate anus, tracheoesophageal fistula, and radial and renal dysplasia and limb anomalies) association, Holt-Oram syndrome, Fanconi pancytopenia, and thrombocytopenia with absence of radius (TAR) syndrome.

Blount Disease

Blount disease refers to excessive medial bowing of the tibias (tibia vara), most commonly occurring during infancy. It is an idiopathic disease but is thought to be related to excessive pressure on the medial metaphysis of the tibia, resulting in delayed endochondral ossification. It can be differentiated from physiologic bowing of the tibias both by the degree

of angulation and the appearance of the medial metaphysis of the tibia. With Blount disease, there is irregularity, fragmentation, and beaking of the medial tibial metaphysis (Fig. 7–51). Severe cases may require tibial osteotomy.

Neurofibromatosis

The nonmusculoskeletal aspects of neurofibromatosis type 1 (NF1) are discussed in Chapter 8. There are many changes that can occur in the bones of patients with NF1, and most of these are thought to be related to mesodermal dysplasia. The bones may demonstrate overgrowth, bowing (Fig. 7–52), areas of sclerosis, and numerous cortical defects. Characteristic findings include pseudoarthrosis formation (see Fig. 7–52), commonly within the tibia, and twisted-appearing (ribbon-like) ribs. The vertebral bodies may demonstrate posterior scalloping from dural ectasia or multiple neurofibromas. There is often kyphoscoliosis.

Clubfoot (Talipes Equinovarus)

Talipes equinovarus, or clubfoot, refers to a common congenital abnormality of the foot. In order to understand both clubfoot and other congenital abnormalities of the foot, it is important to understand the descriptive terminology. *Valgus* and *varus* refer to bowing of a shaft of a bone or at a joint. The name given to the bowing refers to whether the distal part

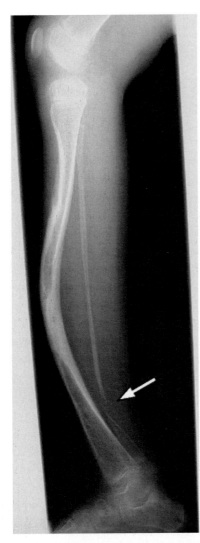

Figure 7–52. Neurofibromatosis in a 7-year-old boy. Radiograph shows marked anterior bowing and patchy sclerosis of the tibia. There is a pseudoarthrosis of the fibula *(arrow)*.

is more lateral or medial than normal. *Valgus* refers to lateral (the "l" in valgus is for lateral) and *varus* refers to medial. *Hindfoot varus* refers to the distal bone of the hindfoot (calcaneus) being angled too far lateral in relation to the more proximal bone of the hindfoot (talus) as seen on the AP view of the foot (Fig. 7–53). Normally, this angle is approximately 30 degrees. This same terminology is also used to describe other parts of the body. Therefore, *genu varum* refers to bowing of the knee, with the distal part (tibia) more medial than normal, and *coxa valgus* refers to bowing at the hip, with the distal part (femur) more lateral than normal. The terms *equinus* and *calcaneus*

refer to the relationship between the ankle (tibia) and the hindfoot (calcaneus) as viewed on the lateral radiograph. *Equinus* refers to fixed plantar flexion of the calcaneus (distal end pointing down, as a deer walks) and *calcaneus* refers to fixed dorsiflexion (distal end of calcaneus pointing up). With clubfoot, or talipes equinovarus, there is hindfoot varus, hindfoot equinus, and forefoot varus (see Fig. 7–53). Normally, a line drawn through the long axis of the talus on an AP view of the foot passes through the first metatarsal bone. With forefoot varus, the distal bone (the first metatarsal) is located more medial to this drawn line.

Tarsal Coalition

Tarsal coalition refers to an abnormal fibrous or bony connection between two of the tarsal bones of the feet. Patients with tarsal coalition can present with chronic foot pain or a propensity for ankle injury. It is a common abnormality affecting approximately 1% of the population and usually presents during adolescence. Although there is debate concerning which of the tarsal coalitions is the most common, talocalcaneal and calcaneonavicular coalitions are by far more common than other types. More than half of cases are bilateral. *Calcaneonavicular coalition* is easily demonstrated on radiographs of the foot. It is best visualized on the oblique view, in which the direct connection (bony coalition) or close proximity and irregularity of the joint margins (fibrous coalition) of the calcaneus and navicular bones can be seen (Fig. 7–54). On the lateral view, the anterosuperior calcaneus appears longer than normal as it extends towards the navicular bone. The appearance has been likened to an anteater's nose (see Fig. 7–54). Rarely, cross-sectional imaging is needed to confirm the diagnosis. In contrast, findings of *talocalcaneal coalition* can be subtle on radiography, and CT is often performed to make the diagnosis. Radiographic findings include secondary signs such as talar beaking, poor visualization of the space within the talocalcaneal joint, and a prominent C-shaped band of overlapping bone overlying the calcaneus (Fig. 7–55). If space can be seen within the talocalcaneal joint on the lateral view, there is not a talocalcaneal coalition. However, this space may not be seen within a normal joint on an oblique film. On coronal (short axis) CT images, the talocalcaneal coalition is visualized

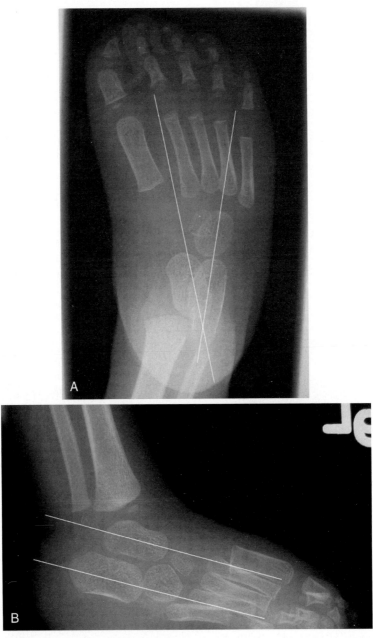

Figure 7–53. Foot angles in clubfoot and a normal foot. *A,* Clubfoot. On frontal view, there is hindfoot varus. The frontal talocalcaneal angle is decreased. There is forefoot varus. A line drawn along the axis of the talus lies medial to the first metatarsal bone. *B,* Clubfoot. On the lateral view, the lateral talocalcaneal angle is decreased. The two bones are almost parallel. There is also equinus (plantar flexion of the hindfoot interrelationship to the tibia).

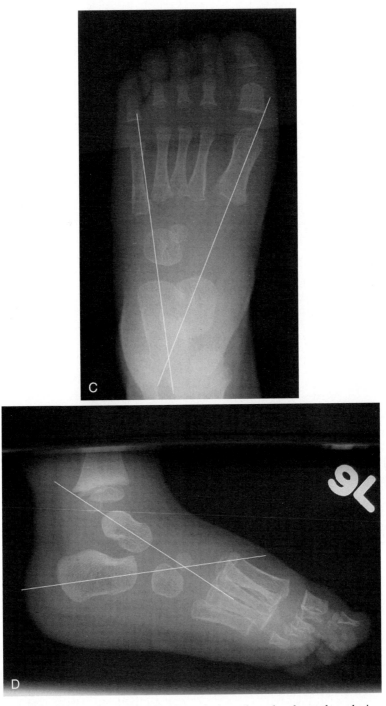

Figure 7–53 *Continued. C,* Normal foot. On the frontal view, the talocalcaneal angle is approximately 30 degrees. A line drawn along the axis of the talus hits the first metatarsal bone. *D,* Normal lateral talocalcaneal relationships.

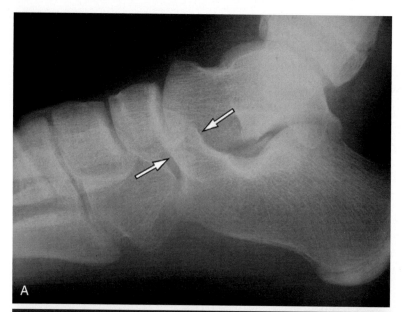

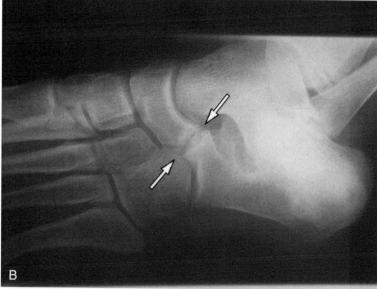

Figure 7–54. Calcaneonavicular coalition. *A,* Lateral radiograph shows the superior calcaneus to be elongated *(arrows)*, appearing like an anteater's nose. *B,* Oblique radiograph demonstrates proximity and irregularity of the margins of the calcaneonavicular joint consistent with fibrous coalition.

as bony fusion or irregularity and close proximity (fibrous coalition) between the middle facet of the talus and the sustentaculum tali of the calcaneus (see Fig. 7–55). Treatment options include surgical excision of the coalition.

DISORDERS PRIMARILY AFFECTING SOFT TISSUES

Vascular Malformations

Vascular malformations and hemangiomas can cause significant morbidity and even mortality in both children and adults. For a number of reasons, there is often confusion regarding these lesions. The classification of and nomenclature used to describe endothelial malformations has been a source of confusion. Historically, lesions were named according to the size of channels within the lesions and the type of fluid the lesion contained. Blood-containing lesions were called *hemangiomas* and lymph-containing lesions were referred to as *lymphangiomas* or *cystic hygromas*. This classification system has been replaced by one described in 1982 by Mulliken and Glowacki. This system separates endothelial malformations into two large groups—hemangiomas and vascular malformations, based on their natural history, cel-

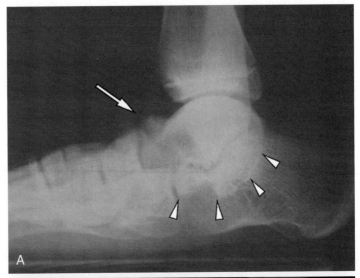

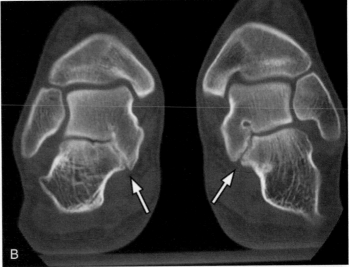

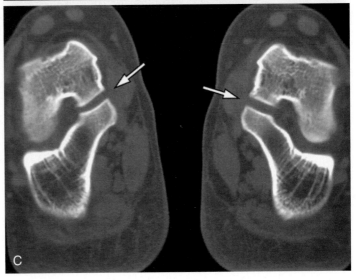

Figure 7–55. Talocalcaneal coalition.
A, Lateral radiograph demonstrates flat foot, talar beaking *(arrow),* and loss of visualization of the talocalcaneal joint. There is a C-shaped overlapping bone *(arrowheads)* superimposed over the calcaneus. *B,* Coronal computed tomographic scan shows irregularity, sclerosis, close proximity, and abnormal oblique orientation of the middle facet of the talocalcaneal joint *(arrows)* consistent with fibrous coalition. *C,* Coronal computed tomographic scan of normal middle facet of talocalcaneal joint shows smooth cortex between talus and sustentaculum tali of calcaneus *(arrows).*

TABLE 7–7. **Differentiating Features of Hemangiomas and Vascular Malformations**

Hemangiomas	Vascular Malformations
Exhibit cellular proliferation	Composed of dysplastic vessels
Small or absent at birth	Present at birth
Rapid growth during infancy	Growth proportional to child
Involution during childhood	No regression

lular turnover, and histologic appearance (Table 7–7).

Infantile Hemangiomas

Hemangiomas are the most common tumor of childhood, occurring in 12% of infants. Hemangiomas undergo a characteristic two-staged process of growth and regression. At birth, the lesions are often small and inconspicuous, with 60% not being present at birth. Shortly after birth, the phase of rapid proliferation occurs and can last over several months. The typical hemangioma begins to involute at approximately 10 months of age, with 50% of lesions being completely resolved by 5 years of age. Most hemangiomas require no therapy. However, potential complications include Kasabach-Merritt syndrome (consumptive coagulopathy), compression of vital structures (e.g., airway, orbital structures), or fissure formation, ulceration, or bleeding. In most cases, the diagnosis of hemangioma can be made on the basis of the temporal growth history and appearance on physical inspection. Therefore, imaging usually is not required. In atypical cases, imaging may be performed to characterize the lesion and evaluate the anatomic extent of disease. MR imaging of proliferating hemangiomas typically shows a discrete lobulated mass that is hyperintense on T2-weighted images (Fig. 7–56) and isointense to muscle on T1-weighted images. Typically, prominent draining veins will be identified as both central and peripheral high-flow vessels. Hemangiomas typically enhance diffusely with gadolinium. Involuting hemangiomas can demonstrate areas of fibrofatty tissue with associated high signal on T1-weighted images and demonstrate less contrast enhancement than do proliferating hemangiomas. Unfortunately,

many of the soft tissue malignancies of infancy, such as fibrosarcoma or rhabdomyosarcoma, can have a similar imaging appearance to proliferative hemangiomas. Therefore, patients who do not exhibit the typical appearance and growth patterns of hemangioma often undergo biopsy to exclude malignancy.

Low-Flow Vascular Malformations

Vascular malformations are always present at birth and enlarge in proportion to the growth of the child. They do not involute and remain present throughout the patient's life. Vascular malformations are subcategorized as lymphatic, capillary, venous, arteriovenous, and mixed malformations based on the histologic make-up of the lesion. Although MR imaging has been used to classify a vascular malformation into one of the previously mentioned categories, a more pertinent issue is classifying vascular malformations as either low-flow or high-flow lesions. Malformations with arterial components are considered high-flow lesions, and those without arterial components are considered low-flow lesions. Low-flow vascular malformations include primarily venous, lymphatic, and mixed malformations.

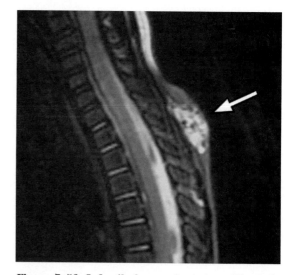

Figure 7–56. Infantile hemangioma in a 15-month-old girl with a palpable lump. Sagittal T2-weighted image shows well-defined lobulated mass (*arrows*) that is isolated to the subcutaneous tissues. The lesion is diffusely high in signal except for several low-signal flow voids within the lesion representing draining veins.

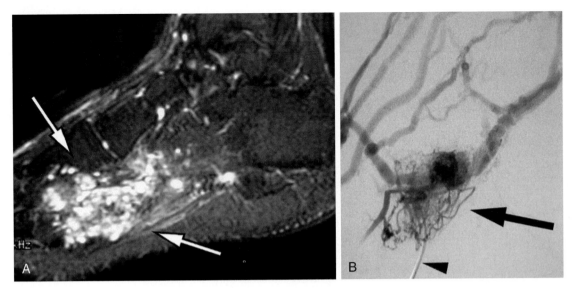

Figure 7–57. Venous malformation of the foot. *A,* Sagittal T2-weighted MR image shows serpentine areas of high signal *(arrows)* within the plantar musculature of the foot. *B,* Venogram performed prior to percutaneous sclerosis shows needle *(arrowhead)* injecting tangle of abnormal vessels *(arrow)* and multiple draining veins.

Venous malformations are dysplasias of small and large venous channels. Many venous malformations cause pain. Often, patients suffer from increasing symptoms in late childhood or early adulthood. Other clinical problems related to venous malformations include decreased range of motion and deformity. Treatment for venous malformations includes elastic compression garments, percutaneous sclerosis, and surgical excision.

Lymphatic malformations consist of chyle-filled cysts lined with endothelium. The most common locations for lymphatic malformations include the neck (75%) and axilla (25%). When lymphatic malformations occur in the neck and axilla, they are often called *cystic hygromas.* Most lymphatic malformations present early in life, with 65% being present at birth and 90% being found by age 2 years. The primary therapy for lymphatic malformations is surgical excision. Another therapeutic option is percutaneous sclerotherapy.

The appearance of a low-flow vascular malformation on MRI is dependent on the composition of lymphatic and venous components. The venous portions of a malformation appear as a collection of serpentine structures separated by septations. These serpentine structures represent slow-flowing blood within the venous channels and appear as high-signal intensities on T2-weighted images and interme-

diate-signal intensities on T1-weighted images (Fig. 7–57). Phleboliths may be present and appear as round, low-signal intensity lesions on MRI. Gadolinium-enhanced T1-weighted images may show enhancement of the slow-flowing venous channels. Lymphatic components of the malformation may contain cystic structures of various sizes, ranging from macrocystic to microcystic (Fig. 7–58). These cystic structures typically appear as high in signal intensity on T2-weighted MR images and do not exhibit central enhancement with gadolinium. Fluid-fluid levels are often present. A characteristic imaging finding of vascular malformations is that they tend to be infiltrative, not respecting fascial planes, and often involve multiple tissue types, such as muscle and subcutaneous fat.

High-Flow Vascular Malformations

Any lesion that has arterial components is considered a high-flow malformation. They include arteriovenous malformations (AVMs) and arteriovenous fistulas. During the proliferating stage, infantile hemangiomas may also be considered high-flow lesions. AVMs represent a direct connection between the arterial and venous systems. The lesions may present in childhood or adulthood and are often exac-

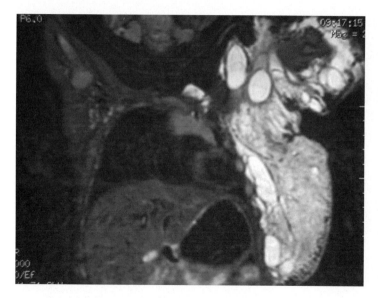

Figure 7–58. Lymphatic malformation of the chest wall in a 4-month-old infant. Coronal T2-weighted image shows extensive, multiloculated, high-signal mass involving the wall of the left side of the chest and left upper extremity.

erbated during puberty or pregnancy. Presenting symptoms include congestive heart failure, embolism, pain, bleeding, and ulceration. High-flow vascular malformations are much less common than are low-flow vascular malformations. On MRI, the lesions appear as a tangle of multiple flow voids (Fig. 7–59) that demonstrate high flow on gradient echographic images. Although the lesions can be associated with surrounding edema or fibrofatty stroma, usually there is no focal discrete soft tissue mass. Color Doppler ultrasonography demonstrates the direct connection between the arterial and venous systems. The most effective treatment for AVMs is transarterial embolization.

Dermatomyositis

Dermatomyositis is an autoimmune disease that involves the skeletal muscle and skin. Children typically present with weakness and rash. MRI has been used to aid in making the diagnosis, directing biopsies to high-yield areas, and monitoring the response to therapy. On T2-weighted fat-saturated images, there is increased signal intensity within the involved muscles, myofascial planes, and subcutaneous tissues (Fig. 7–60). The most commonly involved muscles are those within the anterior compartment of the thigh and those surrounding the hip. There is typically rapid resolution of the abnormal high signal after ther-

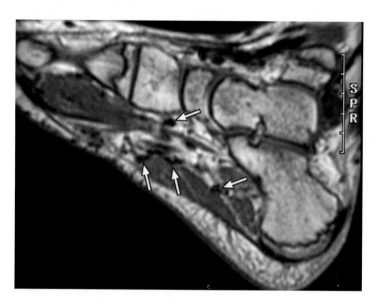

Figure 7–59. High-flow vascular malformation in a 12-year-old boy. Sagittal T1-weighted image shows multiple serpentine flow voids *(arrows)* within the inferior aspect of the foot. No discrete soft tissue mass is present. These findings are consistent with an arteriovenous malformation.

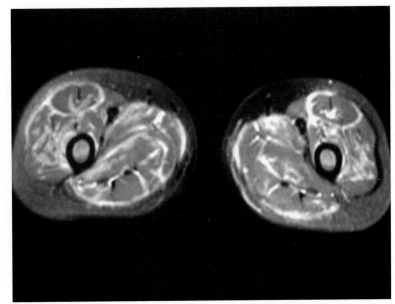

Figure 7–60. Dermatomyositis in a 4-year-old boy. Axial T2-weighted image shows abnormal increased signal within multiple muscle groups and fascial planes of the upper thigh. Normally, all these structures would be low in signal on these images.

apy has been instituted. In patients with chronic dermatomyositis, calcifications may be seen within the soft tissues on radiography.

Soft Tissue Malignancies

Primary malignancies of the soft tissues are not common in children. MRI is the imaging modality of choice for evaluating soft tissue masses. The likely diagnosis is related to the patient's age. In infants, fibrosarcoma is the most common soft tissue malignancy, whereas rhabdomyosarcoma is the most common in older children. Other potential malignancies include primitive neuroectodermal tumors and synovial sarcoma. The latter tends to occur around joints and is notoriously and deceivingly benign-appearing on imaging studies, with smooth, well-defined borders.

Aggressive fibromatosis is a fibroproliferative disorder that is locally aggressive but does not metastasize. The lesions tend to occur in older children in the deep soft tissues. On MRI, despite the fibrous nature, the lesions tend to be high signal on T2-weighted images (Fig. 7–61). After resection, there is a tendency for recurrence along the proximal margin of the resection.

Fibromatosis Coli

Fibromatosis coli should not be confused with the more aggressive fibrotic processes of childhood. It refers to a benign mass of the sternocleidomastoid muscle in neonates who present with torticollis. Typically, ultrasonography is performed to confirm the diagnosis. The ultrasonogram shows asymmetric fusiform thickening of the sternocleidomastoid muscle (Fig. 7–62), the echogenicity of which is typically heterogeneous and asymmetric but may be increased or decreased compared with the contralateral normal muscle. Most symptoms resolve over time with stretching exercises, and surgical division is rarely required.

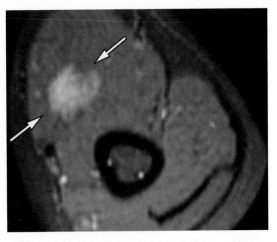

Figure 7–61. Aggressive fibromatosis in a 10-year-old girl. Axial T2-weighted image shows nonspecific, high-signal, intramuscular soft tissue mass *(arrows)* with relatively well-defined borders.

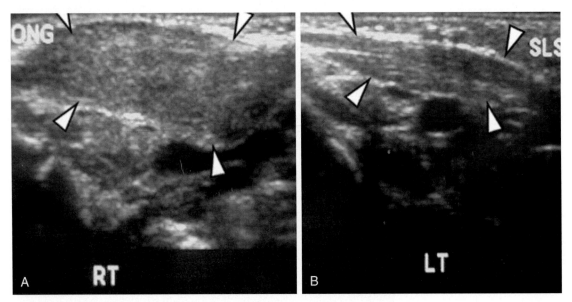

Figure 7–62. Fibromatosis coli in a 1-month old infant with a mass on the right side of the neck and head tilt to the left. Longitudinal ultrasonograms of the right *(A)* and left *(B)* sternocleidomastoid muscles *(arrowheads)*, with the right much thicker than the left.

Suggested Readings

Donnelly LF, Adams DM, Bisset GS III. Centennial dissertation. vascular malformations and hemangiomas: a practical approach in a multidisciplinary clinic. AJR Am J Roentgenol 2000;174:597–608.

Donnelly LF, Bisset GS III, Helms CA, Squire DL. Chronic avulsive injuries of childhood. Skeletal Radiol 1999;78:138–144.

Harcke HT, Grissom LE. Performing dynamic sonography of the infant hip. AJR Am J Roentgenol 1990;155:837–844.

Helms CA. Fundamentals of Skeletal Radiology. 2nd ed. Philadelphia: WB Saunders, 1995.

Keats TE, Joyce JM. Metaphyseal cortical irregularities in children: a new perspective on a multi-focal growth variant. Skeletal Radiol 1984;12:112–118.

Kleinman PK. Diagnostic imaging in infant abuse. AJR Am J Roentgenol 1990;155:703–712.

Kozlowski K. The radiographic clues in the diagnosis of bone dysplasias. Pediatr Radiol 1985;15:1–3.

Mulliken JB, Glowacki J. Hemangiomas and vascular malformations in infants and children: a classification based on endothelial characteristics. Plast Reconstr Surg 1982;69:412–422.

Oestreich AE, Crawford AH. Atlas of Pediatric Orthopedic Radiology. Stuttgart: Thieme, 1985.

Ozonoff MB. Pediatric Orthopedic Radiology. 2nd ed. Philadelphia: WB Saunders, 1992.

Rogers LF, Poznanski AK. Imaging of epiphyseal injuries. Radiology 1994;191:297–308.

Taybi H, Lachman RS. Radiology of Syndromes, Metabolic Disorders, and Skeletal Dysplasias. 4th ed. St. Louis: CV Mosby, 1996.

Chapter

8

Neurologic System

Pediatric neurologic imaging is a distinct subspecialty—probably more than any other organ system in pediatric imaging. Anatomic areas included in neurologic imaging include the skull, brain, meninges, orbits, sinuses, neck, and spine. At many children's hospitals, dedicated neuroradiologists perform and interpret all the neurologic imaging. The large amount of information included in neuroradiology is beyond the scope of this textbook. The following is a review of some of the more commonly encountered entities.

INDICATIONS FOR MAGNETIC RESONANCE IMAGING AND COMPUTED TOMOGRAPHY

In general, magnetic resonance imaging (MRI) has become the definitive test for evaluating intracranial abnormalities. It is the test of choice for evaluating brain involvement by the following: neoplasm, vascular lesions, inflammatory disorders, developmental abnormalities, neurodegenerative disorders, focal seizures, unexplained hydrocephalus, and neuroendocrine disorders. Computed tomography (CT) is typically reserved for trauma and acute neurologic symptoms, such as symptoms of ventriculoperitoneal shunt (VPS) malfunction. Sinus disease, orbital cellulitis, and other indications for head and neck imaging are also often evaluated with CT. Head ultrasonography is reserved for evaluating premature infants and newborns.

Neonatal Head Ultrasonography

Neonatal head ultrasonography is performed through the open anterior fontanelle of neonates and infants using a high-frequency sector transducer. Images are obtained in the sagittal and coronal planes (Fig. 8–1). It is most commonly used to diagnose and follow up intracranial complications in premature infants, for example, germinal matrix hemorrhage and periventricular leukomalacia (PVL). It can also be used to screen for congenital abnormalities or hydrocephalus.

Germinal Matrix Hemorrhage

The germinal matrix is a fetal structure that is a stem source for neuroblasts. It typically involutes by term but is still present in premature infants. The germinal matrix is highly vascular and is subject to hemorrhaging. It lies within the caudothalamic groove (the space between the caudate head and the thalamus). Germinal matrix hemorrhage most commonly occurs in premature infants during the first 3 days after birth. Potential complications include destruction of the precursor cells within the germinal matrix, hydrocephalus, and hemorrhagic infarction of the surrounding periventricular tissues.

Germinal matrix hemorrhage is seen on ultrasonography as an ovoid echogenic mass within the caudothalamic groove (Fig. 8–2). For those not well acquainted with head ultrasonography, there may be confusion in differentiating germinal matrix hemorrhage from the normally echogenic choroid plexus. In contrast to germinal matrix hemorrhage, the normal choroid plexus should never extend as anterior as the caudothalamic groove on a parasagittal view. Hemorrhage may extend into the ventricular system and lead to hydrocephalus. Germinal matrix hemorrhage is categorized into one of four grades (Table 8–1) (Fig. 8–3; see also Fig. 8–2). Intraparenchymal

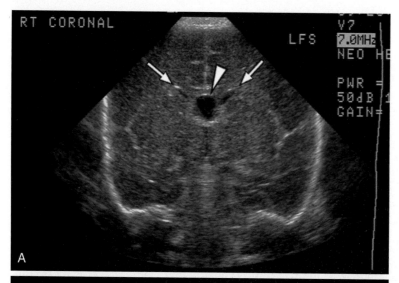

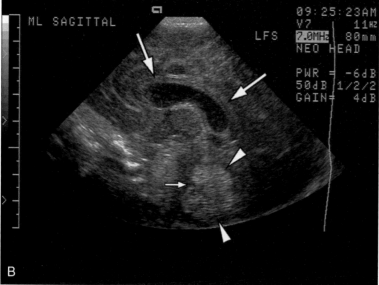

Figure 8–1. Normal findings of a premature neonate on ultrasonography of the head. *A,* Coronal view demonstrates lateral ventricles *(arrows)* and cavum septum pellucidum *(arrowhead).* Note the lack of sulcation at this stage of brain development, with the brain surface appearing smooth. *B,* Midline sagittal view demonstrates normal midline structures, including corpus callosum *(large arrows),* cerebellar vermis *(arrowheads),* and fourth ventricle *(small arrow).*

"hemorrhage" (grade IV) is thought to be secondary to venous infarction rather than to direct extension of hemorrhage. Grade I and grade II hemorrhage tend to have a good prognosis. In contrast, grade III and grade IV hemorrhage tend to have a poor prognosis, with a high incidence of death, neurologic impairment, and hydrocephalus.

Periventricular Leukomalacia

Perinatal partial asphyxia can result in damage to the periventricular white matter, the watershed zone of the premature infant. This is termed *periventricular leukomalacia* (PVL). It most commonly affects the white matter adjacent to the atria and the frontal horns of the lateral ventricles. It is associated with neurologic sequelae such as movement disorders, seizures, and spasticity. On ultrasonography,

TABLE 8–1. **Grades of Germinal Matrix Hemorrhage**

Grade	Morphologic Findings
I	Hemorrhage confined to germinal matrix
II	Intraventricular hemorrhage without ventricular dilatation
III	Intraventricular hemorrhage with ventricular dilatation
IV	Intraparenchymal hemorrhage

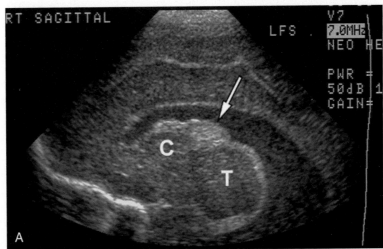

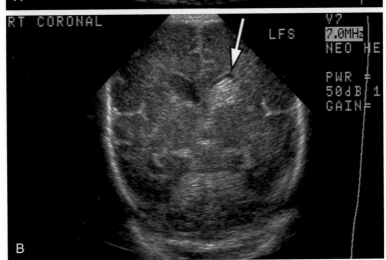

Figure 8–2. Left germinal matrix hemorrhage (grade III) in 28-week gestational age premature infant. *A,* Off-midline sagittal image demonstrates echogenic mass *(arrow)* in left caudal-thalamic groove. There is dilatation of the left lateral ventricle, which contains echogenic debris. *B,* Coronal image shows echogenic mass *(arrow)* and dilatation of the lateral ventricles. C = caudate nucleus; T = thalamus.

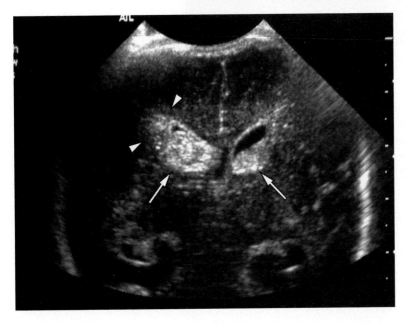

Figure 8–3. Right grade IV and left grade I germinal matrix hemorrhages. On coronal ultrasonography, there are echogenic hemorrhages *(arrows)* in the germinal matrix bilaterally. On the right, abnormally increased echogenicity extends into the adjacent white matter *(arrowheads).*

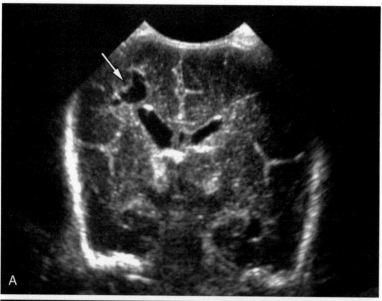

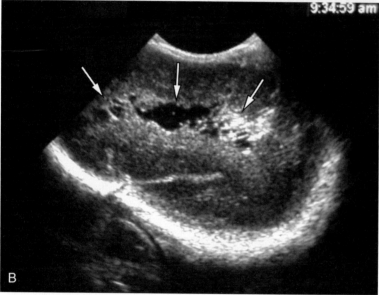

Figure 8–4. Periventricular leukomalacia in a 1-month-old infant who was born prematurely. Coronal *(A)* and sagittal off-midline *(B)* images show cystic changes *(arrows* in *B)* and coarse increased echogenicity within the white matter adjacent to the right lateral ventricle.

increased heterogeneous echogenicity is seen within the periventricular white matter. In severe cases, there may be cystic necrosis and the development of periventricular cysts (Fig. 8–4). With time, there is often volume loss of the involved white matter.

Developmental Abnormalities

Developmental abnormalities can be classified based on the embryologic event that fails, resulting in the abnormality (Table 8–2). Categories include abnormalities of dorsal induction, ventral induction, migration and cortical orga-

nization, neuronal proliferation and differentiation, and myelination. Abnormalities can also result from destruction of already formed structures. The type of developmental lesion often reflects the time that the disturbance to development occurred. Often, multiple distinct developmental abnormalities are present simultaneously.

Chiari Malformations

CHIARI MALFORMATION TYPE I

Chiari I malformation is the presence of an abnormal inferior location of the cerebellar

TABLE 8–2. **Common Developmental and Congenital Abnormalities of the Brain**

Abnormality	Mechanism (Abnormality of)	Description	Associated Imaging Findings
Chiari malformation I	Dorsal induction	Inferior displacement of cerebral tonsils of foramen magnum	Hydrocephalus Hydrosyringomyelia
Chiari malformation II	Dorsal induction	Small posterior fossa with inferior displacement of cerebellum, fourth ventricle, and brainstem into cervical canal—associated with myelomeningocele	Colpocephaly Fenestrated falx Large massa intermedia Tectal beaking Cervicomedullary kink
Holoprosencephaly	Ventral induction	Failure in cleavage of brain into two cerebral hemispheres	Alobar type: Single ventricle Fused thalami Absent corpus callosum and falx
Dandy-Walker malformation	Ventral induction	Complete or partial agenesis of the cerebellar vermis in conjunction with a retrocerebellar cyst communicating with the fourth ventricle	Posterior fossa enlarged (torcula superior to lambdoid) If normal size = D-W variant
Gray matter heterotopia	Migration	Arrested migration of neurons results in heterotopic areas of gray matter within the white matter	Subependymal or subcortical Nodular or laminar appearance Isointense to gray matter
Schizencephaly	Migration	Gray matter–lined cleft extending from lateral ventricle to cerebral surface	Entire cleft lined by gray matter Agenesis of corpus callosum
Lissencephaly (agyria)	Migration	Failure of development of gyri and sulci	Smooth cortical surface Cortical thickening Rarely isolated finding
Pachygyria	Migration	Broad, flat gyri with shallow sulci	Lumpy cortical surface Cortical thickening Rarely isolated finding
Dysgenesis of the corpus callosum	Ventral induction	Complete or partial (anterior part present) absence of the corpus callosum	Squared lateral ventricles Bundles of Probst Colpocephaly High riding third ventricle
Vein of Galen malformation	Unknown	Arteriovenous fistula to vein of Galen resulting in marked dilatation of the vein	Vascular mass in region of posterior third ventricle Hydrocephalus Congestive heart failure
Hydranencepaly	Injury of formed structures	Destruction of the cerebrum secondary to infarct from bilateral internal carotid artery occlusion	Cerebrum replaced by thin-walled sacks of CSF Falx present Thalami separated
Porencephaly	Injury of formed structures	Cyst formation from injury to brain parenchyma during first or second trimester	Thin-walled, CSF cyst No septations

CSF = cerebrospinal fluid.

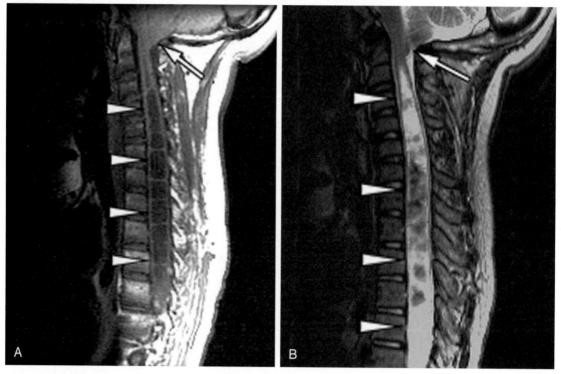

Figure 8–5. Chiari I malformation with associated hydrosyringomyelia. Sagittal T1 *(A)* and T2-weighted *(B)* MR images show the cerebellar tonsils *(arrows)* to be inferiorly located in relation to the foramen magnum. There is a large associated hydrosyringomyelia *(arrowheads)* seen as low signal on T1-weighted images and high signal on T2-weighted images. The heterogeneous signal is related to a pulsation artifact.

tonsils at least 5 mm below the foramen magnum (Fig. 8–5). The medulla and fourth ventricle are in a normal position. Complications of Chiari I malformation include hydrocephalus and hydrosyringomyelia (up to 25% of cases) (see Fig. 8–5). It may be suspected on CT when the foramen magnum appears "full" of soft tissue. It is best visualized on sagittal T1-weighted MR images. The cerebellar tonsils are seen to be positioned inferiorly and typically appear elongated rather than round.

CHIARI MALFORMATION TYPE II

Type II Chiari malformations are almost always associated with myelomeningoceles. Conversely, almost all patients with myelomeningocele have Chiari II malformations. There is a small posterior fossa with associated inferior displacement of the cerebellum, medulla, and fourth ventricle into the upper cervical canal (Fig. 8–6). Associated imaging findings include a kinked appearance of the medulla,

colpocephaly (disproportionate enlargement of the posterior body of the lateral ventricles), fenestration of the falx cerebri associated with interdigitation of gyri across the midline, enlargement of the massa intermedia, inferior pointing of the lateral ventricles, and tectal beaking (a pointed appearance of the quadrigeminal plate). Chiari II malformations are usually associated with hydrocephalus.

Type III and type IV Chiari malformations are rare.

Holoprosencephaly

Holoprosencephaly results from lack of cleavage of the brain into two hemispheres. Although there is a contiguous spectrum of severity, holoprosencephaly is classically classified into one of three distinct groups: alobar, semilobar, or lobar. The severity of the brain abnormality is reflected in the severity of the midline facial abnormality.

Alobar holoprosencephaly is the most severe

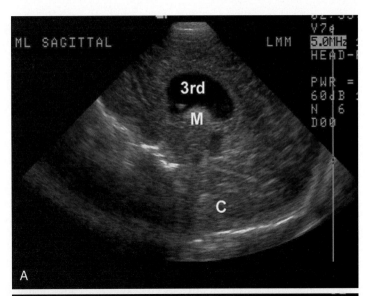

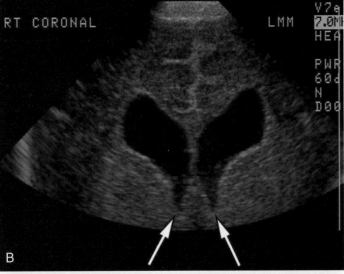

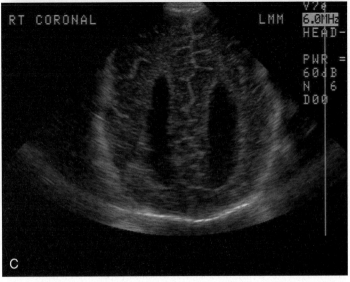

Figure 8–6. Chiari II malformation shown on ultrasonography in a newborn infant with myelomeningocele. *A,* Midline sagittal ultrasonogram shows inferior displacement of the cerebellum (C). The fourth ventricle is effaced and not visualized. There is a prominent massa intermedia (M). The third ventricle is dilated (3rd) secondary to hydrocephalus. *B,* Coronal image shows inferior "pointing" of the lateral ventricles *(arrows).* There is obstructive hydrocephalus, with dilatation of the lateral ventricles. *C,* More posterior coronal image shows interdigitation of the cerebral gyri secondary to fenestration of the falx cerebri.

form and is characterized by a monoventricle. The thalami are fused, and there is no attempt at cleavage of the cerebral hemispheres. There is no falx cerebri or corpus callosum. There is a single anterior cerebral artery. These infants are stillborn or die soon after birth.

With the intermediate form, semilobar holoprosencephaly, the cerebral hemispheres are partially cleaved from each other posteriorly. The temporal horns may be formed, but there is a single ventricle anteriorly. There is partial separation of the thalami. The cerebral hemispheres are partially cleaved posteriorly. Midline structures such as the falx cerebri and corpus callosum may be present posteriorly but not anteriorly.

Lobar holoprosencephaly is the least severe form. The occipital and temporal horns are well formed, but there is failure of cleavage of the cerebral hemispheres frontally (Fig. 8–7). The septum pellucidum is absent, and the corpus callosum may be absent or dysplastic.

Septooptic Dysplasia

Septooptic dysplasia is another type of ventral induction malformation, analogous to mild holoprosencephaly. It is characterized by absence of the septum pellucidum and hypopla-

sia of the optic nerves. It is often associated with schizencephaly, heterotopias, and hypothalamic and pituitary dysfunction. In septooptic dysplasia, the frontal horns of the lateral ventricles have a squared appearance and point inferiorly on coronal MR images.

Posterior Fossa Cystic Malformations

Posterior fossa cystic malformations include a spectrum of abnormalities. They can be divided into four defined groups: Dandy-Walker malformation, Dandy-Walker variant, mega cisterna magna, and arachnoid cyst.

Dandy-Walker malformation is complete or partial agenesis of the cerebellar vermis in conjunction with the presence of a posterior fossa cyst that communicates with the fourth ventricle (Fig. 8–8). The posterior fossa is enlarged so that the torcula is elevated above the lambda (see Fig. 8–8). The falx cerebelli is absent. Often, there are also supratentorial abnormalities, including holoprosencephaly, agenesis of the corpus callosum, polymicrogyria, and heterotopias. Hydrocephalus is common.

Dandy-Walker variant is considered present when not all the criteria for the classic malformation are present. Most commonly, the cere-

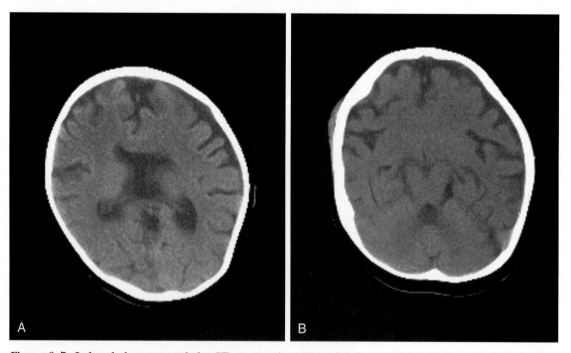

Figure 8–7. Lobar holoprosencephaly. CT at superior *(A)* and inferior *(B)* levels through frontal lobes demonstrates well-formed occipital lobes but fused frontal lobes.

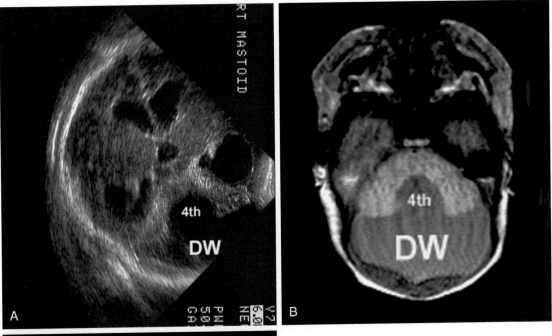

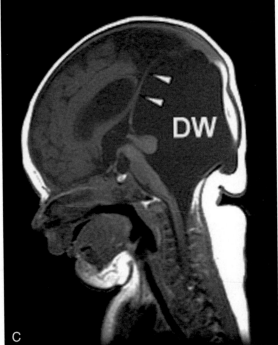

Figure 8–8. Dandy-Walker malformation in a newborn infant. *A,* Ultrasonogram obtained in axial plane, from mastoid approach, demonstrates a large posterior fossa cyst (DW) that communicates with the fourth ventricle (4th). There is dilatation of the lateral and third ventricles as well. *B,* Axial, proton density–weighted MR image shows large posterior fossa cyst (DW) that communicates with the fourth ventricle (4th). *C,* Sagittal, T1-weighted MR image shows large posterior fossa cyst (DW) enlarging the posterior fossa. The cerebellar vermis is absent. The torcula *(arrowheads)* is elevated.

bellar vermis is hypoplastic but present and there is a posterior fossa cyst, but the posterior fossa is not enlarged (Fig. 8–9). When an enlarged posterior fossa cerebrospinal fluid (CSF) cyst is seen in the presence of a fully developed cerebellar vermis, there are two possibilities. If the cyst exhibits no mass effect on the cerebellum, a mega–cisterna magna is considered to be present. If the cyst does exhibit mass effect on the cerebellum, an arachnoid cyst is considered to be present (Fig. 8–10).

Gray Matter Heterotopias

Heterotopias are an abnormality of neuronal migration characterized by arrest in migration

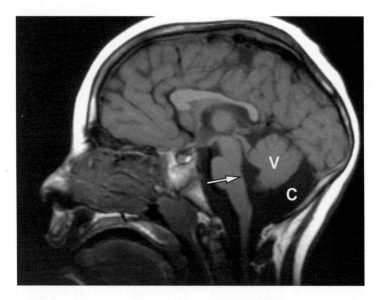

Figure 8–9. Dandy-Walker Variant. Sagittal, T1-weighted, MR image shows posterior fossa cyst (C) that communicates to fourth ventricle *(arrow)*. The vermis (V) is hypoplastic but present. The posterior fossa is not enlarged.

of the neurons from the subependymal area to the cortex. Typically, heterotopias are associated with other migrational disorders, such as schizencephaly, lissencephaly, or polymicrogyria. When heterotopias occur as an isolated abnormality, they typically present with focal seizures. On CT and MRI, the lesions appear as nodular (Figs. 8–11 and 8–12) or linear (Fig. 8–13) areas within the white matter, most typically in the subcortical or subependymal regions. Heterotopias tend to be isointense, with gray matter on all pulse sequences.

Schizencephaly

Schizencephaly is another migrational disorder. The term refers to a gray matter–lined cleft in the cerebral hemisphere. The cleft typically extends from the lateral ventricle to the surface of the brain. On T1-weighted images, the lesion appears as a gray matter–lined cleft (Fig. 8–14). Schizencephaly has been characterized as open or closed lipped. However, this has little clinical relevance. The lesion can be unilateral or bilateral and can occur anywhere in the cerebral hemispheres. In most cases, there is associated agenesis of the corpus callosum.

The presence of gray matter lining the entire cleft is the diagnostic feature that separates schizencephaly from other causes of clefts, such as porencephaly (see further on). In cases of porencephaly, the cleft is lined by (extends through) both gray and white matter.

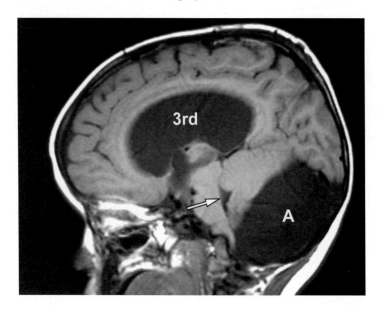

Figure 8–10. Posterior fossa arachnoid cyst. Sagittal T1-weighted MR image shows posterior fossa cyst (A) that does not communicate with the fourth ventricle *(arrow)*. There is mass effect on the cerebellum. The third ventricle (3rd) is markedly dilated.

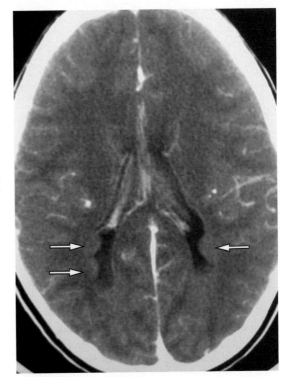

Figure 8–11. Heterotopic gray matter in a 5-year-old boy with seizures. CT shows nodular areas *(arrows)* adjacent to the lateral ventricles. The nodules are the same attenuation as gray matter.

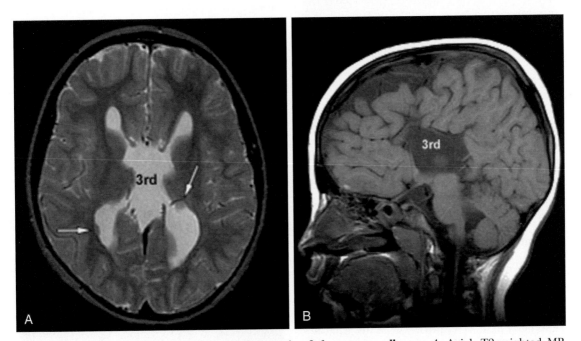

Figure 8–12. Heterotopic gray matter and dysgenesis of the corpus callosum. *A,* Axial, T2-weighted MR image shows nodular areas *(arrows)* adjacent to the lateral ventricles. The nodules are the same signal as gray matter. There is also a high-riding third ventricle (3rd) positioned between the lateral ventricles, suggestive of dysgenesis of the corpus callosum. There is colpocephaly seen as dilatation of the posterior lateral ventricles *(arrows)*. *B,* Sagittal, T1-weighted MR image shows absence of corpus callosum. The third ventricle (3rd) is seen to be superiorly displaced.

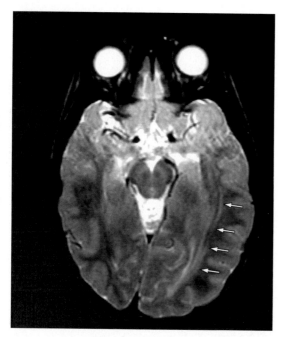

Figure 8–13. Band heterotopia and hemimega-loencephaly in a 6-year-old boy with seizures. Axial, T2-weighted MR image shows heterotopias as multiple linear structures *(arrows)* within the left parietal white matter that are isointense to gray matter. The left hemisphere is larger than the right.

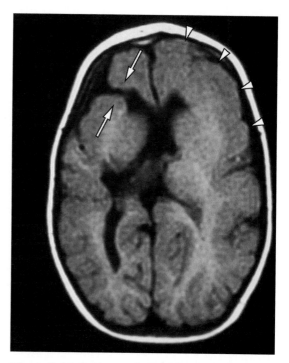

Figure 8–14. Schizencephaly with associated pachygyria in a child with weakness since birth. Axial, T1-weighted image shows gray matter–lined cleft *(arrows)* connecting right lateral ventricle to brain surface. There are also areas of poorly defined, thickened gyri *(arrowheads).*

Lissencephaly

Lissencephaly refers to arrest of migration of neurons resulting in either total failure of development of sulci and gyri (agyria) (Fig. 8–15) or the development of abnormal broad and flat gyri with abnormally shallow sulci (pachygyria) (Fig. 8–16; see also Fig 8–14). Agyria and pachygyria are best visualized with MRI. There is often thickening of the associated cortex. Neither lesion typically appears in isolation. Typically, there are patchy areas of either agyria or pachygyria, or both. These abnormalities are often associated with other migrational abnormalities and also occur as part of a number of rare syndromes.

Polymicrogyria is a similar disorder that results in small, disorganized gyri. It too is usually associated with other migrational abnormalities. There is controversy as to whether polymicrogyria is a disorder of migration or a cortical dysplasia.

Dysgenesis of Corpus Callosum

Dysgenesis of the corpus callosum includes both complete and partial absence. The cor-

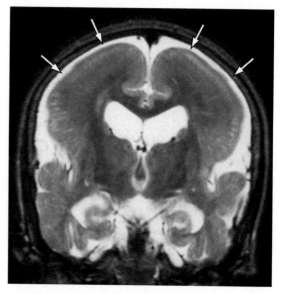

Figure 8–15. Agyria (lissencephaly) in a 10-year-old girl with seizures and developmental delay. Coronal T2-weighted image shows smooth surface of bilateral frontal lobes *(arrows)* without formation of sulci and gyri.

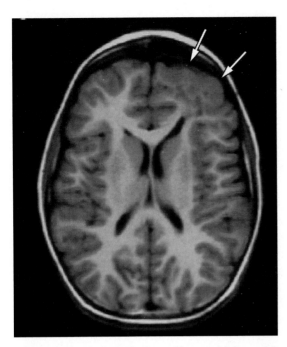

Figure 8–16. Pachygyria in a 10-year-old boy with seizures. Axial, T1-weighted image shows poorly defined, thickened gyri *(arrows)* within the left frontal lobe.

pus callosum normally develops from an anterior to posterior direction. As a result, with partial absence, it is the more anterior part of the corpus callosum that is present. Absence of the corpus callosum can occur as an isolated lesion or in conjunction with many of the other developmental lesions of the brain already described in this chapter (see Fig. 8–12). On coronal MRI, the lateral ventricles are separated and the third ventricle extends more superiorly than normal, being positioned between the lateral ventricles (see Fig. 8–12). The white matter tracts that normally cross the midline via the corpus callosum run along the medial surface of the lateral ventricles and form the bundles of Probst, which can be seen at imaging. Colpocephaly is often present (see Fig. 8–12). Midline masses, such as lipoma and arachnoid cyst, can be associated with this condition.

Vein of Galen Malformations

With vein of Galen malformation (VGMs), also known as *vein of Galen aneurysm,* there is an arteriovenous fistula connecting one or multiple cerebral arteries and the vein of Galen.

Most VGMs present during the neonatal period with congestive heart failure from the associated left-to-right shunting of blood. On chest radiography, there is cardiomegaly, signs of congestive heart failure, and widening of the superior mediastinum secondary to vascular enlargement from the increased blood flow to and from the head. Imaging studies demonstrate a large mass in the region of the posterior third ventricle. Doppler imaging, MR arteriography, or contrast-enhanced CT document the vascular nature of the lesion (Fig. 8–17). On MRI, the prominent arterial structures may be seen feeding the dilated vein. There is often associated hydrocephalus. Most VGMs are treated with arterial embolization. In most cases, lack of treatment results in death.

Sequelae of In Utero Insults

In contrast to developmental abnormalities that result from abnormal formation, other congenital abnormalities may arise from destruction of already developed structures. Most commonly, these are related to vascular ischemia and infarction that can occur secondary to a number of underlying causes. The most commonly encountered lesions are hydranencephaly, porencephaly, and encephalomalacia.

Hydranencephaly

Hydranencephaly refers to destruction of the majority of the cerebral hemisphere secondary to a massive ischemic event thought to be related to bilateral internal carotid artery occlusion. In place of the cerebral parenchyma are large thin-walled cystic structures. The occipital lobes, inferior temporal lobes, thalami, brainstem, and cerebellum are typically intact. These structures remain because they are supplied by the vertebrobasilar arterial system. The presence of the falx cerebri and separation of the thalami seen in hydranencephaly help to differentiate this disorder from severe (alobar) holoprosencephaly. It is sometimes impossible to differentiate hydranencephaly from severe hydrocephalus.

Porencephaly and Encephalomalacia

Before the end of the second trimester, parenchymal injury does not result in glial scar for-

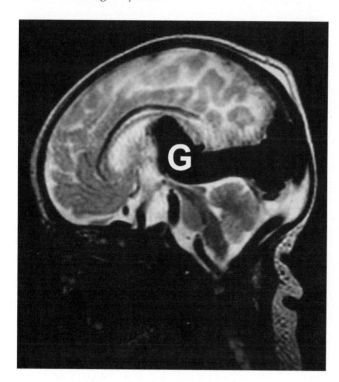

Figure 8–17. Vein of Galen malformation in a newborn infant. Sagittal, T2-weighted MR image shows signal void in aneurysm of vein of Galen (G).

mation. During this time, focal injury results in the development of a fluid-filled space. When such a cyst communicates with the ventricles, it is called a *porencephalic cyst*. On imaging, they appear as thin-walled CSF-containing cysts communicating directly with the ventricles (Fig. 8–18). There are no septations. During the third trimester, parenchymal injury incites glial scar formation. During this period, brain injury results in encephalomalacia, which appears as areas of high T2-weighted signal with multiple septations in the region of injury.

Neurocutaneous Syndromes

The neurocutaneous syndromes (phakomatoses) are a group of related diseases that affect tissues of ectodermal origin, primarily the skin and nervous system. Some of the more common phakomatoses to present in childhood include neurofibromatosis, tuberous sclerosis (TS), and Sturge-Weber syndrome.

Neurofibromatosis

Neurofibromatosis is the most common of the phakomatoses and is divided into a number of subcategories, of which neurofibromatosis type 1 (NF1) and neurofibromatosis type 2 (NF2) are the most common.

NF1 is a autosomal dominant disorder. The diagnostic criteria for NF1 are listed in Table

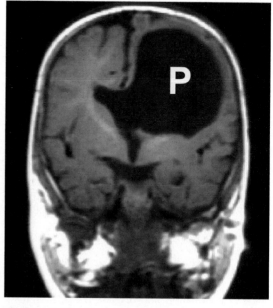

Figure 8–18. Porencephalic cyst. Coronal T1-weighted MR image shows a large CSF cyst (P) that is contiguous with the left lateral ventricle.

TABLE 8–3. **Diagnostic Criteria for Neurofibromatosis Type 1**

Two or more of the following:
1. Six or more café-au-lait macules
2. Two or more neurofibromas or one plexiform neurofibroma
3. Axillary or inguinal freckles
4. Bilateral optic nerve gliomas
5. Two hamartomas of the iris (Lisch nodules)
6. Parent, sibling, or child with NF1

NF = neurofibromatosis.

8–3. The neuroimaging manifestations of NF1 are multiple. The most common central nervous system (CNS) lesion (in up to 95% of patients with NF1) is the "NF1 spots" that appear as high-intensity signal T2-weighted lesions in the globus pallidus (Fig. 8–19), cerebellum, brainstem, internal capsule, splenium, and thalami. The lesions typically arise at 3 years, increase in number and size until 12 years, and then regress. Other lesions of NF1 include optic tract gliomas (Fig. 8–20), cerebral astrocytomas, hydrocephalus, vascular dysplasia (moyamoya secondary to stenosis, aneurysms), dural ectasia, and sphenoid wing dysplasia. NF1 patients can develop cranial nerve schwannomas, peripheral neurofibromas (Fig. 8–21), plexiform neurofibromas (Fig. 8–22), and malignant peripheral nerve sheath tumors. Plexiform neurofibromas are locally aggressive masses that are histologically more disorganized than typical neurofibromas. In the head and neck, they often involve the scalp and orbit. They are often monitored

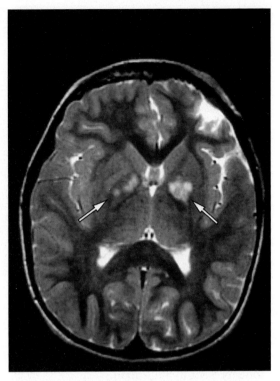

Figure 8–19. Neurofibromatosis type 1 in a 3-year-old girl. Axial, T2-weighted MR image shows NF1 "spots" as abnormally increased signal within the globus pallidus bilaterally *(arrows)*.

with imaging to evaluate findings suspicious for malignant degeneration. Spinal manifestations include posterior vertebral scalloping from dural ectasia, neurofibromas, scoliosis, and lateral meningoceles.

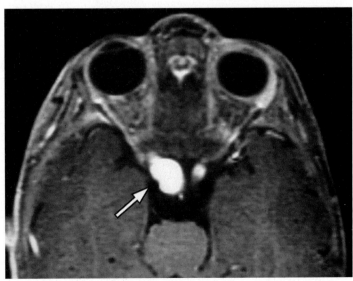

Figure 8–20. Optic nerve glioma in a patient with NF1. Contrast-enhanced, fat-saturated T1-weighted MR image shows enlargement and enhancement of the posterior right optic nerve *(arrow)*.

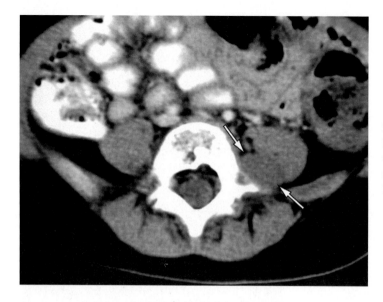

Figure 8–21. Peripheral neurofibroma in a 3-year-old girl with NF1. CT of the abdomen shows well-defined mass *(arrows)* posterior to left psoas muscle.

In contrast, NF2 is characterized by the presence of bilateral acoustic schwannomas. Other associated lesions include meningiomas, gliomas, and neurofibromas. Patients most commonly present in adulthood.

Tuberous Sclerosis

TS is an autosomal dominant syndrome associated with the classic triad of seizures, mental retardation, and adenoma sebaceum (a facial rash that is an angiofibroma of the skin). The

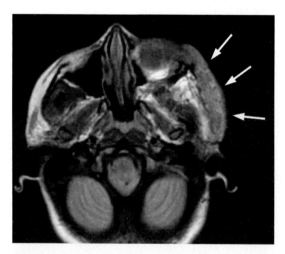

Figure 8–22. Plexiform neurofibroma in a child with NF1. Axial, proton density–weighted MR image shows abnormal high-signal tissue *(arrows)* involving the skin and subcutaneous tissues in the region of the left orbit.

disease affects the skin, CNS, skeletal system, and abdominal organs.

The most common neurologic imaging finding is the presence of tubers, which are hamartomatous lesions that appear as subependymal masses. They typically occur along the lateral ventricles (Fig. 8–23). The signal characteristics are variable and are related to age. In older patients, tubers are often calcified. In older children, the lesions tend to be isointense to gray matter. Most tubers do not enhance. Interval growth and development of contrast enhancement are findings that are associated with malignant degeneration, a rare occurrence. However, enhancement in itself does not imply malignancy. When a tuber near the foramen of Monroe rapidly enlarges, it is referred to as a *giant cell tumor.* Such giant cell tumors frequently lead to hydrocephalus. Patients with TS can also have areas with an abnormally high T2-weighted signal within the white matter secondary to areas of abnormal glial cells (see Fig. 8–23).

Visceral manifestations of TS include renal cysts, renal angiomyelofibromas, cardiac rhabdomyoma, and hamartomas of other organs.

Sturge-Weber Syndrome

Sturge-Weber syndrome, or encephalotrigeminal angiomatosis, is characterized by a low-flow vascular malformation in the distribution of the trigeminal nerve, both intracranially and extracranially. The syndrome manifests with

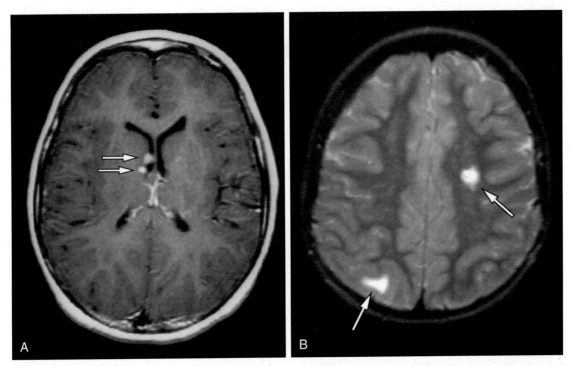

Figure 8–23. Tuberous sclerosis in a 9-year-old boy with seizures. *A,* Contrast-enhanced, T1-weighted MR image shows subependymal masses *(arrows)* consistent with tubers. *B,* Axial, T2-weighted MR image shows areas of abnormally high signal *(arrows)* within the white matter, secondary to abnormal glial cells.

abnormalities of the skin (port wine nevus), leptomeninges, and underlying brain. The altered flow results in chronic ischemic injury to the affected underlying brain. On CT, there is serpiginous calcification, abnormal enhancement, and atrophy of the involved gyri (Fig. 8–24). The cranium is often thickened adjacent to the brain abnormalities. Clinical manifestations include seizures, mental retardation, and hemiparesis.

Normal Myelination

There are great changes in myelination of the brain that occur during the first 24 months of life. Before myelination, white matter is hydrophilic and, because it contains water, appears high in signal on T2-weighted images and low in signal on T1-weighted images (Fig. 8–25). With myelination, the white matter becomes hydrophobic and, because it contains less water, appears low in signal on T2-weighted images and high in signal on T1-weighted images (see Fig. 8–25). Myelination progresses from a caudal to a cranial direction, paralleling neurologic development. During the first 3 months of life, there is progressive myelination of the spinal cord and brainstem, followed

by the cerebellar white matter. The corpus callosum begins to myelinate in the splenium at 2 to 3 months, proceeds anteriorly, and is completely myelinated through the rostrum by 6 to 8 months. The adult pattern of myelination is complete by 18 to 24 months.

Abnormal myelination is a nonspecific finding and can be secondary to a number of causes, including metabolic disease, infection, trauma, hypoxia-ischemia, and malformative syndromes.

Metabolic and Degenerative Disorders

There are a large number of metabolic, degenerative, and toxic disorders that can result in abnormal myelination patterns. Most of these diseases are rare and untreatable. Categories of disease include lysosomal storage disorders, mitochondrial disorders, peroxisomal disorders, and amino acid disorders, among others. On MRI, these disorders typically demonstrate an abnormally increased T2-weighted signal involving portions of white matter or gray matter, or a combination of the two. There may be associated atrophy of the involved structures. The distribution of the abnormal signal

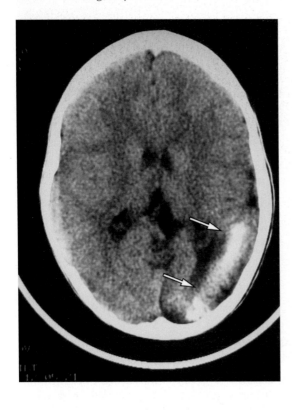

Figure 8–24. Sturge-Weber syndrome in a 9-year-old boy. CT without contrast enhancement shows abnormal calcifications *(arrows)* within the left parieto-occipital region. There is associated atrophy with secondary enlargement of the adjacent lateral ventricle.

can be helpful in narrowing the differential diagnosis (Figs. 8–26 and 8–27). Representative disorders and the associated distribution of abnormality as demonstrated on MRI are listed in Table 8–4.

Infection

Many of the imaging findings of CNS infection (meningitis, cerebritis, empyema, encephalitis, and parenchymal abscess) in children are simi-

TABLE 8–4. **Metabolic and Degenerative Central Nervous System Disorders**

Disorder	Category of Disease	Primary Distribution of Abnormality on Magnetic Resonance Imaging
Leigh disease	Disorder of mitochondria	Deep gray matter
Kearns-Sayre disease	Disorder of mitochondria	Deep gray (primarily globus pallidus) and white matter
Adrenoleukodystrophy	Peroxisomal disorder	White matter (initially central white matter)
Phenylketonuria	Amino acid disorder	White matter (initially central white matter)
Maple syrup urine disease	Amino acid disorder	Deep gray (primarily globus pallidus) and white matter
Mucolipodoses	Lysosomal storage disorders	Cortical gray matter
Mucopolysaccharidoses	Lysosomal storage disorders	Cortical gray matter and white matter
Metachromatic leukodystrophy	Lysosomal storage disorders	White matter (initially central white matter)
Krabbe disease	Lysosomal storage disorders	White matter (initially central white matter)
Canavan disease	Miscellaneous metabolic disorders	Deep gray (primarily globus pallidus) and white matter (initially peripheral white matter)
Alexander disease	Miscellaneous metabolic disorders	White matter (initially peripheral white matter)

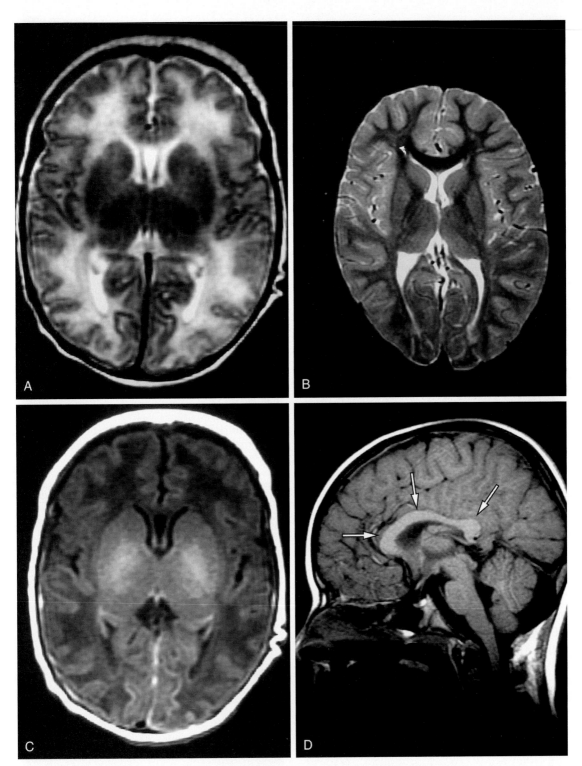

Figure 8–25. Age-related change in MR appearance of white matter related to myelination. *A,* Premyelination T2-weighted appearance in an 8-day-old infant. Axial, T2-weighted MR image shows white matter to be diffusely high in signal. *B,* Postmyelination T2-weighted (adult) appearance in an 8-year-old child. Axial, T2-weighted MR image shows white matter to be diffusely low in signal. *C,* Premyelination T1-weighted appearance in the same 8-day-old infant as shown in *A*. Axial, T1-weighted MR image shows white matter to be diffusely low in signal. *D,* Postmyelination T1-weighted (adult) appearance in same 8-year-old child as shown in *B*. Axial, T1-weighted MR image shows white matter to be higher in signal. Note high signal in corpus callosum *(arrows)*.

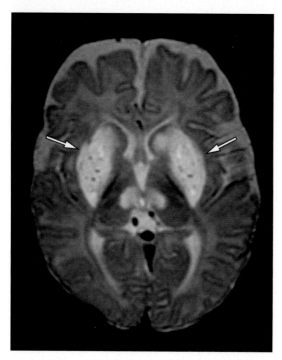

Figure 8–26. Leigh disease in a 5-month-old boy. Axial, T2-weighted MR image shows abnormally increased signal within the deep white matter of the basal ganglia *(arrows)*. There is also atrophy within the frontal lobes.

lar to those seen in adults and are not emphasized here. This section concentrates on several issues unique to children.

CONGENITAL INFECTIONS

There are a number of in utero infections (TORCH [toxoplasmosis, other infections, rubella, cytomegalovirus {CMV} infection, and herpes simplex]; see Chapter 7) that can affect the CNS. They demonstrate unique findings when compared with CNS infection that occurs later in life, because they can affect brain development. The severity of the abnormality often reflects the period of development at which the infection occurred.

CMV infection is the most common TORCH infection to involve the CNS. Imaging findings include periventricular calcifications, migrational abnormalities (cortical dysplasia), cerebellar hypoplasia, and ventricular enlargement (Fig. 8–28). Clinical manifestations include microcephaly, hearing impairment, mental retardation, and developmental delay.

Toxoplasmosis is the second most common

TORCH infection to involve the CNS. The parenchymal calcifications seen in toxoplasmosis are more variable in location than the periventricular calcifications seen with CMV. Other manifestations include hydrocephalus or, in severe cases, hydranencephaly.

With congenital human immunodeficiency virus (HIV) infection, there are abnormalities within the CNS related both to primary involvement with HIV and to secondary complications such as infection and tumor. However, secondary infection and tumor are seen much less commonly in children than in adults. The majority of children with congenital HIV infection have CNS manifestations, typically progressive encephalopathy. Imaging findings include diffuse atrophy, delayed myelination, and calcifications. These calcifications most commonly occur within the basal ganglia and subcortical white matter of the frontal lobes.

ENCEPHALITIS

Encephalitis is inflammation of the brain, sometimes seen in conjunction with menin-

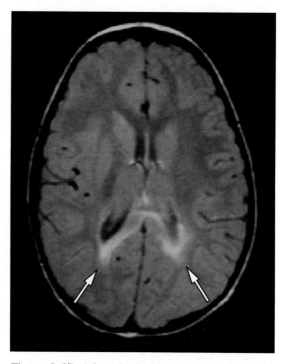

Figure 8–27. Adrenoleukodystrophy in a 9-month-old boy failing milestones. Axial, T2-weighted MR image shows abnormally increased signal *(arrows)* in the central white matter posteriorly.

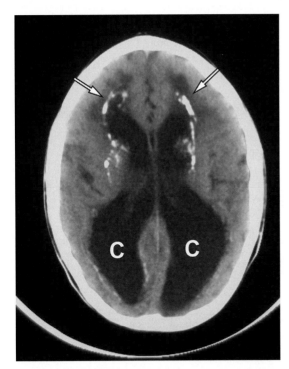

Figure 8–28. Sequelae of cytomegalovirus (CMV) infection. CT shows periventricular calcifications *(arrows)*. There is colpocephaly shown as ventricular dilatation, which is disproportionately greater in the posterior portions of the lateral ventricles (C).

geal inflammation. It can occur secondary to direct viral infection, secondary autoimmune response to a virus or immunization, or as the extension of a meningeal infection. Children typically present with seizures, lethargy, or focal neurologic deficits. Several types of encephalitis that occur predominantly during childhood are listed here.

Herpes simplex caused by herpesvirus 1 can lead to a necrotizing meningoencephalitis. When it occurs secondary to reactivation and migration of a previous, latent infection via the branches of the trigeminal nerve, it typically affects one or both temporal lobes. On MRI, high signal is seen within the cortex of one or both temporal lobes. There are often areas of hemorrhage within the affected areas. In neonates who obtain a systemic infection during birth, any portion of the brain can be affected.

Subacute sclerosing panencephalitis (SSP) is thought to be an encephalitis secondary to reactivation of a latent measles infection. It is a disease of childhood. Imaging demonstrates nonspecific atrophy and an increased T2-

weighted signal within the cerebral white matter (Fig. 8–29).

Acute disseminated encephalomyelitis (ADEM) is an immunologic disease that occurs in response to a recent viral infection or immunization. It typically occurs days to weeks after the preceding stimulus. On MRI, areas of increased T2-weighted signal are typically seen in the white matter (Fig. 8–30), the brainstem, and the cerebellum. The treatment consists of steroids, and some children may recover completely.

Tumors

Tumors of the CNS are the most common solid malignancy of childhood. When imaging to determine the differential diagnosis, it is easiest to categorize tumors by their anatomic location: posterior fossa, supratentorial (cerebral or region of the third ventricle), extraaxial, and head and neck tumors.

Posterior Fossa Tumors

Tumors of the posterior fossa are more common in childhood than in adulthood. The

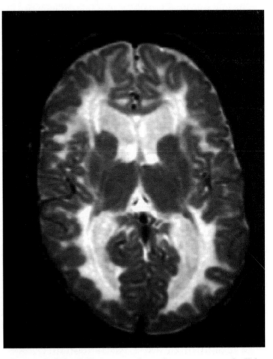

Figure 8–29. Subacute sclerosing panencephalitis. Axial, T2-weighted MR image shows abnormally increased signal throughout the periventricular white matter. There is associated volume loss with dilatation of the lateral ventricles.

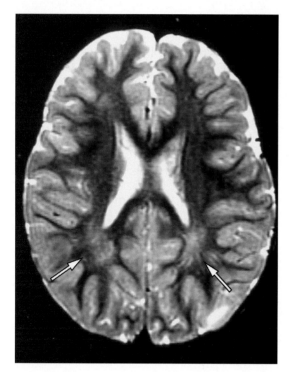

Figure 8–30. Acute disseminated encephalomyelitis (ADEM) in a 3-year-old with seizures. Axial, T2-weighted MR image shows abnormally increased signal *(arrows)* in the white matter posterior to the lateral ventricles.

TABLE 8–5. **Posterior Fossa Tumors**

Tumor	Imaging Characteristics
Cerebellar astrocytoma	Cystic or solid Mural nodule common when cystic Solid—heterogeneous signal density Well defined Fourth ventricle displaced anteriorly with well-defined interface No calcification or hemorrhage
Medulloblastoma	Arises from roof of fourth ventricle—poorly defined interface Homogeneous signal on MRI Poorly defined CSF metastasis
Brainstem glioma	Circumferential enlargement or exophytic mass of brainstem (most commonly pons) Nonenhancing Fourth ventricle pushed anteriorly Hydrocephalus uncommon
Ependymoma	Arises from floor of fourth ventricle—poorly defined interface Heterogeneous on CT and MRI (hemorrhage, necrosis) Well-defined lobulated margins Calcification 70%

MRI = magnetic resonance imaging; CSF = cerebrospinal fluid; CT = computed tomography.

most common tumors of the posterior fossa in children include medulloblastoma, cerebellar astrocytoma, brainstem glioma, and ependymoma (Table 8–5). As previously discussed, other nonneoplastic conditions that are associated with a posterior fossa mass include Dandy-Walker malformation, arachnoid cyst, and mega cisterna magna. Extraaxial tumors, such as meningiomas, can also occur. Posterior fossa tumors often present with obstructive hydrocephalus secondary to compression of the fourth ventricle.

Cerebellar Astrocytoma

Cerebellar astrocytoma is the most common type of posterior fossa tumor. It is a low-grade malignancy (pilocytic subtype) and has the best prognosis of any CNS malignancy. Most require only surgical resection. The lesion typically occurs in the vermis or cerebellar hemispheres. There is a wide spectrum of appearances on imaging. Cerebellar astrocytomas can be predominantly cystic or completely solid in

appearance. There can be an enhancing mural nodule associated with the cystic lesions (Fig. 8–31). The margins of the lesions are usually well defined. The fourth ventricle is displaced

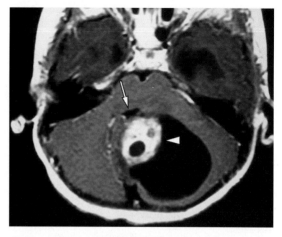

Figure 8–31. Cerebellar astrocytoma. Contrast enhanced T1-weighted MR image shows a predominantly cystic mass displacing the fourth ventricle *(arrow)* anteriorly. There is an enhancing mural nodule *(arrowhead)*.

anteriorly and the margin between the lesion and the fourth ventricle is typically well defined. Unlike medulloblastoma or ependymoma, cerebellar astrocytoma usually does not demonstrate areas of calcification or hemorrhage. The solid lesions enhance heterogeneously.

Medulloblastoma

Medulloblastoma is the second most common posterior fossa tumor in children and is the most malignant. It is considered a primitive neuroectodermal tumor and typically arises from the granular layer of the inferior medullary velum of the vermis. The neoplasm invades the fourth ventricle. On imaging, the lesion appears as a poorly defined mass filling the fourth ventricle (Fig. 8–32). Because it arises from the "roof" of the fourth ventricle, the border between the vermis and the lesion as seen on a sagittal MR image is poorly defined (see Fig. 8–32). On CT, the lesion may appear as hyperdense and enhance diffusely and homogeneously. On MRI, the lesions tend to be more homogeneous in signal than either cerebellar astrocytomas or ependymomas. Medulloblastomas tend to be hypointense to mildly hyperintense on T2-weighted images. There is a propensity for seeding within the intracranial and intraspinal CSF spaces.

Brainstem Glioma

Brainstem gliomas are most commonly astrocytomas of moderate aggressiveness. They occur most frequently in the pons. Unlike other posterior fossa masses, the lesions tend to present with cranial nerve abnormalities, pyramidal tract signs, or cerebellar dysfunction, rather than with signs of hydrocephalus. The lesions may cause circumferential enlargement of the brainstem (Fig. 8–33) or grow in an exophytic fashion. On MRI, the lesions tend to demonstrate a homogeneous high signal on T2-weighted images (see Fig. 8–33). Enhancement is rare before treatment, with the exception of exophytic lesions. Approximately 10% have a cystic component. If displaced, the fourth ventricle is pushed posteriorly (see Fig. 8–33). Complete surgical resection is not possible in many of these tumors. Radiation therapy remains the primary mode of therapy.

Ependymoma

Ependymomas are relatively slow-growing, typically benign tumors that arise from ciliated ependymal cells. Two thirds occur in the fourth ventricle. When they occur in the fourth ventricle, ependymomas arise and have a broad connection with the floor of the fourth ventricle, opposite the roof involvement

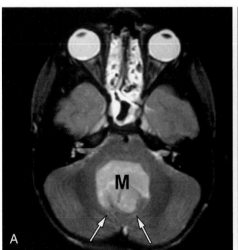
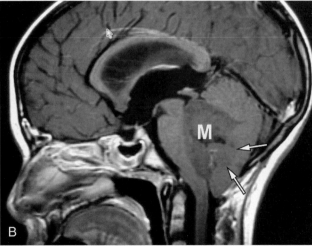

Figure 8–32. Medulloblastoma in an 11-year-old boy. *A,* Axial, T2-weighted MR image shows homogeneous high-signal mass filling the fourth ventricle. The border between the mass (M) and the vermis is poorly defined *(arrows)*. *B,* Sagittal, T1-weighted MR image shows mass filling the fourth ventricle. The poorly defined border *(arrows)* between the mass (M) and the vermis is more easily appreciated.

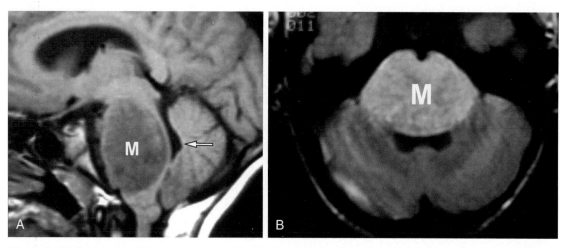

Figure 8–33. Brainstem glioma in a 7-year-old girl who presented with seventh nerve palsy. *A,* Sagittal, T1-weighted MR image shows mass (M) within brainstem. The mass is homogeneous in signal. The fourth ventricle *(arrow)* is displaced posteriorly. *B,* Axial, T2-weighted MR image shows homogeneous high-signal mass (M) in pons.

seen with medulloblastoma. Therefore, the border between the lesion and the floor of the fourth ventricle is often poorly defined (Fig. 8–34). The lesions may fill and grow out of the fourth ventricle via the foramina into the cisterna magna and spinal canal (see Fig. 8–34). The lesions appear heterogeneous on CT and MRI. Calcification is seen on CT in 70% of cases. Enhancement is heterogeneous on CT and MRI. The lesions have well-defined, lobulated margins.

Cerebral Tumors

Cerebral tumors in children are much less common than are those of the posterior fossa. Most cerebral tumors affecting children are glial in origin (astrocytoma, oligodendroglioma, or glioblastoma). These tumors range in appearance from well circumscribed to infiltrative (Fig. 8–35). The imaging appearance does not always correlate with the histologic grade. Less common tumors include em-

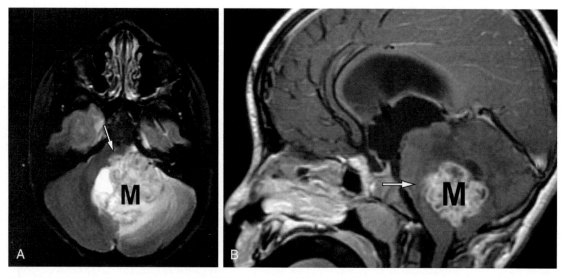

Figure 8–34. Ependymoma in a 9-year-old boy. *A,* Axial, T2-weighted MR image shows heterogeneous mass (M) filling the fourth ventricle. The border *(arrow)* between the brainstem and mass is poorly defined. *B,* Sagittal, contrast-enhanced, T1-weighted MR image shows mass (M) with heterogeneous enhancement. Again, the border *(arrow)* between the brainstem and mass is poorly defined.

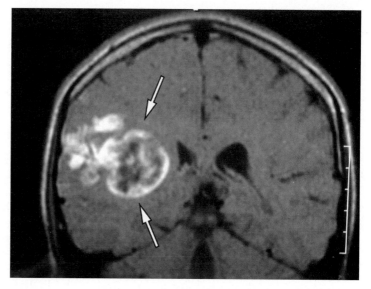

Figure 8–35. Glioblastoma in a 13-year-old girl with headaches. Coronal, contrast-enhanced, T1-weighted MR image shows heterogeneously enhancing, poorly defined mass *(arrows)*.

bryonal tumors (PNET), ependymoma, and choroid plexus tumors. The latter tumors occur most frequently in the lateral ventricles. They are benign and slow growing in most cases. However, there are malignant choroid plexus sarcomas (Fig. 8–36). These lesions are markedly vascular and demonstrate marked enhancement at imaging.

Suprasellar and Other Tumors Around the Third Ventricle

Tumors that occur in the region of the third ventricle include those that arise in the su-

prasellar region, those in the region of the pineal gland, and intraventricular tumors. Although there is a long list of tumors that can occur in this region, the most common tumors in children include optic glioma, hypothalamic glioma, craniopharyngioma, and germ cell tumor. There are also several pineal tumors that are unique to childhood.

OPTIC GLIOMA

Optic glioma is one of the most common causes of suprasellar tumors in childhood. It

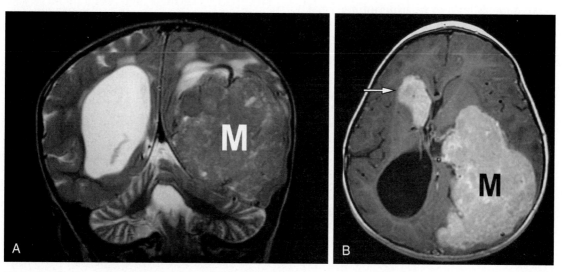

Figure 8–36. Choroid plexus sarcoma in a 4-year-old girl. *A,* Coronal T2-weighted image shows heterogeneous signal mass (M) distending left lateral ventricle. The mass is isointense to gray matter. There is hydrocephalus. *B,* Axial, contrast-enhanced, T1-weighted MR image shows mass (M) in left lateral ventricle as well as extension into the frontal horn of the right lateral ventricle *(arrow)*. There is diffuse enhancement of the mass.

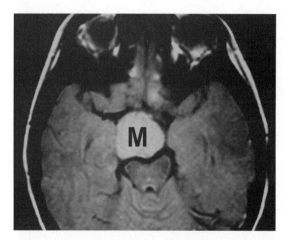

Figure 8–37. Hypothalamic glioma in a 4-year-old boy with seizures. Axial, T2-weighted MR image shows mass (M) in region of hypothalamus. The mass is homogeneously high in T2-weighted signal.

is typically an astrocytic tumor and can involve any or all portions of the visual pathways: optic nerves, chiasm, and hypothalami. Lesions range from benign hamartomatous lesions to aggressive malignancy. There is an increased incidence in patients with NF1. Optic nerve involvement is demonstrated as bulbous enlargement of the optic nerves on MRI (see Fig. 8–20). It is often difficult to differentiate optic gliomas of the chiasm from hypothalamic gliomas (Fig. 8–37) on MRI. Tumors arising in either location often extend to the other location. Both hypothalamic and optic nerve gliomas tend to be hyperintense on T2-weighted images and demonstrate diffuse enhancement with gadolinium.

GERM CELL TUMORS

Germ cell tumors of the CNS most commonly occur in the region of the pineal gland, hypothalamus, or third periventricular region. The most common histologic type is germinoma. Other types include teratoma, embryonal carcinoma, and choriocarcinoma. There may be hemorrhage in the lesions and the MRI signal and CT density are variable. Teratomas may demonstrate fatty tissue or calcifications related to tumor, bone, or teeth.

PINEAL TUMORS

Primary pineal tumors range from benign pineocytomas to pineoblastomas. The latter are highly malignant tumors, histologically similar to PNET. They occur almost exclusively in childhood. On imaging of either pineocytoma or pineoblastoma, a pineal mass is seen that demonstrates enhancement. There is almost always hydrocephalus.

CRANIOPHARYNGIOMA

Craniopharyngiomas arise from persistence and proliferation of squamous epithelial cells within the tract of an embryologic structure, the craniopharyngeal duct. They account for 7% of all intracranial tumors in children. Typically, they are intrasellar and suprasellar in location (Fig. 8–38). They are benign and slow-growing lesions. Calcifications are present in up to 80% of cases. Typically, CT shows a large, calcified suprasellar mass. The solid portions tend to enhance. There is often a cystic component. On MRI, the cystic components tend to be high signal on all sequences, because they contain proteinaceous and cholesterol-laden fluid (see Fig. 8–38). The signal characteristics of the solid portions are variable on MRI.

Trauma

The evaluation of significant pediatric head trauma should be performed with CT. Skull radiographs obtained to rule out skull fracture are grossly overused and result in increased cost and radiation and little useful information. The presence of a skull fracture does not necessarily mean that intracranial injury exists, and the absence of a skull fracture certainly does not exclude it. Finally, the presence or absence of a skull fracture usually does not affect the management of a child with head trauma.

Most of the computed tomographic findings of intracranial trauma, including the appearance of subdural hematoma, epidural hematoma, subarachnoid hemorrhage, and parenchymal contusion, are similar in appearance in both adults and children.

Abuse

For the most part, the imaging appearance of intracranial trauma that occurs secondary to abuse is similar to that seen with accidental trauma. Intracranial injury is the number one

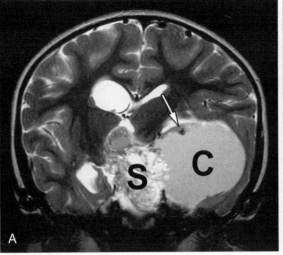
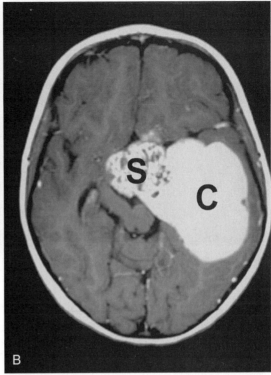

Figure 8–38. Craniopharyngioma. *A,* Coronal T2-weighted image shows heterogeneous signal mass in the suprasellar region. There are cystic (C) and solid (S) components. There is a low-signal area consistent with calcification *(arrow).* There is hydrocephalus. *B,* Axial, contrast-enhanced, T1-weighted MR image shows solid portion of mass (S) to enhance heterogeneously. The cystic component (C) is high in signal.

cause of death in abused children. Types of injury that should increase the degree of suspicion for abuse include interhemispheric subdural hematoma (from shaking) and the combination of a subdural hematoma in association with anoxic-ischemic injury (a result of suffocation and strangulation) (Fig. 8–39). Subdural hemorrhages of varying ages, as demonstrated by signal characteristics on MRI, are also suggestive.

Hydrocephalus and Ventriculoperitoneal Shunts

Hydrocephalus can be secondary to one of the many problems previously listed in this chapter: developmental anomaly, tumor, after hemorrhage, or after infection. It is a common problem encountered in pediatric neurologic imaging. These patients are often treated with ventricular shunts. The most commonly used shunt is the VPS, in which the proximal portion of the shunt is positioned in one of the lateral ventricles and the distal end is positioned in the peritoneal cavity. When patients with VPSs present with headaches, vomiting, or lethargy, increased cranial pressure from shunt malfunction is investigated. Imaging includes radiographs of the shunt from cranium to abdomen to ensure that there is no evidence of shunt disconnection or kinking. The most common site for shunt dislocation is at the connections between the shunt tubing and the shunt chamber, which usually overlies the cranium. Familiarity with the different types of commercially available shunts is important, because some types have radiolucent portions that could be mistaken for areas of disconnection.

A computed tomographic scan of the head is also obtained to look for any interval change in the size of the cerebral ventricles (Fig. 8–40). Symptoms are most often related to insufficient shunting and an interval increase in ventricular size but occasionally can be secondary to overshunting, which produces slit-like ventricles. An abdominal pseudocyst surrounding and obstructing the intraabdominal tip of the VPS is also a possible cause of ob-

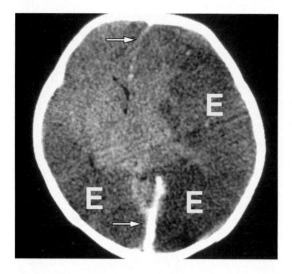

Figure 8–39. Fatal child abuse in an infant. Nonenhanced computed tomographic scan shows diffuse low attenuation (E) throughout the majority of the brain consistent with edema and infarction from strangulation. There is a resultant rightward midline shift. There is also high attenuation along the falx *(arrows)* consistent with subarachnoid hemorrhage.

struction. These may be suspected when interval radiographs demonstrate a static position of the distal shunt tubing. Further investigation for VPS pseudocyst is usually performed with ultrasonography.

Craniosynostosis

Craniosynostosis refers to premature closure of the sutures of the skull. It can occur as an idiopathic primary condition or secondary to

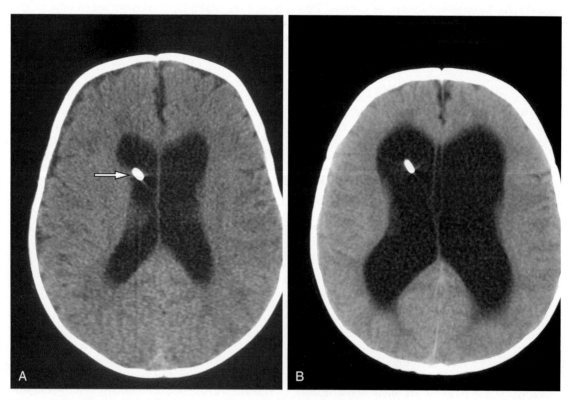

Figure 8–40. Changes on CT suggestive of ventriculoperitoneal shunt malfunction in a vomiting child. *A,* CT obtained 4 months before demonstrates dilated lateral ventricles and high-density shunt tubing *(arrow)*. *B,* Computed tomographic scan at time of presentation shows interval increase in size of lateral ventricles, consistent with increased hydrocephalus. The sulci are now effaced.

a number of genetic or metabolic disorders. Primary craniosynostosis is typically present at birth and occurs more often in boys than in girls. The sagittal suture is most commonly involved. Because the skull stops growing in the direction of the closed suture and contin-

ues to grow in the direction of the open sutures, craniosynostosis of a particular suture leads to a predictable head shape on physical examination and radiography. With sagittal suture synostosis, the head becomes long and narrow (dolichocephaly) (Fig. 8–41). With co-

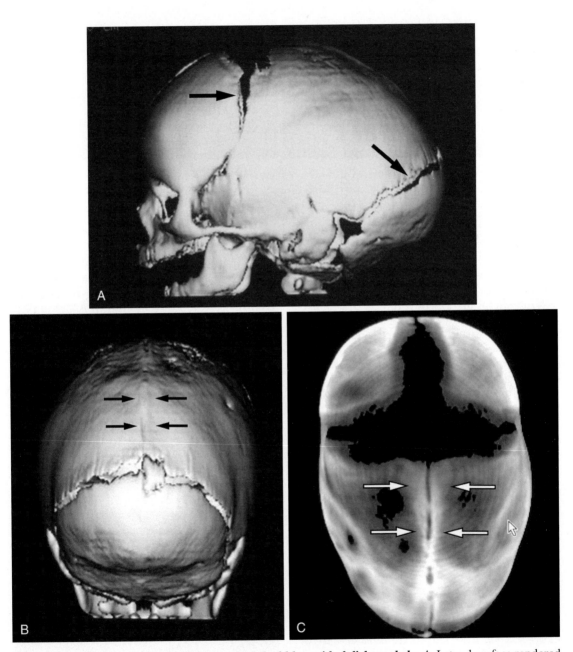

Figure 8–41. Sagittal suture synostosis in a 6-week-old boy with dolichocephaly. *A,* Lateral surface-rendered three-dimensional computed tomographic scan shows a long, narrow skull (dolichocephaly). The coronal and lambdoid sutures *(arrows)* are patent. *B,* Posterior surface–rendered three-dimensional computed tomographic scan shows fusion of the sagittal suture *(arrows).* *C,* Maximum integrity projection (MIP) image, as shown from above, demonstrates narrowing of the posterior portion of the sagittal suture with perisutural sclerosis *(arrows).* (Ignore small arrow.)

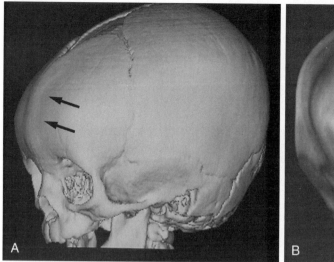 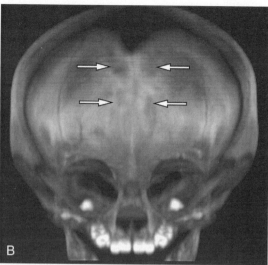

Figure 8–42. Metopic suture synostosis in an 8-week-old boy with trigonocephaly. *A,* Lateral surface–rendered three-dimensional computed tomographic scan shows a pointed appearance *(arrows)* to the forehead (trigonocephaly). The metopic suture is not visualized as a patent space. *B,* MIP image, as shown from the front, demonstrates narrowing of the metopic suture with perisutural sclerosis *(arrows).*

ronal suture synostosis, the head becomes short from anterior to posterior and wide from left to right. The orbits assume an oval, oblique lateral margin referred to as a "harlequin eye" appearance. With metopic craniosynostosis, the forehead assumes a pointed or triangular appearance (trigonocephaly) (Fig. 8–42). Synostosis of all the sutures results in cloverleaf skull (kleeblattschädel). There is severe deformity of the skull, with bulging in the squamosal areas and in the bregma. It is associated with thanatophoric dwarfism.

The screening examination for craniosynostosis remains radiography. On radiographs, in addition to the characteristic skull shapes, the involved suture will demonstrate bony bridging, perisutural sclerosis, or sutural narrowing. Many institutions perform three-dimensional helical CT of the head (see Figs. 8–41 and 8–42) using surface-rendered or maximal intensity projection (MIP) three-dimensional images.

Lacunar Skull

Lacunar skull, also known as *lückenschädel,* is the term used to describe a defect in mesenchymal formation of the skull associated with myelomeningocele. The radiographic findings include multiple oval lucencies that occur secondary to thinning of the intertable of the skull (Fig. 8–43). It is more prominent in the

occipital and parietal regions. It is present in all patients with myelomeningocele younger than 3 months, and the imaging findings are typically resolved by 6 months. It is always associated with myelomeningocele. It is said that lacunar skull should not be confused with the skull changes of increased intracranial pressure (Fig. 8–44). With increased intracranial pressure, there is marked accentuation of the

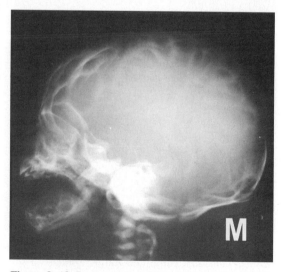

Figure 8–43. Lacunar skull in an infant with encephalocele. Radiograph shows multiple oval lucencies. The encephalocele can be seen as a subtle posterior soft tissue mass (M).

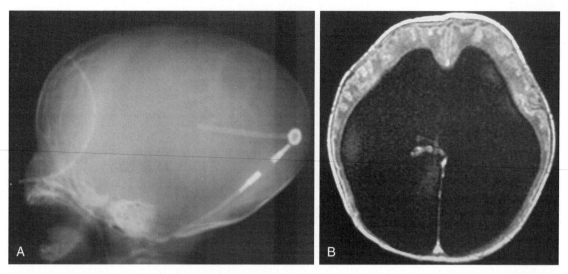

Figure 8–44. Skull changes of increased intracranial pressure. *A,* Radiograph shows accentuation of convolutional markings. Note ventriculoperitoneal shunt. *B,* Axial, T1-weighted MR image shows massive dilatation of the lateral ventricles.

normal convolutional markings. The appearance has been likened to hammer-beaten silver. Personally, I think they appear rather similar, with lacunar skull appearing more severe. Other findings of increased intracranial pressure include sutural diastasis, sellar enlargement, and demineralization.

Orbital Cellulitis

Orbital cellulitis is the most common abnormality of the pediatric orbit. It is usually a bacterial infection and arises from extension of sinus infection. The more common infectious agents include *Staphylococcus, Streptococcus,* and *Pneumococcus.* Orbital cellulitis is categorized anatomically as being preseptal or postseptal based on the relationship of the inflamed tissue to the orbital septum. When inflammation extends posterior to the septum, it is considered postseptal and is typically extraconal and subperiosteal in location (Fig. 8–45). Almost all cases of postseptal cellulitis are associated with ethmoid sinus disease. The inflammatory process is categorized as celluli-

Figure 8–45. Preseptal and postseptal cellulitis in a 4-year-old girl. Axial, contrast-enhanced computed tomographic scan shows marked thickening of the preseptal soft tissues *(arrows).* There is asymmetric thickening of the medial rectus muscle (M). There is abnormal extraconal soft tissue *(arrowheads)* between the medial rectus muscle and the bony wall of the orbit. There is no evidence of drainable abscess. There is ethmoid sinus opacification. A line drawn through the anterior bony confines of the orbit defines tissue as preseptal and postseptal.

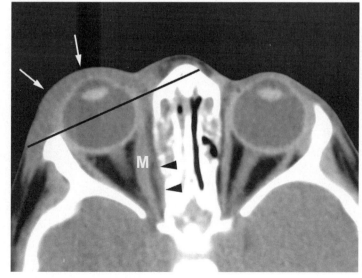

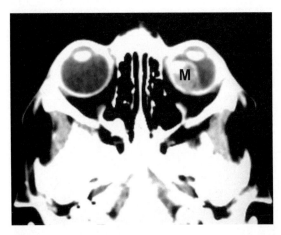

Figure 8–46. Retinoblastoma in a 1-year-old girl. CT shows calcified mass (M) within the posterior aspect of left globe.

tis or abscess. The presence of a drainable abscess is suggested on CT when rim enhancement is present surrounding an area of fluid attenuation or gas. Drainable abscesses are typically treated surgically. Cellulitis is treated with antibiotics alone.

Retinoblastoma

Retinoblastoma is a tumor that arises in the retina. It presents in patients younger than 5 years. It is bilateral in up to 25% of cases and can also rarely involve the pineal region (triretinoblastoma). In bilateral cases, there is often a genetic predisposition. Patients with retinoblastoma are also predisposed to secondary osteosarcoma after radiation therapy. On

TABLE 8–6. **More Common Causes of Pediatric Orbital Masses**

Orbital cellulitis-abscess
Orbital pseudotumor
Hemangioma
Lymphatic-venous malformation
Optic nerve glioma
Rhabdomyosarcoma
Lymphoma-leukemia
Retinoblastoma
Langerhans cell histiocytosis
Metastatic neuroblastoma
Hematoma

CT, there is a calcified intraocular mass (Fig. 8–46). MRI demonstrates a heterogeneous intraocular mass of variable enhancement. There are a variety of other causes of intraorbital masses, the most common of which are listed in Table 8–6. The differential diagnosis can be limited based on the location of the mass: global, intraconal, or extraconal (Fig. 8–47).

Neck Masses

There are a large number of causes of pediatric neck masses (Table 8–7). The most common cause of a mass in the neck of a child is suppurative lymphadenopathy (Fig. 8–48). This can occur secondary to systemic viral infection or focal bacterial infection. Lymph nodes greater than 1 to 1.5 cm within the neck are considered abnormal. Sometimes a purulent lymph node will develop into a drainable abscess.

Five percent of pediatric malignancies occur

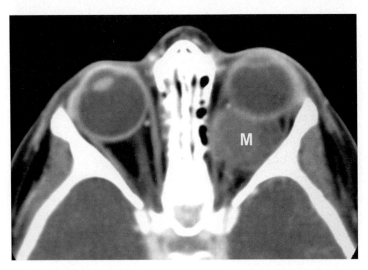

Figure 8–47. Orbital lymphatic malformation in a 2-year-old boy with proptosis. Contrast-enhanced computed tomographic scan shows well-defined, nonenhancing mass (M) posterior to the left globe.

TABLE 8–7. **More Common Causes of**
Pediatric Neck Masses

Congenital	Neoplastic
Thyroglossal duct cyst	Rhabdomyosarcoma
Brachial cleft cyst	Lymphoma
Lingual thyroid	Metastatic disease
Dermoid-epidermoid	
	Vascular
Inflammatory	Venous malformation
Suppurative	Lymphatic malformation
lymphadenitis	
Abscess	
Inflamed salivary gland	
Ranula	

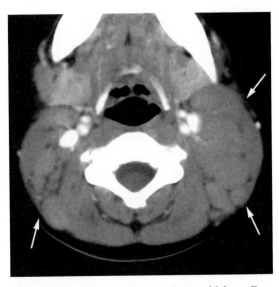

Figure 8–49. Lymphoma in a 5-year-old boy. Contrast-enhanced computed tomographic scan shows bulky lymphadenopathy *(arrows)* bilaterally; it is greater on the left than on the right.

in the head and neck. Most malignant lesions present as a painless mass. The head and neck is one of the most common sites, along with the genitourinary tract, for rhabdomyosarcoma to occur. Rhabdomyosarcoma typically presents in the preschool-aged child. In older children, lymphoma is the most common cause of malignant lymphadenopathy (Fig. 8–49).

There are a number of congenital lesions that can present as palpable neck masses. They include branchial cleft cyst (Fig. 8–50), thyroglossal duct cyst (Fig. 8–51), lingual thyroid, laryngocele, and dermoid-epidermoid. Brachial cleft cysts can persist from any of the developmental brachial arches, but those arising from the second brachial cleft are the most common. Typically, second brachial cleft cysts occur at the angle of the mandible (see Fig. 8–50). Midline neck masses are most likely to

be dermoid-epidermoid, thyroglossal duct cysts (see Fig. 8–51), mucous retention cysts, and lymph nodes. Off-midline masses are more likely to be brachial cleft cysts.

Congenital Vertebral Anomalies

There are a number of fairly common anomalies of the vertebral bodies that occur from

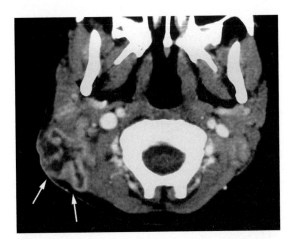

Figure 8–48. Suppurative lymphadenopathy with abscess formation. Contrast-enhanced computed tomographic scan shows matted lymph nodes, with areas of fluid attenuation with rim enhancement *(arrows).*

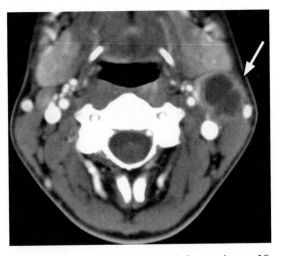

Figure 8–50. Second brachial cleft cyst in an 18-year-old girl with a tender mass. Computed tomographic scan shows low-attenuation cystic lesion *(arrow)* just inferior to the left angle of the mandible. The lesion has an enhancing rim.

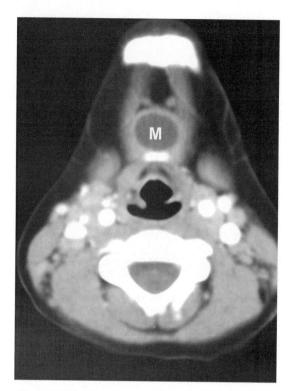

Figure 8–51. Thyroglossal duct cyst in a 2-year-old boy. Contrast-enhanced computed tomographic scan shows well-defined, nonenhancing mass (M) in the midline, just inferior to the base of the tongue.

TABLE 8–8. **Common Types of Spinal Dysraphism**

Open spinal dysraphism
  Myelomeningocele
  Myelocele

Closed (occult) spinal dysraphism
  Lipomyelomeningocele
  Dermal sinus tract
  Tethered cord syndrome

and neuronal tissues fail to fuse. The types of abnormalities are categorized as open (neural tissue exposed through bony and skin defect: spina bifida aperta) and closed (abnormality covered by skin: spina bifida occulta) (Table 8–8). Spinal dysraphism is the most common congenital abnormality of the CNS.

The most common of the open dysraphisms are myelomeningocele and meningocele. The lesions are defined by the contents of the herniated sac. Meningoceles contain meninges but not neural tissue (Fig. 8–53). Myelomeningoceles contain portions of the spinal cord or nerve roots. Although the lesions are most common in the lower lumbar spine, they can occur at any level. Cephaloceles occur through

abnormal development. There may be lack of fusion of the two cartilaginous centers of the vertebral bodies that results in a cleft in the sagittal plane. This is referred to as a *butterfly vertebra* (Fig. 8–52). When one of the lateral cartilaginous centers fails to form, a hemivertebra results. These anomalies may be associated with scoliosis, rib anomalies, and other vertebral anomalies. Anterior and posterior hemivertebrae are also possible. If there is failure of separation of two or more adjacent vertebral bodies, a block vertebra is formed. Klippel-Feil anomaly refers to the fusion of multiple cervical vertebral bodies. There are a number of associated anomalies seen with Klippel-Feil syndrome. These include low posterior hairline, short webbed neck, genitourinary anomalies, and congenital heart disease. A Sprengel deformity (high-riding scapula) in association with a bridging omovertebral bone is present in 25% of patients with Klippel-Feil syndrome.

Spinal Dysraphism

Spinal dysraphism refers to a group of disorders of the spine in which the posterior bony

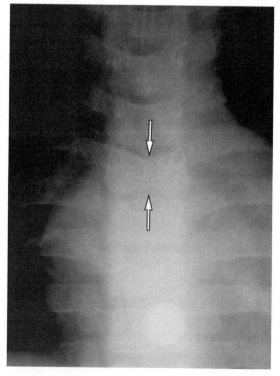

Figure 8–52. Butterfly vertebral body. A narrow central portion *(arrows)* is seen, with normal height at both lateral aspects in this radiograph of the spine.

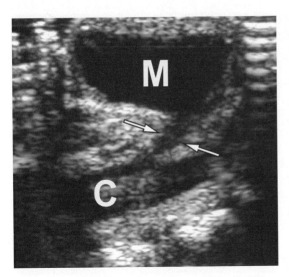

Figure 8–53. Meningocele in a newborn. Midline, sagittal ultrasonogram shows meningocele as cystic structure (M). There is a hypoechoic tract *(arrows)* connecting the cyst to the spinal canal (C).

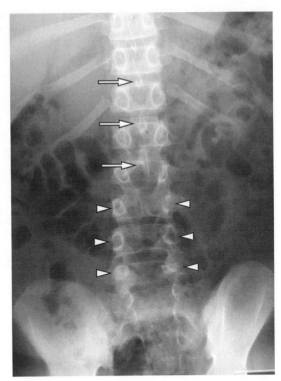

Figure 8–54. Dysraphic changes within the lumbar and sacral spine. Radiograph shows absence of the posterior elements and widening of the interpeduncular distance *(arrowheads)*. The posterior elements superior to the level of dysraphism appear normal *(arrows)*.

defects in the cranium. Myelomeningoceles are associated with multiple other congenital anomalies. As discussed previously, essentially all patients with myelomeningocele (but not meningoceles) have associated Chiari II malformations. Hydrocephalus occurs in up to 90% of these patients. Hydrosyringomyelia, or dilatation of the central canal of the spinal cord, is also often present. On radiography, the absent posterior elements of the spine are apparent in association with widening of the spinal canal and interpediculate distances (Fig. 8–54). There may be associated congenital vertebral anomalies. Typically, multiple contiguous vertebral levels are involved. MRI is often used to look for delayed complications such as syrinx, dermoid, or postoperative tethering.

With the closed dysraphisms, children may be asymptomatic or may present with a subcutaneous mass or dermal tract, bladder dysfunction, lower extremity neurologic abnormalities, or orthopedic deformities of the feet or legs. The closed dysraphisms represent a spectrum of findings. Components include tethered cord, congenital dermal sinus, and lipomyelomeningocele.

In infants who demonstrate a sacral dimple, patch of hair, or other findings suspicious for an occult dysraphism, the initial screening examination is often ultrasonography. In the normal infant, the conus medullaris is located at or more superior to the level of L2-3 (Fig. 8–55). The cord and nerve roots are seen to

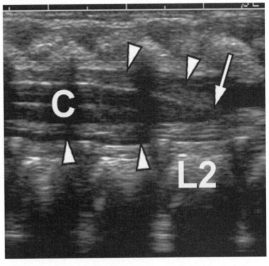

Figure 8–55. Normal spine ultrasonogram. Midline sagittal ultrasonogram shows tip of conus medullaris *(arrow)* to be located at the level of L2, the normal position. The cord (C) is shown as a hypoechoic structure, and the surrounding nerve roots *(arrowheads)* are more echogenic.

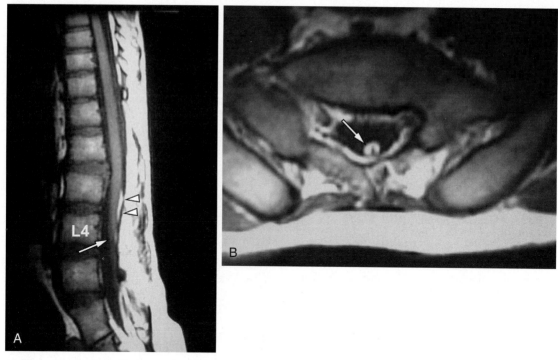

Figure 8–56. Tethered cord. *A,* Sagittal T1-weighted image shows the tip of the conus medullaris *(arrow)* to lie abnormally low, at the level of L4. There is high signal *(arrowheads)* along the distal cord and filum terminale consistent with lipomatous infiltration. *B,* Axial, T1-weighted MR image shows fat surrounding filum terminale *(arrow).* The filum is positioned posteriorly.

be free moving at real-time ultrasonographic evaluation. In tethered cord syndrome, the tip of the spinal cord is low lying, below the level of L2-3 (Fig. 8–56). Tethered cord may occur as a primary problem or in association with other components of spinal dysraphism, such as lipomyelomeningocele or a dermoid tract. With a tethered cord, the filum terminale may be short and abnormally thick (>2 mm). On real-time ultrasonographic examination, the cord and nerve roots do not float freely in the CSF space and may be positioned posteriorly.

When ultrasonographic evaluation is performed, posterior developmental masses should also be excluded. These include lipomyelomeningocele, a contiguous dermal sinus tract, or other posterior developmental masses such as lipoma or dermoid. Lipomyelomeningocele is the most common of the occult myelodysplasias. When present, a lipomatous mass extends inferior and posterior from the incompletely fused spinal cord through a defect in the dura and bone and is contiguous with the subcutaneous fat. A palpable mass may be present, but the overlying skin is intact. A dermal sinus is an epithelium-lined tract that extends from the skin to the deep soft tissues. It

may connect to the spinal canal or end in a dermoid, epidermoid, or lipoma. The tracts are usually identifiable on ultrasonography and appear as a low signal intensity tract on T1-weighted MR images. When findings of occult dysraphism either are found on ultrasonography or are highly suspected clinically, definitive evaluation is performed with MRI.

Spinal Trauma

Injury to the spine is much less common in infants and young children than it is in adults. Most injuries that occur in older children and teenagers have the same appearance and locations as those seen in adults and will not be discussed here. In infants and young children, the majority of cervical spine injuries involve the superior cervical spine, as opposed to the lower cervical spine, as seen with injuries in adults. This is thought to be related to the relatively large head size of young children and the immaturity of the spinal column. As with all cervical spine trauma, the technical factors and interpretation of radiographs must be diligent.

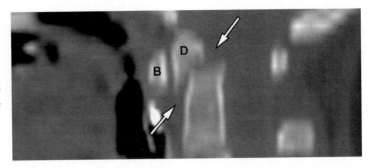

Figure 8–57. Fracture through base of dens. Sagittal reconstructed computed tomographic scan shows fracture line *(arrows)* through base of dens with anterior displacement of dens (D) and anterior button of C1 (B) in relationship to the base of C2.

Fractures of the upper cervical spine in infants and young children often involve the atlas and axis. With flexion injuries, there can be a fracture through the base of the dens (at the synchondroses between the dens and the body of C2) (Fig. 8–57). With this injury, there is typically anterior displacement of C1 in association with soft tissue swelling. Extension injuries of this region may result in fractures of the posterior arch of C1, the dens, or a "hangman's fracture" (fracture through the posterior arch of C2). Atlantooccipital disloca-

tions can also occur (Fig. 8–58). Atlantooccipital dislocation is a severe injury that often results in death. On radiographs, the distance between the occiput and C1 is increased, and there is marked soft tissue swelling. Atlantoaxial instability can also occur and is discussed further on.

Lap belt injuries occur in children who are restrained by a lap belt but not a shoulder belt. Anterior compression fractures of the lumbar vertebral bodies may occur in association with disruption of the posterior processes (Chance

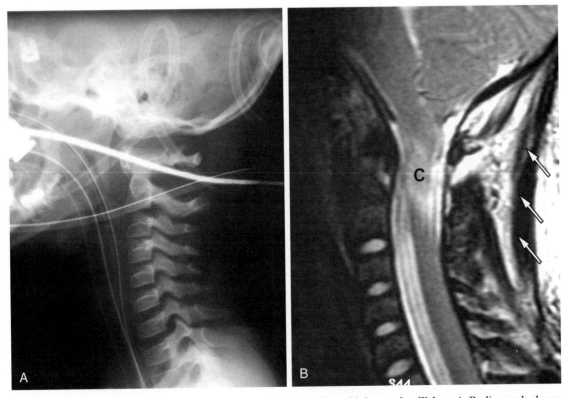

Figure 8–58. Craniocervical dislocation in a 5-year-old boy after a high-speed collision. *A,* Radiograph shows increased distance between the skull base and the C1 vertebral body. *B,* Sagittal T2-weighted MR image shows high signal within the cord (C) representing a cord contusion. There is high-signal edema within the posterior soft tissues *(arrows)* secondary to ligamentous injury.

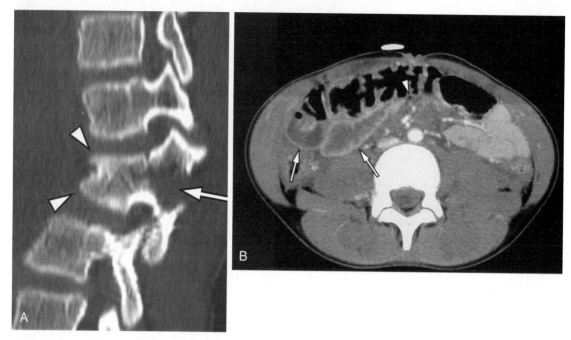

Figure 8–59. Chance fracture with associated bowel injury in a 12-year-old girl wearing a lap belt during a high-speed collision. *A,* Sagittal, reconstructed computed tomographic scan shows anterior compression *(arrowheads)* and fracture through the posterior processes *(arrow)* of the lumbar vertebral body. *B,* Computed tomographic scan shows fluid-filled bowel loops *(arrows)* with enhancing rim. There is also extraluminal gas *(arrowhead)* and hemorrhage within the mesentery. The patient had a small bowel perforation shown at surgery.

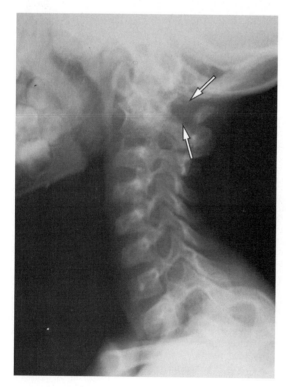

Figure 8–60. Congenital absence of the posterior portion of C1. This is seen by the lucent area *(arrows)* on radiograph.

fracture) (Fig. 8–59). These fractures are not commonly associated with neurologic injury but are frequently associated with intraabdominal injuries, particularly bowel injury (see Fig. 8–59).

Normal Variants and Congenital Anomalies of the Cervical Spine

Another difficulty in interpreting pediatric cervical spine radiographs for trauma is recognizing normal variants and differentiating these normal variants from trauma. One of the more common normal variants that may lead to confusion is cervical pseudosubluxation. In normal children, there may be slight anterior positioning of C2 in relation to C3. However, in contrast to ligamentous injury, with pseudosubluxation, the posterior cervical line (a line drawn along the anterior aspect of the posterior processes) will remain straight. Pseudosubluxation may also be seen at the C3-4 level.

There are a number of age-related variations of C1 and C2. The three ossification centers that make up the atlas fuse laterally by 3 years and posteriorly by 1 year. Before fusion, a lucent synchondrosis is seen radiographically. In

addition, there may be a congenital defect in the posterior portion of C1 that should not be confused with a fracture (Fig. 8–60). C2 also has multiple ossification centers. These nonossified synchondroses should not be mistaken for fractures. The synchondrosis between the dens and body of C2 typically fuses between 3 and 6 years. Before fusion, the lucent synchondrosis is seen through the base of the dens. The ossiculum terminale (tip of the dens) fuses to the body of the dens by 12 years. The dens normally may also be tilted slightly posteriorly in young children.

Atlantoaxial Instability

The atlantoaxial joint, or articulation between C1 and C2 vertebral bodies, is a unique joint that provides the ability for lateral rotation of the cervical spine. The joint is stabilized by a number of ligaments. The transverse ligament is responsible for stabilizing the relationship between the dens of C2 and anterior arch of C1. In children, the space between the dens and anterior arch of C1 should not exceed 5 mm. Atlantoaxial subluxation leads to an abnormal increase in this distance (Fig. 8–61).

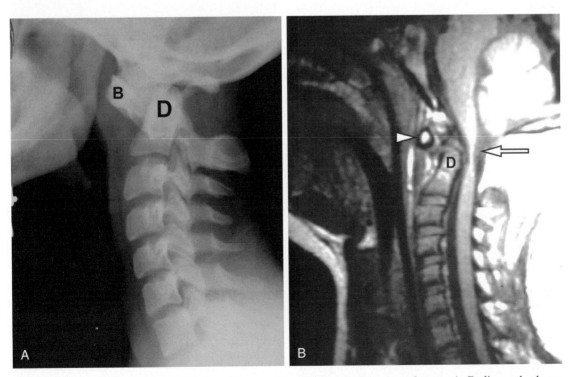

Figure 8–61. Atlantoaxial instability in a 20-year-old patient with Down syndrome. *A,* Radiograph shows increased distance between the anterior button of C1 (B) and the dens of C2 (D). *B,* Sagittal T1-weighted MR image again shows increased distance between the anterior button of C1 *(arrowhead)* and the dens of C2 (D). There is also marked narrowing of the spinal canal, with severe spinal cord compression *(arrow).*

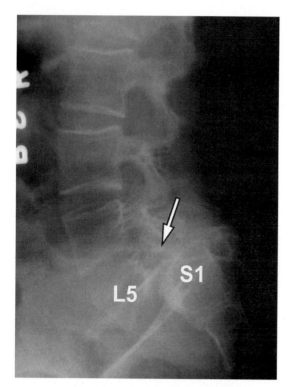

Figure 8–62. L5-S1 Spondylolysis with grade 5 spondylolisthesis. Lateral radiograph shows marked anterior displacement of the L5 vertebral body in relation to the S1 vertebral segment. Since L5 is completely anterior to S1, this is a grade 5 spondylolisthesis. There is lucency through the pars *(arrows)* consistent with the spondylolysis.

Unfortunately, it also leads to a decrease in the diameter of the spinal canal and can cause cord compression (see Fig. 8–61). Causes of atlantoaxial instability include trauma, inflammation (juvenile rheumatoid arthritis, retropharyngeal abscess), or congenital predisposition (Down syndrome, hypoplasia of the dens, absence of the anterior arch of C1). Patients with Down syndrome are typically screened for atlantoaxial instability before participation in physical activities.

Spondylolysis and Spondylolisthesis

The most common abnormality identified on radiography in children who present with lower back pain is spondylolysis. *Spondylolysis* refers to a defect in the pars interarticularis of the posterior vertebral arch. It usually occurs

bilaterally and at a single level. The overwhelming majority of cases (93%) occur at the L5-S1 level, with the second most common location being L4-5. It is a common lesion, affecting approximately 7.1% of adolescents. Many are asymptomatic. Symptoms usually present in late childhood. There is debate concerning whether the cause is traumatic or congenital, or some combination of the two. Spondylolisthesis refers to anterior displacement of the more superior vertebral body on the inferior vertebral body (Fig. 8–62). Spondylolisthesis is graded 1 to 5 based on increments of one quarter of the vertebral body. Grade 1 refers to anterior displacement up to one quarter of the anterior vertebral body beyond the anterior border of the inferior vertebral body. Grade 2 is up to one half and grade 4 is up to the entire vertebral body. Grade 5 is complete anterior displacement and inferior migration so that the superior vertebral body

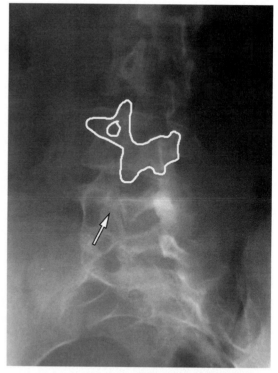

Figure 8–63. L5-S1 spondylolysis shown on oblique radiograph. The defect through the pars at the L5-S1 level is demonstrated as a lucency *(arrow)*, likened to a broken neck of a "Scotty dog." The normal "Scotty dog" (without a lucent broken neck) is outlined at the more superior normal level.

is anterior and inferior to the inferior vertebral body (see Fig. 8–62).

On lateral radiographs, spondylolysis appears as a lucent defect through the region of the pars with or without associated anterior slippage. Oblique views demonstrate the lucency through the pars. The pars defect has been likened to a lucent, broken neck of what appears like a Scottish terrier on the oblique views (Fig. 8–63). Personally, I think the defect is often easier to see on the straight lateral films. When confirmation is necessary, CT can be used.

Suggested Reading

Ball WS Jr. Pediatric Neuroradiology. Philadelphia: Lippincott-Raven, 1997.

Barkovich AJ. Pediatric Neuroimaging. 2nd ed. New York: Raven Press, 1995.

Robertson RL, Ball WS II, Barnes PD. Skull and brain. In: Kirks DR, ed. Practical Pediatric Imaging of Infants and Children. 3rd ed. Philadelphia: Lippincott-Raven, 1998.

Robson CD, Kim FM, Barnes PD. Head and neck. In: Kirks DR, ed. Practical Pediatric Imaging of Infants and Children. 3rd ed. Philadelphia: Lippincott-Raven, 1998.

Young Poussaint T, Barnes PD, Ball WS II. Skull and brain. In: Kirks DR, ed. Practical Pediatric Imaging of Infants and Children. 3rd ed. Philadelphia: Lippincott-Raven, 1998.

Index

Note: Page numbers in *italics* refer to illustrations; page numbers followed by t refer to tables.

A

AAIIMM take pneumonic, 112–113, 113t
Abscess, lung, 52, *53*
  retropharyngeal, 8, *9*
  atlantoaxial instability and, 262
Abuse, child. See *Child abuse.*
Accordion sign, of pseudomembranous colitis, 135, *135*
Acetabulum, trident, 196–197, *198*
Achondroplasia, 196, *196*, 197, *197*, *198*, 199t
  acetabular angle and, *198*, 203
Acute chest syndrome, of sickle cell anemia, 54–55, *57*
Acute disseminated encephalomyelitis (ADEM), 243, *244*
Acute respiratory distress syndrome (ARDS), 30. See also *Respiratory distress syndrome.*
Adenitis, mesenteric, 123, *124*
Adrenoleukodystrophy, 240t, *242*
Adult polycystic kidney disease, 158
Age, patient. See also *Child(ren).*
  antibiotics and, 47–48
  bladder capacity and, 142
  brain myelination and, 3, 239, *241*
  cervical spine variation and, *260*, 261
  computed tomography and, 2, 2t
  differential diagnosis and, 3
  hip pain and, 204t
  infection and, 47–48, *47–49*
  left-to-right cardiac shunt and, 82
  organ development and, 2–3
  thymus development and, 60
Agyria, 227t, 234, *234*
  heterotopias and, 232
Airway, 5, *7*

Airway *(Continued)*
  lower, obstruction of, 10, 12
    intrinsic, 19, *19*
  upper, obstruction of, acute, 5–8, *6*, *7–11*
    chronic, 8, 10, *11*
Alpha-fetoprotein, in differential diagnosis, 126
Aneurysm, ascending aortic, *12*, *94*
  autosomal dominant polycystic kidney disease and, 158
  sinus of Valsalva, *94*
  vein of Galen, 227t, 235, *236*
Angiography, aortic stenosis on, *85*
  coronary arteries on, *84*
Angiomatosis, encephalotrigeminal, 238–239, *240*
Angiomyelofibroma, 161, *162*
  tuberous sclerosis and, 238
Aorta, aneurysm of, *12*, *94*
  coarctation of, 87, *87–89*
Aortic arch, double, 14, *14–15*
  right-sided, 74, *74*
Aortic stenosis, 83, *85*
  supravalvular, 83, *86*
Apophyseal irregularity, 171, *171*, 173
Appendicitis, 113–114, *113–115*
Arachnoid cyst, 231, *232*
Arteriovenous malformations (AVMs), 219–220, *220*
Arteriovenous shunt, *79*
Arthritis, juvenile rheumatoid, 204t, 209, *210*
  atlantoaxial instability and, 262
  septic, 203, 204t, 205–206, *205–206*
Asplenia, 72–73, *74*
Astrocytoma. See also *Glioma.*
  cerebellar, 244–245, *244*, 244t
Atelectasis, 48, *49*
Atresia, biliary, 123–124, *125*
  hepatoblastoma and, 126
  duodenal, neonatal, 99–100, 99t, *100*
  esophageal, 109

Atresia *(Continued)*
  postoperative complications of, 109–110, *109*, *120*
  ileal, 106
  pulmonary, intact septum with, 77, *77*
  tricuspid, 81, *81*
Avulsion, apophyseal, 176, 178, *178–179*
  of medial epicondyle, 176, *177*
  of patellar tendon, 179, *180*
  of tibial tuberosity, 179, *180*

B

Bladder, capacity of, patient age and, 142
Blount disease, 212, *212*
Bochdalek hernia, 39
Bone. See also *Craniosynostosis; Fracture(s); Periosteal reaction; Skull.*
  constitutional disorders of, 195
  lesions of, focal sclerotic, 188t
    multifocal, 194, 194t
    permeative, 183, 183t
  skeletal, patient age and, 3
  tumor, 193
Brain, development of, TORCH infections and, 242
  developmental abnormalities of, 226, 227t. See also specific abnormalities.
  myelination of, patient age and, 3, 239, *241*
Bronchiectasis, 52, *56*
Bronchogenic cysts, 44, *45*, *64–65*
Bronchopulmonary dysplasia (BPD), 33, *34*, 35
  ventilation and, 33
  versus pulmonary interstitial emphysema, 30

C

Caffey disease, 183, *184*

265